Vascular Anomalies

Cameron C. Trenor III • Denise M. Adams
Editors

Vascular Anomalies

A Guide for the Hematologist/ Oncologist

Springer

Editors
Cameron C. Trenor III
Dana-Farber Cancer Institute
Boston Children's Hospital
Boston, MA
USA

Division of Hematology/Oncology
Vascular Anomalies Center
Harvard Medical School
Boston Children's Hospital
Boston, MA
USA

Denise M. Adams
Dana-Farber Cancer Institute
Boston Children's Hospital
Boston, MA
USA

Division of Hematology/Oncology
Vascular Anomalies Center
Harvard Medical School
Boston Children's Hospital
Boston, MA
USA

ISBN 978-3-030-25622-7 ISBN 978-3-030-25624-1 (eBook)
https://doi.org/10.1007/978-3-030-25624-1

This Springer imprint is published by the registered company Springer Nature Switzerland AG
The registered company address is: Gewerbestrasse 11, 6330 Cham, Switzerland

We dedicate this book to those who have provided support and inspiration in the field of vascular anomalies, primarily the patients, families, family support groups, and other collaborators.

Our patients are truly heroes, and they provide the needed resilience and drive to accomplish much of our efforts to seek diagnoses and develop the best treatment options. They inspire collaboration and our desire to develop interdisciplinary education and the development of vascular anomaly centers. The steady encouragement and inquisitive nature of this cohort help stipulate continuous feedback and modifications to the delivery of care. Their willingness to participate in vital research studies has fostered an environment of unity as we strive to forward our mutual goals of best practices and distinction in care. Their desire to expand the awareness of this mission through lobbying of federal agencies and donors to support and provide resources for continuous exploration of treatments is noteworthy. For without these dedicated individuals, we would not be achieving results for the betterment of our field/patients. We are forever grateful for this support.

Preface

This book was conceptualized by two pediatric hematologists/oncologists, bringing complementary experience - one from oncology and one from hematology - to a shared passion for vascular anomalies. The purpose was to enhance the education of pediatric hematologist/oncologists in the field of vascular anomalies and entice their interest in joining the growing numbers of "vascular anomalists." It is an exciting time with new discoveries and opportunities in medical therapies and comprehensive care of patients with vascular anomalies.

Surgeons and radiologists were the first professionals to form groups to study vascular anomalies. Initial investigation of vascular anomalies was led by Dr. Judah Folkman, the founder of angiogenesis. He mentored Dr. John Mulliken, the founder of the Vascular Anomalies Center at Boston Children's Hospital. These are two of our luminaries in the field.

Twenty years ago, Dr. Mulliken and colleagues reported a simple classification of vascular anomalies (tumors and malformations). Pattern recognition was the basis for diagnostic classification and was best performed by astute clinicians. Most treatment options were surgical and interventional, and there were limited medical options with no clinical trials. There were no consortiums or cooperative groups for the organization of clinical trials. In contrast, 20 years ago in Pediatric Hematology/Oncology, clinicians worked together in cooperative groups. There were multiple active clinical trials. Diseases were risk-stratified and outcome measures were being studied. Furthermore, the start of genetic discovery was changing treatment paradigms.

Thanks to warm mentorship from the pioneers in this field, pediatric hematologist/oncologists with an interest in vascular anomalies were actively deemed "having the vascular anomaly gene" and were welcomed as partners into vascular anomaly centers. We are forever grateful for the guidance and support of Drs. Judah Folkman and John Mulliken.

Currently, the classification system for vascular anomalies was revised by the scientific committee of the International Society for the Study of Vascular Anomalies (ISSVA), including significant contributions from hematologist/oncologists on this committee. There are better standards of practice for vascular anomalies; some of these are medical practices formulated by pediatric hematologists/oncologists. Today, hematologists/oncologists have a central role in many vascular anomaly centers. Furthermore, there are precise phenotypes of disease that can be linked to genotypes. This genotype/phenotype partnering has led to treatment options and clinical trials that are improving the outcomes for patients with vascular anomalies. Translational and clinical providers are teaming with basic scientists to continue to move this field forward. An interdisciplinary approach is essential in the treatment and care of vascular anomalies, and this collaboration is essential.

This book exemplifies this interdisciplinary collaboration. We are honored that today's leaders in the field of vascular anomalies agreed to contribute their expertise and content - and even more honored to call these international experts our friends. We hope that this book sparks the interest of other hematologists/oncologists who have "the gene" to join this exciting bandwagon and help improve the outcomes for these patients.

Boston, MA, USA

Cameron C. Trenor III
Denise M. Adams

Contents

Contributors

Denise M. Adams, MD Dana-Farber Cancer Institute, Boston Children's Hospital, Boston, MA, USA

Division of Hematology/Oncology, Vascular Anomalies Center, Harvard Medical School, Boston Children's Hospital, Boston, MA, USA

Ahmad Alomari Department of Radiology, Boston Children's Hospital, Harvard Medical School, Boston, MA, USA

Francine Blei Department of Pediatrics, Vascular Anomalies Program, Lenox Hill Hospital of Northwell Health, New York, NY, USA

Laurence M. Boon Human Molecular Genetics, de Duve Institute, Brussels, Belgium

Center for Vascular Anomalies, Cliniques Universitaires Saint-Luc, Catholic University of Louvain, Brussels, Belgium

Leonardo R. Brandão Division of Haematology/Oncology, The Hospital for Sick Children, Toronto, ON, Canada

Patricia E. Burrows Department of Radiology, Medical College of Wisconsin, St. Petersburg, FL, USA

Gulraiz Chaudry Department of Radiology, Boston Children's Hospital, Harvard Medical School, Boston, MA, USA

Roshni Dasgupta Division of Pediatric General and Thoracic Surgery, Cincinnati Children's Hospital Medical Center, Hemangioma and Vascular Malformation Center, Cincinnati, OH, USA

Belinda Dickie Department of Surgery, Boston Children's Hospital, Boston, MA, USA

Vascular Anomalies Center, Harvard Medical School, Boston, MA, USA

Steven J. Fishman Department of Surgery, Vascular Anomalies Center, Harvard Medical School, Children's Hospital Boston, Boston, MA, USA

Ilona J. Frieden Departments of Dermatology and Pediatrics, University of California, San Francisco, San Francisco, CA, USA

Amy Geddis Department of Pediatrics, Cancer and Blood Disorders Clinic, Seattle Children's Hospital, Seattle, WA, USA

Arin K. Greene Department of Plastic and Oral Surgery, Boston Children's Hospital, Harvard Medical School, Boston, MA, USA

Anita Gupta Department of Pathology, Cincinnati Children's Hospital Medical Center, Cincinnati, OH, USA

Adrienne M. Hammill Division of Hematology, Hemangioma and Vascular Malformation Center, University of Cincinnati College of Medicine, Cincinnati Children's Hospital Medical Center, Cincinnati, OH, USA

Ionela Iacobas Pediatric Cancer and Hematology Centers, Texas Children's Hospital/Baylor College of Medicine, Houston, TX, USA

Michael R. Jeng, MD Department of Pediatrics, Stanford University School of Medicine, Lucile Packard Children's Hospital, Palo Alto, CA, USA

Ann M. Kulungowski Division of Pediatric Surgery, Vascular Anomalies Center, University of Colorado School of Medicine, Children's Hospital Colorado, Aurora, CO, USA

Margaret T. Lee Division of Pediatric Hematology/Oncology/Stem Cell Transplantation, Columbia University Medical Center, New York, NY, USA

Anna Lillis Department of Radiology, The Ohio State University College of Medicine, Columbus, OH, USA

Department of Radiology, Nationwide Children's Hospital, Columbus, OH, USA

Joana M. Mack Vascular Anomalies Center, Division of Hematology/Oncology, Cancer and Blood Disorders Program, Arkansas Children's Hospital, Little Rock, AR, USA

Sheilagh Maguiness Dermatology, University of Minnesota, Minneapolis, MN, USA

Taizo A. Nakano Center for Cancer and Blood Disorders, Children's Hospital Colorado, University of Colorado School of Medicine, Aurora, CO, USA

Ha-Long Nguyen Human Molecular Genetics, de Duve Institute, Brussels, Belgium

Manish N. Patel Department of Radiology and Medical Imaging, Hemangioma and Vascular Malformation Center, University of Cincinnati School of Medicine, Cincinnati Children's Hospital Medical Center, Cincinnati, OH, USA

Kiersten W. Ricci Hemangioma and Vascular Malformation Center, Division of Hematology, Cincinnati Children's Hospital Medical Center and University of Cincinnati College of Medicine, Cincinnati, OH, USA

Kristen Snyder Cancer Center, Children's Hospital of Philadelphia, Philadelphia, PA, USA

Samantha A. Spencer Orthopedic Center, Boston Children's Hospital, Harvard Medical School, Boston, MA, USA

Clifford M. Takemoto Department of Hematology, St. Jude Children's Research Hospital, Memphis, TN, USA

Megha M. Tollefson Division of Pediatric Dermatology, Mayo Clinic, Rochester, MN, USA

Cameron C. Trenor III Dana-Farber Cancer Institute, Boston Children's Hospital, Boston, MA, USA

Division of Hematology/Oncology, Vascular Anomalies Center, Harvard Medical School, Boston Children's Hospital, Boston, MA, USA

Miikka Vikkula Human Molecular Genetics, de Duve Institute, Brussels, Belgium

Center for Vascular Anomalies, Cliniques Universitaires Saint-Luc, Catholic University of Louvain, Brussels, Belgium

Nomenclature of Vascular Anomalies: Evolution to the ISSVA 2018 Classification System

1

Francine Blei

The term "vascular anomalies" embraces a heterogeneous group of vascular lesions, involving one or more vessel type (capillary, artery, vein, and/or lymphatic). This chapter will focus on the historical context of "birthmarks" and evolution of the current most updated comprehensive classification of vascular anomalies. Detailed descriptions of diagnoses (clinical, radiologic, and pathologic features) and their treatment are discussed in subsequent chapters of this book.

Clinically, "vascular anomalies" represent a spectrum of disorders, from a simple cutaneous "birthmark" to life-threatening entities that may be associated with a high incidence of morbidity and mortality. Recognition of temporal and physical patterns of presentation has contributed to the identification of *syndromic* vascular anomalies (e.g., segmental hemangiomas associated with PHACE and LUMBAR syndromes and CLOVES, Proteus, and hereditary hemorrhagic telangiectasia syndromes with vascular malformations), enabling appropriate preemptive evaluation, patient/parent education, and treatment [1–5].

Historically, the field of vascular anomalies has been absent in medical training syllabi, and knowledge was acquired when physicians rotated in centers with recognized vascular anomalies programs (which attracted a broad range of vascular anomalies patients of varying complexity). As more physicians have become exposed to and interested in this field, there has been a quantum increase in vascular anomalies practitioners.

Purported causes of birthmarks are wrought with folklore (in Jewish, Greek, Christian, and Indian cultures) and negative connotations, from ancient times to the present [6]. Birthmarks were attributed to "constellations in human form," supernatural influences, or a result of parental (usually maternal) "impression" – due to images seen or thoughts at the time of conception or during pregnancy affecting

F. Blei (✉)
Department of Pediatrics, Vascular Anomalies Program,
Lenox Hill Hospital of Northwell Health, New York, NY, USA
e-mail: fblei@northwell.edu

C. C. Trenor III, D. M. Adams (eds.), *Vascular Anomalies*,
https://doi.org/10.1007/978-3-030-25624-1_1

fetal development. Despite scientific interest in embryologic development and teratology, throughout the nineteenth and early twentieth century, the notion of maternal/parental impression persisted [7–9] and https://embryo.asu.edu/pages/teratogens#sthash.6Ow0mlSl.dpuf. Terms for "birthmark" often convey a negative context. In Italy, the term for birthmark is "voglia di fragole" or "desire for strawberries," reflecting the perception that the birthmark in the child was due to the mother's craving for strawberries during pregnancy. Similarly, the French term for birthmark, "envie," is thought to refer to the mother's unsatisfied desires during pregnancy. Similarly, in German "muttermal" means "mother's mark." The Finnish translation of Nathaniel Hawthorne's haunting short story, *The Birthmark*, is *Paholainen käsikirjoituksessa* meaning "The devil in the script" [10].

Despite the early recognition of birthmarks, descriptive categories did not emerge until the late eighteenth and early nineteenth centuries, with treatises by Virchow, Plenck, Willan, and then Alibert, and reviewed in great detail in the first chapter of *Mulliken and Young's Vascular Birthmarks* [11]. In the 1960s, Malan and Puglionisi described arterial, venous, and lymphatic dysplasias in the extremities [12, 13]. In 1988, the Hamburg classification divided vascular malformations into "truncular" (containing major axial vessels) or "extratruncular" (comprising branches of major vessels) [14]. Dr. John Mulliken and Dr. Anthony Young began a series of workshops in 1976, subsequently occurring every other year, to discuss vascular anomalies among various subspecialists with similar interests. This evolved and was formalized into the International Society for the Study of Vascular Anomalies (ISSVA) in 1992, after an International Workshop in Vascular Anomalies, which occurred 2 years earlier. From a handful of physicians, this group currently has over 290 active members (05/2019) from 5 continents representing multiple medical subspecialties, clinicians, and researchers (http://www.issva.org/). ISSVA has emerged from obscurity and is now a sought after professional organization, attracting new members at an increased rate.

Mulliken and Glowacki were first to clearly separate vascular anomalies into two distinct categories based on endothelial characteristics and clinical features [15], with further refinement based on in vitro, biologic, and radiologic differences [15, 16]. In this classification, vascular anomalies are divided into hemangiomas or vascular malformations, the former having a proliferative phase and the latter representing simple (with one vessel type) or complex (with two or more vessel types) vascular abnormalities (Table 1.1). The framework for an ISSVA classification of vascular anomalies, which built upon the Mulliken and Glowacki classification, was

Table 1.1 1982 Classification of vascular anomalies – Mulliken and Glowacki [15]

Hemangioma	Vascular malformation
Proliferative phase	Simple
Involuting phase	Capillary
	Venous
	Arterial
	Lymphatic
	Combined
	Capillary venous
	Arteriovenous
	Capillary venous/lymphatic

established at the 1996 ISSVA workshop and later published by Enjolras et al. (Table 1.2) [17]. This updated classification included newly recognized entities and separated vascular malformations into slow- or fast-flow lesions. Proliferative lesions in this classification scheme included subcategories of hemangiomas: infantile hemangiomas (GLUT-1 positive), congenital hemangiomas (rapidly involuting congenital hemangiomas (RICH) and noninvoluting congenital hemangiomas (NICH)), tufted angiomas, kaposiform hemangioendothelioma, pyogenic granuloma, and rare hemangioendotheliomas and acquired dermatologic vascular tumors. Syndromic vascular malformations and those with known genetic mutations at the time were included. This taxonomy provided a framework for updated nomenclature and characterized vascular anomalies, which could help direct evaluation and management. Further updates and refinements to this classification are discussed in the latter portion of this chapter.

Table 1.2 1996 ISSVA classification of vascular anomalies

Vascular tumors	Vascular malformations
Infantile hemangiomas **(Hemangiomas of infancy)** **(GLUT-1 positive)**	*Slow-flow vascular malformations:* Capillary malformation (port-wine stain, telangiectasia, angiokeratoma) Venous malformation(VM) (common sporadic VM, Bean syndrome, familial cutaneous and mucosal VM, glomovenous malformation, Maffucci syndrome) Lymphatic malformation
Congenital hemangiomas **RICH (rapidly involuting congenital hemangioma)** **NICH (noninvoluting congenital hemangioma)**	*Fast-flow vascular malformations* Arterial malformation, arteriovenous fistula, arteriovenous Malformation
Tufted angioma (with or without Kasabach-Merritt syndrome)	*Complex-combined vascular malformations:* CVM, CLM, LVM, CLVM, AVM-LM, CM-AVM
Kaposiform hemangioendothelioma (with or without Kasabach-Merritt syndrome)	
Spindle cell hemangioendothelioma	
Other rare hemangioendotheliomas (epitheliod, composite, retiform, polymorphous, Dabka tumor, lymphangioendothelioma, etc.)	
Dermatologic acquired vascular tumors (pyogenic granuloma, targetoid hemangioma, glomeruloid hemangioma, microvenular hemangioma, etc.)	

Enjolras et al. [17]

C capillary, *V* venous, *L* lymphatic, *AV* arteriovenous, *M* malformation, *GLUT1* erythrocyte glucose transporter protein 1

[a]International Society for the Study of Vascular Anomalies

In addition to the classification updates, staging systems may help guide management decisions. Examples include the Schobinger staging of arteriovenous malformations based on clinical aggressiveness and staging systems for cervicofacial lymphatic malformations corresponding to anatomic location and extent [18, 19].

Patients with vascular anomalies may have focal aberrations of vascular development (in vascular malformations) or vascular proliferation (in hemangiomas). Syndromic vascular anomalies, a "developmental field defect," include the blood/lymphatic vessels as well as skeletal, soft tissue, and/or organ involvement. The cardiovascular system is the first functioning organ in the developing fetus. Research in the past decades has elucidated factors mediating the differentiation and development of normal blood and lymphatic vessels. Over time, a more complex series of well-orchestrated intricate processes continues to emerge, defining a myriad of growth and transcription factors, rheologic influences, and molecular signaling pathways involved in normal vascular development [20–23].

In recent years, additional breakthroughs have been published, defining molecular and genetic mechanisms implicated in the development of vascular anomalies. Germline genetic mutations causing inherited vascular anomalies (e.g., HHT, RASA-1, EPH4, FLT4, TIE2, KRIT1, PTEN, Glomulin) [5, 24–33] or genetic mutations expressed mosaically in somatic, affected tissue (e.g., GNAQ, PIK3CA, AKT1, KRAS, NRAS) [34–44] have been identified, providing insight into potential mechanisms implicated in the development of vascular anomalies and allowing for more targeted therapies for prevention and/or treatment [45–49].

Since 1996, there has been an increase in the quantity and quality of clinical, basic, and genetic research in vascular anomalies, along with the identification of new therapies (e.g., propranolol for hemangiomas and sirolimus for some vascular malformations and kaposiform hemangioendothelioma, advanced sclerotherapy procedures), which have drawn attention and interest to the field. Typically, more than one subspecialist is involved with the evaluation and management of patients with vascular anomalies, and Vascular Anomalies Centers, which centralize physicians of many disciplines, have become a model for multidisciplinary care and research. It is essential that all team members be fluent in the updated nomenclature.

Despite clearly different clinical presentations, chronological course, and symptoms, terminology for vascular anomalies has been fraught with errors, and patients are frequently misdiagnosed and diagnostic inaccuracies have dominated this field. Most frequently, the term "hemangioma" inaccurately used to describe any benign vascular lesion in a patient of any age, irrespective of the lesion's clinical appearance and behavior. One study found "terminological imprecision" in medical journals, incorrectly using the word "hemangioma" in the majority of manuscripts reviewed [50]. Additionally, diagnoses of patients referred to vascular anomalies centers are often incorrect [51]. Some of these nomenclature misnomers are historic in nature - experienced pathologists, radiologists and other diagnostic clinicians may be unaware of the evolution of newer subdivided classification systems for vascular anomalies, leading to continued use of outdated terminology. Aligning the vocabulary among providers, educators, and researchers is essential, and use of a comprehensive updated classification system is indispensable.

The 1996 ISSVA classification became outdated, since new diagnoses, causative genes, and syndromes have been recognized [39, 46, 52–58]. The classification was updated and approved by the ISSVA Board and membership in 2014 and is published in a comprehensive manuscript [59]. The original stratification of proliferative (tumor) vs malformation remains; however, two new categories were added – malformations of individually named vessels ("truncular" in the Schobinger classification) and lesions of unclear etiology (tumor vs malformation). The ISSVA classification is increasingly referred to in peer-reviewed publications, and a further update was approved in 2018 (issva.org/classification) [60–63].

An interactive PowerPoint® version of the classification is available for download and reference (issva.org/classification). Each slide is summarized in Table 1.3.

Table 1.3 Detailed table of ISSVA 2018 classification, http://www.issva.org → CLASSIFICATION, or http://www.issva.org/UserFiles/file/ISSVA-Classification-2018.pdf

Slide #	Title of slide	Entitles included
1	Overview vascular anomalies	Most general separation of vascular tumors and vascular malformations
2	Benign vascular tumors 1	Hemangioma subtypes, other
3	Benign vascular tumors 2	Hobnail hemangioma, other
4	Locally aggressive and malignant vascular tumors	Kaposiform hemangioendothelioma, etc. Angiosarcoma, epithelioid hemangioendothelioma
5	Simple vascular malformations I	Capillary malformations
6	Simple vascular malformations IIa	Lymphatic malformation subtypes Generalized lymphatic anomaly, kaposiform lymphangiomatosis, Gorham's disease, channel-type lymphatic malformation
7	Simple vascular malformations IIb	Primary lymphedema (link to genetic mutations)
8	Simple vascular malformations III	Venous malformations (link to genetic mutations and different types of cerebral cavernous malformations)
9	Simple vascular malformations IV	Arteriovenous malformations Arteriovenous fistulae (link to Genetic mutations)
10	Combined vascular malformations	CM +/− VM +/− LM +/−AVM combinations
11	Anomalies of major named vessels	Affected vessel Anomaly type
12	Vascular malformations associated with other anomalies	Syndromic vascular malformations (link to genetic mutations)
13	Provisionally unclassified vascular malformations	(link to genetic mutations)
14	Appendix 1	Abbreviations used (excluding gene names)
15	Appendix 2-a	Causal genes
16	Appendix 2-b	Causal genes
17	Appendix 2-c	Causal genes
18	Appendix 3	Infantile hemangioma Pattern of distribution, type, syndromes
19	Appendix 4	Vascular anomalies possibly associated with platelet count/coagulation disorders
20	Appendix 5	PIK3CA-related overgrowth spectrum

The first slide of the updated ISSVA classification (ISSVA PowerPoint) expands the original framework of Mulliken and Glowacki's schema (Table 1.1), replacing "hemangioma" with "vascular tumors" and maintaining "vascular malformations" as the main headings. Clicking on the underlined blue word or abbreviation links to another slide, which provides further information (e.g., subcategories of the diagnostic category or the known genetic mutation) for the respective entity.

References

1. Haggstrom AN, Garzon MC, Baselga E, Chamlin SL, Frieden IJ, Holland K, et al. Risk for PHACE syndrome in infants with large facial hemangiomas. Pediatrics. 2010;126(2):e418–26.
2. Iacobas I, Burrows PE, Frieden IJ, Liang MG, Mulliken JB, Mancini AJ, et al. LUMBAR: association between cutaneous infantile hemangiomas of the lower body and regional congenital anomalies. J Pediatr. 2010;157(5):795–801 e1-7.
3. Kulungowski AM, Alomari AI, Chawla A, Christison-Lagay ER, Fishman SJ. Lessons from a liver hemangioma registry: subtype classification. J Pediatr Surg. 2012;47(1):165–70.
4. Cohen MM Jr. The AKT genes and their roles in various disorders. Am J Med Genet A. 2013;161A(12):2931–7.
5. McDonald J, Wooderchak-Donahue W, VanSant Webb C, Whitehead K, Stevenson DA, Bayrak-Toydemir P. Hereditary hemorrhagic telangiectasia: genetics and molecular diagnostics in a new era. Front Genet. 2015;6:1.
6. Doniger W, Spinner G. Misconceptions: parental imprinting. In: Galison P, Graubard S, Mendelsohn E, editors. Science in culture. Somerset: Transaction Publishers; 2001. p. 233.
7. Barrow V. A brief history of teratology to the early 20th century. Teratology. 1971;4:119–29.
8. Tantibanchachai C. Teratogens. The embryo project encyclopedia (2014-01-22) [Internet]. 2014. Available from: http://embryo.asu.edu/handle/10776/7510.
9. Brener M. Reincarnation, maternal impression, and epigenesis: XLIBRIS; 2016.
10. Hawthorne N. The birthmark. online: CreateSpace Independent Publishing Platform; 2016.
11. Mulliken JB, Young A. Vascular birthmarks: hemangiomas and malformations. 1st ed. Philadelphia: W.B. Saunders; 1988.
12. Malan E, Puglionisi A. Congenital Angiodysplasias of the extremities. I. Generalities and classification; venous dysplasias. J Cardiovasc Surg. 1964;5:87–130.
13. Malan E, Puglionisi A. Congenital angiodysplasias of the extremities. II. Arterial, arterial and venous, and haemolymphatic dysplasias. J Cardiovasc Surg. 1965;6(4):255–345.
14. Belov S. Anatomopathological classification of congenital vascular defects. Semin Vasc Surg. 1993;6(4):219–24.
15. Mulliken JB, Glowacki J. Hemangiomas and vascular malformations in infants and children: a classification based on endothelial characteristics. Plast Reconstr Surg. 1982;69(3):412–22.
16. Burrows PE, Mulliken JB, Fellows KE, Strand RD. Childhood hemangiomas and vascular malformations: angiographic differentiation. AJR Am J Roentgenol. 1983;141(3):483–8.
17. Enjolras O, Wassef M, Chapot R. Color atlas of vascular tumors and vascular malformations. Cambridge: Cambridge University Press; 1996.
18. de Serres LM, Sie KC, Richardson MA. Lymphatic malformations of the head and neck. A proposal for staging. Arch Otolaryngol Head Neck Surg. 1995;121(5):577–82.
19. Gilbert P, Dubois J, Giroux MF, Soulez G. New treatment approaches to arteriovenous malformations. Semin Intervent Radiol. 2017;34(3):258–71.
20. Gaengel K, Genove G, Armulik A, Betsholtz C. Endothelial-mural cell signaling in vascular development and angiogenesis. Arterioscler Thromb Vasc Biol. 2009;29(5):630–8.
21. Hogan BM, Schulte-Merker S. How to plumb a pisces: understanding vascular development and disease using zebrafish embryos. Dev Cell. 2017;42(6):567–83.

22. Marcelo KL, Goldie LC, Hirschi KK. Regulation of endothelial cell differentiation and specification. Circ Res. 2013;112(9):1272–87.
23. Ribatti D, Nico B, Crivellato E. The development of the vascular system: a historical overview. Methods Mol Biol. 2015;1214:1–14.
24. Boon LM, Mulliken JB, Vikkula M. RASA1: variable phenotype with capillary and arteriovenous malformations. Curr Opin Genet Dev. 2005;15(3):265–9.
25. Revencu N, Boon LM, Mulliken JB, Enjolras O, Cordisco MR, Burrows PE, et al. Parkes Weber syndrome, vein of Galen aneurysmal malformation, and other fast-flow vascular anomalies are caused by RASA1 mutations. Hum Mutat. 2008;29(7):959–65.
26. Amyere M, Revencu N, Helaers R, Pairet E, Baselga E, Cordisco M, et al. Germline loss-of-function mutations in EPHB4 cause a second form of capillary malformation-arteriovenous malformation (CM-AVM2) deregulating RAS-MAPK signaling. Circulation. 2017;136(11):1037–48.
27. Connell FC, Gordon K, Brice G, Keeley V, Jeffery S, Mortimer PS, et al. The classification and diagnostic algorithm for primary lymphatic dysplasia: an update from 2010 to include molecular findings. Clin Genet. 2013;84(4):303–14.
28. Vikkula M, Boon LM, Carraway KL 3rd, Calvert JT, Diamonti AJ, Goumnerov B, et al. Vascular dysmorphogenesis caused by an activating mutation in the receptor tyrosine kinase TIE2. Cell. 1996;87(7):1181–90.
29. Wouters V, Limaye N, Uebelhoer M, Irrthum A, Boon LM, Mulliken JB, et al. Hereditary cutaneomucosal venous malformations are caused by TIE2 mutations with widely variable hyper-phosphorylating effects. Eur J Hum Genet. 2010;18(4):414–20.
30. Riant F, Bergametti F, Ayrignac X, Boulday G, Tournier-Lasserve E. Recent insights into cerebral cavernous malformations: the molecular genetics of CCM. FEBS J. 2010;277(5):1070–5.
31. Tan WH, Baris HN, Burrows PE, Robson CD, Alomari AI, Mulliken JB, et al. The spectrum of vascular anomalies in patients with PTEN mutations: implications for diagnosis and management. J Med Genet. 2007;44(9):594–602.
32. Brouillard P, Boon LM, Mulliken JB, Enjolras O, Ghassibe M, Warman ML, et al. Mutations in a novel factor, glomulin, are responsible for glomuvenous malformations (“glomangiomas”). Am J Hum Genet. 2002;70(4):866–74.
33. Brouillard P, Boon LM, Revencu N, Berg J, Dompmartin A, Dubois J, et al. Genotypes and phenotypes of 162 families with a glomulin mutation. Mol Syndromol. 2013;4(4):157–64.
34. Shirley MD, Tang H, Gallione CJ, Baugher JD, Frelin LP, Cohen B, et al. Sturge-Weber syndrome and port-wine stains caused by somatic mutation in GNAQ. N Engl J Med. 2013;368(21):1971–9.
35. Ayturk UM, Couto JA, Hann S, Mulliken JB, Williams KL, Huang AY, et al. Somatic activating mutations in GNAQ and GNA11 are associated with congenital hemangioma. Am J Hum Genet. 2016;98(4):789–95.
36. Thomas AC, Zeng Z, Riviere JB, O'Shaughnessy R, Al-Olabi L, St-Onge J, et al. Mosaic activating mutations in GNA11 and GNAQ are associated with Phakomatosis Pigmentovascularis and extensive dermal melanocytosis. J Invest Dermatol. 2016;136(4):770–8.
37. Keppler-Noreuil KM, Sapp JC, Lindhurst MJ, Parker VE, Blumhorst C, Darling T, et al. Clinical delineation and natural history of the PIK3CA-related overgrowth spectrum. Am J Med Genet A. 2014;164A(7):1713–33.
38. Martinez-Lopez A, Blasco-Morente G, Perez-Lopez I, Herrera-Garcia JD, Luque-Valenzuela M, Sanchez-Cano D, et al. CLOVES syndrome: review of a PIK3CA-related overgrowth spectrum (PROS). Clin Genet. 2017;91(1):14–21.
39. Lindhurst MJ, Sapp JC, Teer JK, Johnston JJ, Finn EM, Peters K, et al. A mosaic activating mutation in AKT1 associated with the Proteus syndrome. N Engl J Med. 2011;365(7):611–9.
40. Nikolaev SI, Vetiska S, Bonilla X, Boudreau E, Jauhiainen S, Rezai Jahromi B, et al. Somatic activating KRAS mutations in arteriovenous malformations of the brain. N Engl J Med. 2018;378(3):250–61.
41. Couto JA, Huang AY, Konczyk DJ, Goss JA, Fishman SJ, Mulliken JB, et al. Somatic MAP2K1 mutations are associated with extracranial arteriovenous malformation. Am J Hum Genet. 2017;100(3):546–54.

42. Manevitz-Mendelson E, Leichner GS, Barel O, Davidi-Avrahami I, Ziv-Strasser L, Eyal E, et al. Somatic NRAS mutation in patient with generalized lymphatic anomaly. Angiogenesis. 2018;21(2):287–98.
43. Lim YH, Douglas SR, Ko CJ, Antaya RJ, McNiff JM, Zhou J, et al. Somatic activating RAS mutations cause vascular tumors including pyogenic granuloma. J Invest Dermatol. 2015;135(6):1698–700.
44. Greene AK, Goss JA. Vascular anomalies: from a clinicohistologic to a genetic framework. Plast Reconstr Surg. 2018;141(5):709e–17e.
45. Happle R. Lethal genes surviving by mosaicism: a possible explanation for sporadic birth defects involving the skin. J Am Acad Dermatol. 1987;16(4):899–906.
46. Nguyen HL, Boon LM, Vikkula M. Genetics of vascular malformations. Semin Pediatr Surg. 2014;23(4):221–6.
47. Nguyen HL, Boon LM, Vikkula M. Vascular anomalies caused by abnormal signaling within endothelial cells: targets for novel therapies. Semin Intervent Radiol. 2017;34(3):233–8.
48. Venot Q, Blanc T, Rabia SH, Berteloot L, Ladraa S, Duong JP, et al. Targeted therapy in patients with PIK3CA-related overgrowth syndrome. Nature. 2018;558(7711):540–6.
49. Al-Olabi L, Polubothu S, Dowsett K, Andrews KA, Stadnik P, Joseph AP, et al. Mosaic RAS/MAPK variants cause sporadic vascular malformations which respond to targeted therapy. J Clin Invest. 2018;128(4):1496–508.
50. Hassanein AH, Mulliken JB, Fishman SJ, Greene AK. Evaluation of terminology for vascular anomalies in current literature. Plast Reconstr Surg. 2011;127(1):347–51.
51. Greene AK, Liu AS, Mulliken JB, Chalache K, Fishman SJ. Vascular anomalies in 5,621 patients: guidelines for referral. J Pediatr Surg. 2011;46(9):1784–9.
52. Alomari AI, Spencer SA, Arnold RW, Chaudry G, Kasser JR, Burrows PE, et al. Fibro-adipose vascular anomaly: clinical-radiologic-pathologic features of a newly delineated disorder of the extremity. J Pediatr Orthop. 2014;34(1):109–17.
53. Uller W, Fishman SJ, Alomari AI. Overgrowth syndromes with complex vascular anomalies. Semin Pediatr Surg. 2014;23(4):208–15.
54. Kurek KC, Luks VL, Ayturk UM, Alomari AI, Fishman SJ, Spencer SA, et al. Somatic mosaic activating mutations in PIK3CA cause CLOVES syndrome. Am J Hum Genet. 2012;90(6):1108–15.
55. Keppler-Noreuil KM, Rios JJ, Parker VE, Semple RK, Lindhurst MJ, Sapp JC, et al. PIK3CA-related overgrowth spectrum (PROS): diagnostic and testing eligibility criteria, differential diagnosis, and evaluation. Am J Med Genet A. 2015;167A(2):287–95.
56. Nozaki T, Matsusako M, Mimura H, Osuga K, Matsui M, Eto H, et al. Imaging of vascular tumors with an emphasis on ISSVA classification. Jpn J Radiol. 2013;31(12):775–85.
57. Revencu N, Boon LM, Dompmartin A, Rieu P, Busch WL, Dubois J, et al. Germline mutations in RASA1 are not found in patients with Klippel-Trenaunay syndrome or capillary malformation with limb overgrowth. Mol Syndromol. 2013;4(4):173–8.
58. Revencu N, Boon LM, Mendola A, Cordisco MR, Dubois J, Clapuyt P, et al. RASA1 mutations and associated phenotypes in 68 families with capillary malformation-arteriovenous malformation. Hum Mutat. 2013;34(12):1632–41.
59. Wassef M, Blei F, Adams D, Alomari A, Baselga E, Berenstein A, et al. Vascular anomalies classification: recommendations from the International Society for the study of vascular anomalies. Pediatrics. 2015;136(1):e203–14.
60. Dasgupta R, Fishman SJ. ISSVA classification. Semin Pediatr Surg. 2014;23(4):158–61.
61. Eivazi B, Werner JA. Extracranial vascular malformations (hemangiomas and vascular malformations) in children and adolescents - diagnosis, clinic, and therapy. GMS Curr Top Otorhinolaryngol Head Neck Surg. 2014;13:Doc02.
62. Nassiri N, Thomas J, Cirillo-Penn NC. Evaluation and management of peripheral venous and lymphatic malformations. J Vasc Surg Venous Lymphat Disord. 2016;4(2):257–65.
63. Muller-Wille R, Wildgruber M, Sadick M, Wohlgemuth WA. Vascular anomalies (Part II): interventional therapy of peripheral vascular malformations. Fortschr Röntgenstr 2018; 190(10): 927–37.

Diagnosis of Vascular Anomalies

2

Amy Geddis, Anna Lillis, and Anita Gupta

Abbreviations

CLOVES	Congenital lipomatous overgrowth, vascular malformations, epidermal nevi, scoliosis/skeletal/spinal anomalies
D2-40	Podoplanin
FAO	Fibroadipose overgrowth
GLUT-1	Glucose 1 transporter protein -1
HHML	Hemihyperplasia-multiple lipomatosis
HHT	Hereditary hemorrhagic telangiectasia
MCAP	Megalencephaly-capillary malformation
MPPH	Megalencephaly-polymicrogyria-polydactyly-hydrocephalus
PHACE syndrome	Posterior fossa malformations, hemangiomas, arterial anomalies, cardiac defects and coarctation of the aorta, and eye anomalies
TRICKS	Time-resolved MRA sequences

A. Geddis (✉)
Department of Pediatrics, Cancer and Blood Disorders Clinic, Seattle Children's Hospital, Seattle, WA, USA
e-mail: Amy.Geddis@seattlechildrens.org

A. Lillis
Department of Radiology, The Ohio State University College of Medicine, Columbus, OH, USA

Department of Radiology, Nationwide Children's Hospital, Columbus, OH, USA
e-mail: Anna.Lillis@NationwideChildrens.org

A. Gupta
Department of Pathology, Cincinnati Children's Hospital Medical Center, Cincinnati, OH, USA
e-mail: Anita.Gupta@cchmc.org

C. C. Trenor III, D. M. Adams (eds.), *Vascular Anomalies*,
https://doi.org/10.1007/978-3-030-25624-1_2

Clinical Features

As with any patient, the diagnosis of vascular anomalies starts with a careful history. Vascular anomalies present with a variety of symptoms, including a mass or effects of that mass on involved structures, effusions, bleeding, or thrombosis. Overlying skin changes, including a vascular "stain," blebs, brownish or bluish discoloration may be present. Consideration of the age at presentation, the rate of growth or factors related to growth such as trauma or hormonal changes, characteristics and location of the lesion, and associated clinical or laboratory features can aid in the diagnosis of vascular anomalies. Increasing evidence points to a genetic component to many vascular malformations and the family history may provide clues to an inherited syndrome.

Age at Presentation The age at presentation is a key consideration in the diagnosis of vascular anomalies. Capillary and lymphatic malformations are typically diagnosed at birth. Infantile hemangiomas may be initially inconspicuous but grow rapidly in the first weeks to months of life. Kaposiform hemangioendothelioma is most common in infants and young children, but presentation can range from in utero [1] to young adulthood [8]. Venous and arteriovenous malformations are present at birth but often become more apparent in late childhood or with puberty. Lymphatic malformations are generally diagnosed at birth but may enlarge in association with trauma, hemorrhage or infection, or at puberty. Telangiectasias in hereditary hemorrhagic telangiectasia (HHT) typically do not appear until adulthood.

Growth Vascular anomalies are mainly classified into tumors and malformations based on growth characteristics. Vascular tumors (e.g., hemangiomas, hemangioendotheliomas, angiosarcomas) grow rapidly due to vascular proliferation. Most are benign, though they may be locally invasive (kaposiform hemangioendothelioma), and rare tumors can metastasize (angiosarcoma, epithelioid hemangioendothelioma). Vascular malformations, in contrast, represent developmental anomalies; they are present at birth and grow in proportion to the child. However, injury, inflammatory stimuli, or hormonal changes may stimulate growth, and, thus, some malformations may become more apparent in late childhood or adolescence.

Physical Exam Findings and Location The color of the lesion should be noted; a red color is most commonly associated with hemangiomas and capillary malformations, whereas venous malformations may appear bluish if superficial. Lymphatic malformations are often flesh-colored, unless acutely inflamed, but they may appear red or bluish if there has been hemorrhage into a macrocyst. Lesions can be flat, plaque- or mass-like, with borders that are discrete or infiltrating. Capillary malformations are flat and well-demarcated, whereas vascular tumors tend to be plaque- or mass-like (Fig. 2.1a). A compressible lesion that fills when in a dependent position suggests a venous malformation. The presence of an overlying bruit, thrill or warmth suggests a high-flow component as in an arteriovenous malformation (Fig. 2.1b). However, the appearance of a lesion can be affected by its depth or presence of additional vascular components, and can change with growth of the lesion or with intralesional hemorrhage or thrombosis.

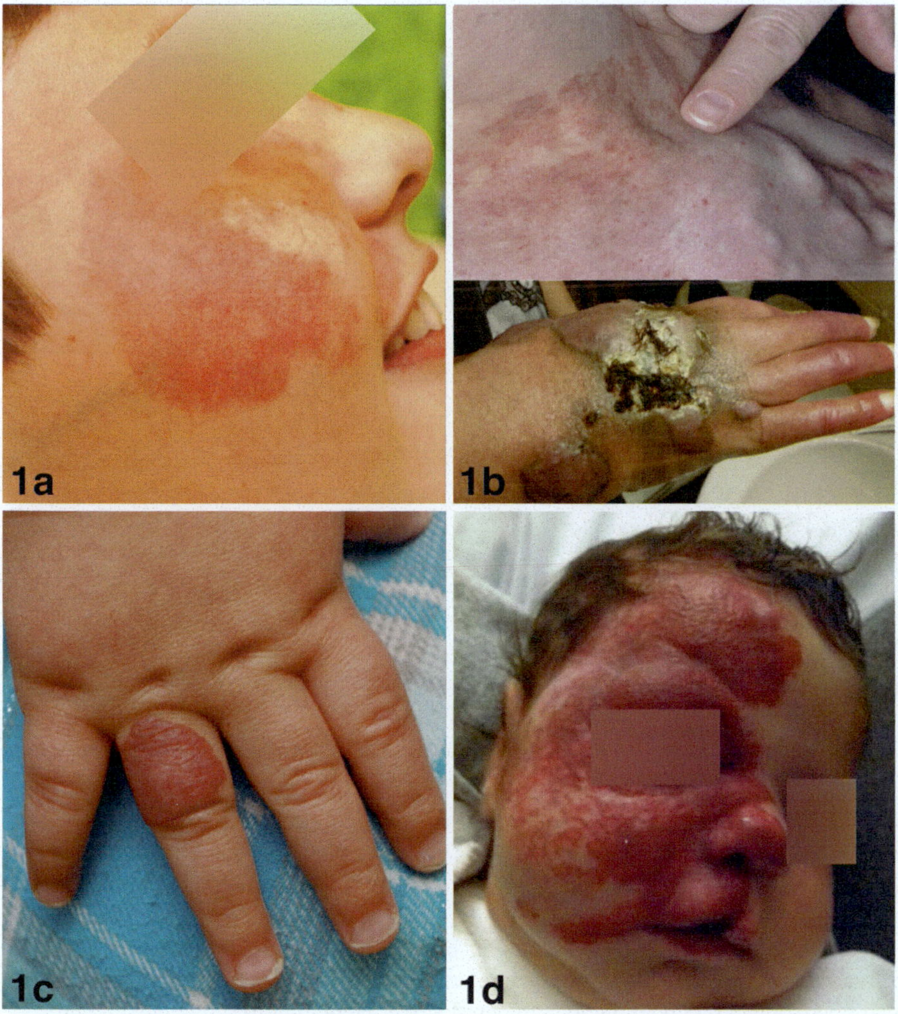

Fig. 2.1 (**a**) Capillary malformation. (**b**) Arteriovenous malformation. (**c**) Infantile hemangioma. (**d**) Infantile segmental hemangioma

In addition to the appearance of the lesion, the location of the vascular anomaly may influence presenting symptoms and provide clues to the diagnosis as well as trigger a search for associated features or syndromes. Infantile hemangiomas are commonly found in the head and neck region or less often the trunk and limbs (Fig. 2.1c). Periorbital and orbital hemangiomas in infants may affect development of visual acuity; even if they only partially obstruct vision [18]. Blockage of the tear duct may also occur. PHACE syndrome (posterior fossa malformations, hemangiomas, arterial anomalies, cardiac defects and coarctation of the aorta, and eye anomalies) should be considered if any hemangioma is >5 cm and segmental (Fig. 2.1d). Capillary malformations involving the face in the distribution of the first branch of the trigeminal nerve

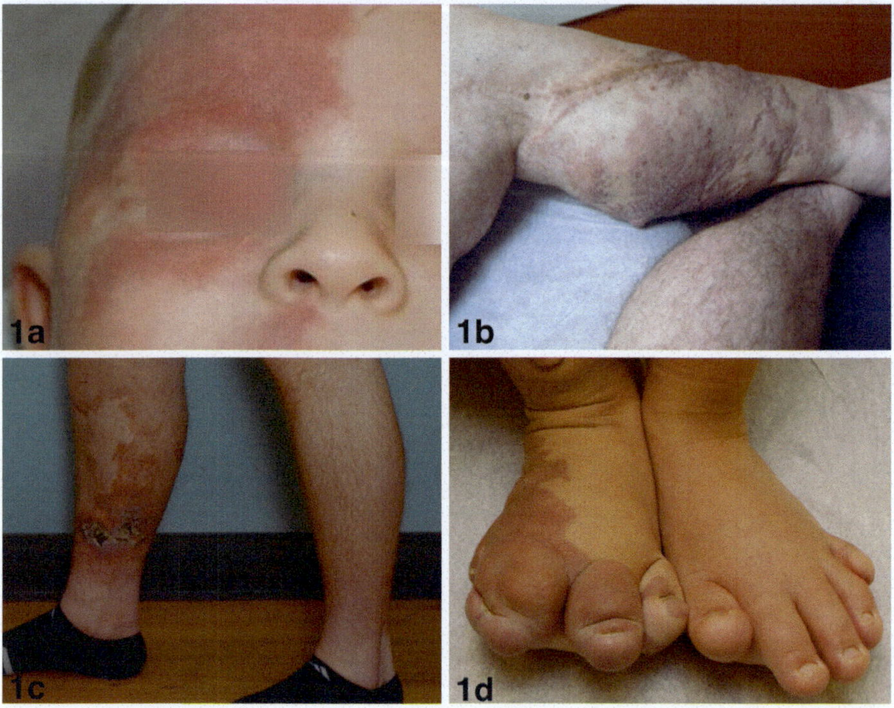

Fig. 2.2 (**a**) Sturge-Weber. (**b**) Klippel-Trenaunay syndrome. (**c**) Parkes Weber. (**d**) CLOVES

are often associated with leptomeningeal angiomas, choroidal hemangioma, and glaucoma (Sturge-Weber syndrome) (Fig. 2.2a). Airway obstruction may complicate vascular anomalies in the head and neck region. Infantile hemangiomas in the "beard" distribution (preauricular areas, chin, anterior neck, and lower lip) have a propensity to compress the airway as they enlarge, or they may be associated with additional subglottic lesions [13, 14]. Infantile hemangiomas in the midline lumbosacral region can be associated with spinal dysraphism [5, 10]. Hemangiomas may also be present in viscera, most commonly the liver. The presence of multiple (5 or more) cutaneous infantile hemangiomas increases the likelihood of hepatic involvement [16]. Large hepatic congenital or multifocal infantile hemangiomas are associated with an increased risk of high-output cardiac failure and diffuse hepatic infantile hemangioma may cause consumptive hypothyroidism [7]. Lymphatic malformations frequently involve the head and neck, including oral structures such as the tongue, which can also lead to airway obstruction. In addition, lymphatic malformations that involve the neck, axillary, or intrathoracic sites may be associated with pleural effusions. Mediastinal involvement is less common in lymphatic malformation, but is the most common location for kaposiform lymphangiomatosis [3]. Bony lesions are characteristic of generalized lymphatic anomaly and Gorham-Stout disease; involvement of the appendicular skeleton is more common in the former. Pelvic and lower extremity involvement is common in the mixed capillary lymphaticovenous malformations of Klippel-Trenaunay syndrome, as well as in primary lymphedema. Limb overgrowth and megalencephaly may be a complication of multiple vascular malformation syndromes including Klippel-Trenaunay syndrome (Fig. 2.2b); Parkes Weber syndrome (Fig. 2.2c); congenital lipomatous overgrowth, vascular malformations, epidermal nevi, spinal/skeletal/scoliosis anomalies (CLOVES) (Fig. 2.2d); fibroadipose overgrowth (FAO); hemihyperplasia-multiple lipomatosis (HHML); Proteus syndrome; megalencephaly-capillary malformation (MCAP); and megalencephaly-polymicrogyria-polydactyly-hydrocephalus (MPPH) [19].

Associated Clinical Laboratory Features Coagulopathy and thrombosis are frequent complications in slow-flow vascular anomalies. Kasabach-Merritt syndrome is a life-threatening coagulopathy with severe thrombocytopenia, hypofibrinogenemia, and elevated D-dimers associated with kaposiform hemangioendotheliomas or tufted angiomas. Venous malformations or mixed malformations with a venous component may also have localized intralesional coagulopathy with mild to moderate thrombocytopenia, hypofibrinogenemia, and elevated D-dimers [11]. Phleboliths, round calcified thrombi, may be noted on imaging and are often painful. Venous thrombosis and pulmonary embolism can occur, especially in Klippel-Trenaunay and CLOVES syndrome where there may be failure of regression of large embryonic veins and/or abnormal development of the deep venous system of the lower limbs; valvular defects, phlebectasia, and hypoplasia are frequently present [12, 15]. In particular, the persistence of the embryonic lateral marginal vein is a potential site for development of thrombi that may propagate to the deep veins in the thigh and pelvis and subsequently embolize to the lungs. Pulmonary hypertension and embolic stroke may occur as a complication of pulmonary arteriovenous malformations [2]. Bleeding can also be associated with vascular lesions, even in the absence of coagulopathy. Patients with hereditary hemorrhagic telangiectasia suffer from recurrent severe epistaxis and can bleed from intestinal telangiectasia as well; iron deficiency should alert the clinician to the possibility of gastrointestinal hemorrhage. Chronic intestinal bleeding and iron deficiency may also complicate blue rubber bleb syndrome and cutaneovisceral angiomatosis with thrombocytopenia. Rectal bleeding, hemorrhoids, and hematuria can be seen in Klippel-Trenaunay syndrome with pelvic involvement [17]. Finally, intra-articular venous malformations can lead to hemarthrosis.

Family History Genetic mutations have been described in several of the vascular malformation syndromes, and in general, three patterns have emerged. Affecting the majority of patients, Somatic mutations have been identified in abnormal vascular tissue from patients with capillary malformations and segmental overgrowth syndromes, sporadic venous malformations, and lymphatic malformations. Chromosomal translocations have been identified in tumor tissue from patients with epithelioid and pseudomyogenic hemangioendothelioma. Germline inherited mutations are the basis of familial syndromes such as hereditary hemorrhagic telangiectasia, some lymphedema syndromes, hereditary venous malformations, capillary malformation-arteriovenous malformation, and Proteus syndromes. A familial predisposition with incomplete penetrance, due to the inheritance of one mutated allele and the somatic acquisition of a second mutation within the abnormal vascular tissue, is seen in patients with glomuvenous and cerebral cavernous malformations.

Diagnostic Evaluation

The diagnosis of a vascular anomaly often depends largely on the clinical history and exam. Blood work, radiographic imaging, and biopsy may, in different situations, help define the type of vascular anomaly or rule out alternative diagnoses. More recently, genetic testing may facilitate diagnosis and counseling. A multidisciplinary approach is required, especially for malformations that are complex or have associated syndromic features.

The *clinical history and exam* will take into account the patient's age at presentation, growth characteristics, appearance and location of the lesion(s), and associated features. It is important to identify symptoms that demand acute management as well as those that inform the differential diagnosis (see above). Digital photos of the lesions are a helpful addition to the medical record.

Laboratory studies useful in the evaluation of vascular anomalies include a complete blood count and coagulation studies (PT, aPTT, fibrinogen, and D-dimers); this will identify associated complications such as Kasabach-Merritt syndrome or localized intralesional coagulopathy. Severe thrombocytopenia (platelet counts <50 K) strongly suggests Kasabach-Merritt syndrome, consistent with the diagnosis of Kaposiform hemangioendothelioma or tufted angioma. D-dimers are also frequently elevated in slow-flow lesions with a venous component, but rarely in pure lymphatic malformations and arteriovenous malformations [4]. If microcytic anemia is present, iron studies should be performed. In infants with liver lesions, the concomitant presence of cutaneous hemangiomas favors diagnosis of infantile hepatic hemangioma. Serum alpha fetoprotein should be obtained in those children in whom hepatoblastoma is suspected; however, since AFP is elevated at birth, serial AFPs monitoring the rate of fall with age may be required in order to interpret the results. Thyroid studies (T4, TSH) should be obtained in infants with hepatic hemangiomas to screen for consumptive hypothyroidism.

Radiographic imaging is useful for defining the extent of the lesion and to identify fast flow or slow flow as well as lymphatic components. Imaging is also important in the evaluation of complications such as thrombosis and in the planning of interventional approaches. Additional studies may be indicated in vascular lesions with syndromic associations to identify occult vascular and nonvascular abnormalities. Ultrasound is frequently employed as a first step in imaging because it does not expose the patient to radiation and often does not require sedation. Ultrasound is especially sensitive for identification of cystic or fluid filled spaces and, in combination with Doppler, can distinguish high- and low-flow lesions as well as areas of impaired flow due to thrombosis. Fast flow is characteristic of arteriovenous malformations and hemangiomas, whereas slow flow is seen in venous and capillary malformations. Ultrasound may also identify pleural effusions or ascites. In young infants, ultrasound of the spine can detect spinal dysraphism. Magnetic resonance imaging provides a cross-sectional overview of the lesion and is the most frequently used modality in the evaluation of large or complex vascular anomalies. Enhancement characteristics can identify lymphatic components (T2-bright, non-enhancing) versus venous, arterial, or capillary components (enhance with contrast). Additional sequences, such as time-resolved MRA sequences "TRICKS" or "TWIST" can identify lesions as "fast" or "slow" flow by measuring the rate at which contrast enters, dwells, and then is washed out of a vascular lesion. Phleboliths, which are small, rounded, calcified structures having evolved from chronic clot, typically indicate a venous component. Lymphoscintigraphy may be used in the evaluation of lymphedema; this involves the injection of Tc99m-labeled antimony sulfur or albumin distally into the web space between the first and second digit of the affected area and tracing the flow of the labeled colloid proximally through the lymphatics [9]. CT may be useful in specific circumstances to define bony involvement. An echocardiogram should be obtained if there is a risk of high-output cardiac failure, especially in children with large hepatic lesions or with AVMs.

Biopsy is not always required to make a diagnosis and may be contraindicated in the face of severe coagulopathy or some anatomic locations. In addition, biopsy of lymphatic rib lesions is discouraged as it can lead to the formation of a chronic pleural effusion. Nevertheless, when the diagnosis is unclear, biopsy can provide useful information to aid the diagnosis and rule out alternative processes. In addition to morphologic review [6], immunohistochemical stains can differentiate between different types of vascular anomalies. GLUT-1 (glucose 1 transporter protein-1) is expressed in infantile hemangiomas and not expressed in other cutaneous vascular anomalies of infancy, congenital hemangiomas and pyogenic granulomas. PROX-1 and/or podoplanin (i.e., D2-40) immunostains are reactive in lymphatic malformations and kaposiform hemangioendothelioma and negative in venous malformations. Smooth muscle actin highlights glomus cells lining venous channels. In addition, tissue can be analyzed for somatic genetic mutations (see below). Pleural effusions or ascites should be tapped, which may provide diagnostic information as well as therapeutic benefit. Pleural or ascitic fluid with elevated triglycerides and lymphocytes indicates a chylous effusion and suggests dysfunction of the central conducting lymphatics.

Genetic testing for a number of germline and somatic mutations may be clinically available and facilitate diagnosis. Somatic mosaic mutations can be assayed from biopsied tissue, whereas genomic mutations are typically assayed from peripheral blood leukocytes. Clinical testing is currently available for a number of genetic mutations associated with vascular anomalies including ACVRL1, AKT1, AKT2, AKT3, ENG, GNAQ, GLMN, MTOR, PIK3CA, PIK3R2, PTEN, RASA1, and SMAD4. The field is rapidly changing; current information can be found on the website GeneTests.org.

In summary, the approach to an accurate vascular anomalies diagnosis requires a comprehensive clinical assessment, thorough personal and family history, complete blood count and coagulation studies, correlation with imaging, biopsy, or resection of the lesion in some cases, and increasingly, genetic testing.

References

1. Calvo-Garcia MA, Kline-Fath BM, Adams DM, Gupta A, Koch BL, Lim FY, et al. Imaging evaluation of fetal vascular anomalies. Pediatr Radiol. 2015;45(8):1218–29. https://doi.org/10.1007/s00247-014-3248-x.
2. Circo S, Gossage JR. Pulmonary vascular complications of hereditary haemorrhagic telangiectasia. Curr Opin Pulm Med. 2014;20(5):421–8. https://doi.org/10.1097/MCP.0000000000000076.

3. Croteau SE, Kozakewich HP, Perez-Atayde AR, Fishman SJ, Alomari AI, Chaudry G, et al. Kaposiform lymphangiomatosis: a distinct aggressive lymphatic anomaly. J Pediatr. 2014;164(2):383–8. https://doi.org/10.1016/j.jpeds.2013.10.013.
4. Dompmartin A, Ballieux F, Thibon P, Lequerrec A, Hermans C, Clapuyt P, et al. Elevated D-dimer level in the differential diagnosis of venous malformations. Arch Dermatol. 2009;145(11):1239–44. https://doi.org/10.1001/archdermatol.2009.296.
5. Drolet BA, Chamlin SL, Garzon MC, Adams D, Baselga E, Haggstrom AN, et al. Prospective study of spinal anomalies in children with infantile hemangiomas of the lumbosacral skin. J Pediatr. 2010;157(5):789–94. https://doi.org/10.1016/j.jpeds.2010.07.054.
6. Gupta A, Kozakewich H. Histopathology of vascular anomalies. Clin Plast Surg. 2011;38(1):31–44. https://doi.org/10.1016/j.cps.2010.08.007.
7. Huang SA, Tu HM, Harney JW, Venihaki M, Butte AJ, Kozakewich HP. Severe hypothyroidism caused by type 3 iodothyronine deiodinase in infantile hemangiomas. N Engl J Med. 2000;343(3):185–9.
8. Lyons LL, North PE, Mac-Moune Lai F, Stoler MH, Folpe AL, Weiss SW. Kaposiform hemangioendothelioma: a study of 33 cases emphasizing its pathologic, immunophenotypic, and biologic uniqueness from juvenile hemangioma. Am J Surg Pathol. 2004;28(5):559–68.
9. Maclellan RA, Greene AK. Lymphedema. Semin Pediatr Surg. 2014;23(4):191–7. https://doi.org/10.1053/j.sempedsurg.2014.07.004.
10. Maugans T, Sheridan RM, Adams D, Gupta A. Cutaneous vascular anomalies associated with neural tube defects: nomenclature and pathology revisited. Neurosurgery. 2011;69(1):112–8. https://doi.org/10.1227/NEU.0b013e3182134360.
11. Mazoyer E, Enjolras O, Bisdorff A, Perdu J, Wassef M, Drouet L. Coagulation disorders in patients with venous malformation of the limbs and trunk: a case series of 118 patients. Arch Dermatol. 2008;144(7):861–7. https://doi.org/10.1001/archderm.144.7.861.
12. Oduber CE, van der Horst CM, Hennekam RC. Klippel-Trenaunay syndrome: diagnostic criteria and hypothesis on etiology. Ann Plast Surg. 2008;60(2):217–23. https://doi.org/10.1097/SAP.0b013e318062abc1.
13. O-Lee TJ, Messner A. Subglottic hemangioma. Otolaryngol Clin N Am. 2008;41(5):903–11, viii-ix. https://doi.org/10.1016/j.otc.2008.04.009.
14. Orlow SJ, Isakoff MS, Blei F. Increased risk of symptomatic hemangiomas of the airway in association with cutaneous hemangiomas in a "beard" distribution. J Pediatr. 1997;131(4):643–6.
15. Reis J 3rd, Alomari AI, Trenor CC 3rd, Adams DM, Fishman SJ, Spencer SA, Shaikh R, Lillis AP, Surnedi MK, Chaudry G. Pulmonary thromboembolic events in patients with congenital lipomatous overgrowth, vascular malformations, epidermal nevi, and spinal/skeletal abnormalities and Klippel-Trénaunay syndrome. J Vasc Surg Venous Lymphat Disord. 2018;6(4):511–6. https://doi.org/10.1016/j.jvsv.2018.01.015.
16. Rialon KL, Murillo R, Fevurly RD, Kulungowski AM, Zurakowski D, Liang M, et al. Impact of screening for hepatic hemangiomas in patients with multiple cutaneous infantile hemangiomas. Pediatr Dermatol. 2015;32(6):808–12. https://doi.org/10.1111/pde.12656.
17. Sreekar H, Dawre S, Petkar KS, Shetty RB, Lamba S, Naik S, et al. Diverse manifestations and management options in Klippel-Trenaunay syndrome: a single centre 10-year experience. J Plast Surg Hand Surg. 2013;47(4):303–7. https://doi.org/10.3109/2000656X.2013.766201.
18. Stass-Isern M. Periorbital and orbital infantile hemangiomas. Int Ophthalmol Clin. 2014;54(3):73–82. https://doi.org/10.1097/IIO.0000000000000039.
19. Uller W, Fishman SJ, Alomari AI. Overgrowth syndromes with complex vascular anomalies. Semin Pediatr Surg. 2014;23(4):208–15. https://doi.org/10.1053/j.sempedsurg.2014.06.013.

The Genetic Basis of Vascular Anomalies

3

Ha-Long Nguyen, Laurence M. Boon, and Miikka Vikkula

Introduction

Vascular anomalies are localized lesions that arise from aberrant regulation and establishment of the vasculature. There are two categories of vascular anomalies: vascular tumors and malformations. Vascular tumors are characterized by an overactive endothelium and consist mainly of hemangiomas. The endothelium of vascular malformations is more quiescent, and this category comprises a large number of subtypes. Based on clinical, radiological, and histological evaluations, they are subdivided according to the vessel type affected as venous, arteriovenous, capillary, lymphatic, and combined lesions (e.g., capillary-venous malformation). Additionally, vascular malformations may be a major or minor part of the phenotype in syndromes. For example, in Klippel-Trenaunay syndrome (KTS), extensive capillary-lymphatico-venous malformation (CLVM) is associated with hypertrophy, whereas in PTEN hamartoma tumor syndrome (PHTS), variable defects, from macrocephaly to penile freckles, are accompanied by abnormally vascularized lesions.

The mode of development (familial vs. sporadic) of each vascular anomaly varies widely; however, knowledge of this trait influences the treatment regimen and patient education provided. In some cases, the most frequent form of the disease is familial (e.g., glomuvenous malformation and hereditary hemorrhagic telangiectasia). Therefore, special consideration must be given to evaluation of risk

H.-L. Nguyen
Human Molecular Genetics, de Duve Institute, Brussels, Belgium

L. M. Boon · M. Vikkula (✉)
Human Molecular Genetics, de Duve Institute, Brussels, Belgium

Center for Vascular Anomalies, Cliniques Universitaires Saint-Luc, Catholic University of Louvain, Brussels, Belgium
e-mail: miikka.vikkula@uclouvain.be

C. C. Trenor III, D. M. Adams (eds.), *Vascular Anomalies*,
https://doi.org/10.1007/978-3-030-25624-1_3

to develop the disease in a (not-yet-born) family member and management of follow-up to detect newly developing lesions. In other instances, the disease seems to occur exclusively sporadically (e.g., KTS or CLVM; Sturge-Weber syndrome; lymphatic malformation). Thus, management is largely done on a case-by-case basis. For the majority of vascular anomalies, the lesions predominantly appear sporadically, though a variable fraction (1–20%) may be familial forms (e.g., capillary malformation, venous malformation, cerebral cavernous malformations).

The extent of disease most likely reflects the level of dysregulation caused by the mutations. Weak effects can be present in all cells and from the single cell stage onward (as in germline mutations of inherited forms), whereas mutations with strong effects are likely incompatible with life in the heterozygous stage. This may be due either to embryonic vascular defects critical to early embryogenesis or to more widespread defects if present in all cell types and not only restricted to a limited number/type of cells (e.g., endothelial cells).

The familial or inherited vascular anomalies were crucial in providing the first insights into the pathogenesis of vascular anomalies. The first somatic mutations were identified in sporadically occurring venous malformations. They were point mutations in the TIE2 receptor encoding gene *TEK* [1] (Fig. 3.1). This was based on traditional Sanger sequencing of DNA extracted from resected lesions. As less than 50% of the alleles were mutant (often only around 10%, the minimum detection level of Sanger sequencing), RNA-based screens were done to enrich for the endothelial-specific TIE2 transcripts. This allowed enhanced sensitivity for mutation detection and pointed out the heterogeneity of the causative mutation within affected tissues. It also highlighted the need for extremely sensitive mutation detection in various vascular anomaly tissues to find causative (or associated) changes [2].

With the advancement of massively parallel sequencing, it is now possible to perform high-throughput screens on tissue samples. Targeted panels allow sequencing thousands of times a limited number of genes (high vertical coverage) and result in a sensitive detection rate of 1% for mutant alleles. In tandem, digital droplet PCR (ddPCR) does the same in a performance- and cost-efficient manner for known mutations, on the basis of specific probes synthesized for each variant to be tested. This vastly improved the ability to reveal causative or associated nucleotide variants (mutations) in lesional tissues that account for most of the venous, capillary, lymphatic malformations, and arteriovenous malformations.

The different types of vascular lesions are now known to be largely due to disrupted (endothelial) receptor intracellular signaling pathways. Mutations have been identified in proteins such as receptor tyrosine kinases, G-protein-coupled receptor adaptor molecules, and various proteins involved in the PI3kinase(K)–AKT, MAPK, and SMAD signaling pathways (Fig. 3.1). This has opened a new era of potential for the management of vascular anomalies that could only be dreamed of 25 years ago, when all these studies were initiated. We can now start to hypothesize, develop, and test targeted molecular therapies, and the first reports show promising efficacy in ameliorating patients' quality of life [3, 4].

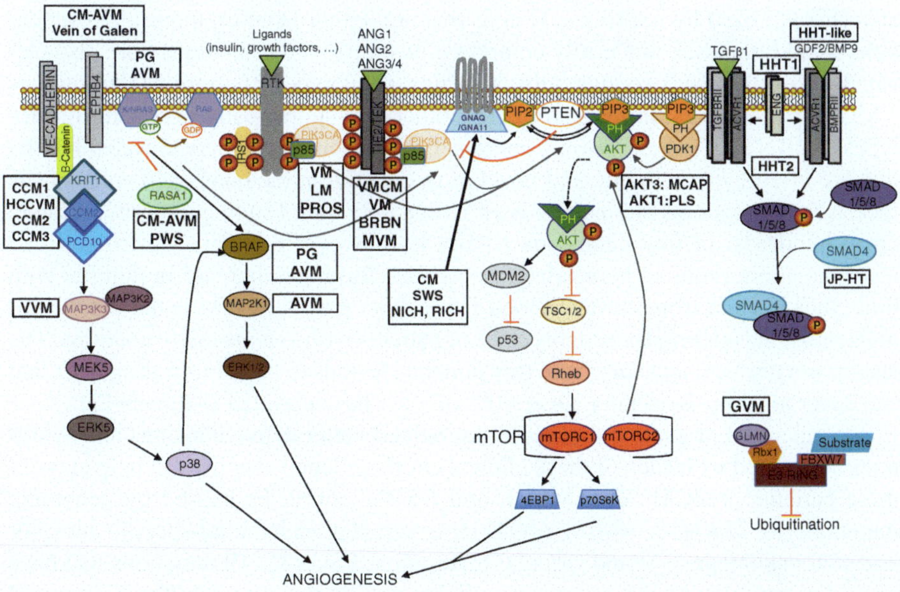

Fig. 3.1 Summary of vascular anomalies and associated syndromes that are linked to molecules of essential signaling pathways within the vasculature. Mutations within genes that code for proteins that are involved in the MAPK pathways have been found for capillary malformation (CM), arteriovenous malformation, AVM, CM-AVM, Vein of Galen, cerebral cavernous malformation (CCM)1–3, hyperkeratotic cutaneous capillary-venous malformation (HCCVM), verrucous venous malformation (VVM), pyogenic granuloma (PG), Parkes-Weber syndrome (PWS), Sturge-Weber syndrome, rapidly involuting congenital hemangiomas (RICH), and noninvoluting congenital hemangiomas (NICH). Meanwhile, for venous malformation (VM), lymphatic malformation (LM), PIK3CA-related overgrowth spectrum (PROS), mucocutaneous VM (VMCM), multifocal VM (MVM), blue rubber bleb nevus syndrome (BRBN), megalencephaly-CM (MCAP), and Proteus syndrome (PLS), the PI3K/AKT signaling is affected. Hereditary hemorrhagic telangiectasia (HHT) results from dysregulation of TGF-β superfamily signaling, more specifically via the BMP ligands. Glomuvenous malformations (GVM) are linked to glomulin, a protein that may have a more generalized role as a part of the machinery involved in FBW7-mediated protein ubiquitination and degradation

Venous Malformations

Venous anomalies exemplify the benefits of revealing causative mutations. There are at least five distinguishable entities: the autosomal dominantly inherited glomuvenous malformation (GVM), mucocutaneous venous malformation (VMCM; MIM 600195), sporadically occurring venous malformation (VM; MIM 600221), multifocal venous malformation (MVM), and blue rubber bleb nevus syndrome (BRBN; MIM 112200). GVMs account for about 5% of venous anomaly patients, and there is a clear family history. GVMs are classically present as multifocal small dark-blue cutaneous lesions, which are usually hyperkeratotic [5]. Rarer VMCM is also characterized by multifocal lesions that are lighter in color, more often subcutaneous and mucosal, and easily compressible on palpation. D-dimers are also elevated. From the three sporadically occurring phenotypes, the rare MVM mimics VMCM, yet lacks a family history. The other two sporadically occurring phenotypes, BRBN and VM are distinct entities. BRBN includes rubbery elevated lesions that are often hyperkeratotic and develop frequently on the hands and soles of the feet. Affected patients are usually born with a *dominant* lesion and grow multiple, up to hundreds, of tiny cutaneous BRBN lesions over time [6]. Gastrointestinal lesions that are prone to hemorrhaging can also form and increase in number with time; thus anemia from chronic blood loss is also prevalent. VM is the most common entity, accounting for roughly 95% of patients with venous malformations. The lesions are unifocal and vary from tiny punctate lesions to large infiltrating ones that can cover an entire extremity. Over 40% of VMs have elevated D-dimers [7].

Identification of genetic mutations has helped better define the signs and symptoms associated with each of these clinical entities. Genetic testing can help classify these patients. VMCM, VM, MVM, and BRBN can all be caused by activating mutations in *TEK/TIE2* (MIM 600221), a vascular endothelial-specific receptor essential in angiogenesis and vascular maturation (Fig. 3.1). All mutations that have been discovered are within the intracellular part of the receptor (the kinase and kinase insert domains or the carboxy-terminal tail) and lead to increased ligand-independent receptor autophosphorylation. The predominant mutation in VMs (of which 60% are due to a TIE2 mutation) is a somatic leucine 914-to-phenylalanine (L914F) change [1, 8]. In contrast, the most common inherited mutation in VMCM is an arginine 849-to-tryptophan substitution (R849W) [1, 6]. This weakly activating germline mutation needs somatic second hits in TIE2 to induce lesion formation [1, 6]. MVM patients have an underlying *de novo* mosaic mutation detectable in their blood, and superposed somatic mutations, often occurring on the same allele (in cis) [6]. Double cis somatic changes in TEK are also detected in BRBN. As they have equal frequencies and identities in separate lesions from distant sites within the same patient, activated dissemination of lesions seems to occur in these patients.

PI3K/AKT signaling is the canonical TIE2 signaling pathway, and it is also affected downstream in response to the overactive TIE2 (Fig. 3.1). Human umbilical vein endothelial cells (HUVEC) transfected with the mutations resulted in dysregulation of angiogenic factors linked to this pathway and abnormal EC morphology. This opened the possibility to use sirolimus, which inhibits mTOR downstream of PI3K/AKT signaling, to counteract the effects with very promising preclinical and Phase II clinical data [4, 9]. The importance of the deregulation of this pathway in VM pathogenesis was underscored by the recent discovery that another 20% of VMs are due to activating PIK3CA mutations [10] (Fig. 3.1). These mutations cause inappropriate PI3K activation, and *in vitro* treatment of PIK3CA- and TIE2-mutant cells with a PI3K inhibitor, BYL719, normalized the cells [10]. Thus, this signaling pathway has become a favorable target (in particular PI3K, AKT, and mTOR) for therapeutic intervention. Consequently, Phase III clinical trials have begun using sirolimus. Sirolimus effectively ameliorates patients' quality of life as symptoms become less pronounced, and early data demonstrate reduction in lesional volume in some patients (Boon et al., unpublished). Similar effects were seen in a compassionate use BYL719 study in PIK3CA-related overgrowth syndromes associated with a vascular anomaly [11].

Glomuvenous malformations (GVM) are caused by loss-of-function mutations in the *glomulin* gene (GLMN; MIM 601749) [12] (Fig. 3.1). The most common change is found in 45% of patients, yet most of the mutations are specific to a single family [13]. Forty different mutations have so far been reported in 162 GVM families. Akin to VMCM, the multifocality of GVM is explained by the principle of paradominant inheritance. The most common "second hit" is an acquired uniparental isodisomy [14]. The exact function of GLMN, particularly in the vasculature, is unknown. It appears to play a major role in regulating differentiation of vascular smooth muscle cells (vSMC), based on the specificity of the GVM phenotype. In vitro studies suggest that it may interact with the transforming growth factor-β (TGF-β) and hepatocyte growth factor (HGF) signaling pathways [15–17]. GLMN may also have a more generalized role in FBW7-mediated protein ubiquitination and degradation [18].

Arteriovenous Malformations

Arteriovenous malformations (AVM) have fast arterial flow, making them more progressive and destructive than other vascular anomalies. They have a strong angiogenic potential, as partial resection often leads to severe deterioration of the lesion with time. The majority of AVMs arises sporadically and may affect any organ. Yet, AVMs are also a prominent feature in patients affected by two inherited disorders: hereditary hemorrhagic telangiectasia (HHT; MIM 187300, 600376, and 175050) and capillary malformation-arteriovenous malformation (CM-AVM; MIM 608354 and 618196).

HHT and CM-AVM have incidences estimated at 1/5000, and 1/10,000, respectively. Based on the identified genes, two major signaling pathways are involved in pathogenesis: TGF-β/SMAD (HHT) and MAPK/ERK (CM-AVM) pathways. However, despite the AVMs having overlapping clinical characteristics, mechanistic cross talk between the two pathogenic pathways regulating angiogenesis has remained elusive.

In HHT, a diagnosis is made by two methods: (1) clinically, if a patient presents with at least three of the four Curaçao criteria, or (2) by using genetic testing, as long as the patient carries a mutation in one of the known 3 HHT genes [19]. There are two other types of HHT, mapped to chromosomes 5 (HHT3; MIM 601101) and 7 (HHT4; MIM 610655) [20, 21], but the causative genes have yet to be identified. The known genes encode proteins of the TGF-β signaling superfamily: the endothelial co-receptor endoglin (ENG; MIM 131195) (HHT1; MIM 187300), the type I receptor activin kinase-like-1 (MIM 601284) (ACVRL1/HHT2; MIM 600376), and the intracellular co-mediator SMAD4 (MIM 600993) [22, 23] (Fig. 3.1). About 80% of patients have a mutation in the first two genes. Over 500 variants for each HHT1 and HHT2 have been reported, with pathological ones (~67 and 50%, respectively) leading to loss of function [24]. Patients that possess SMAD4 mutations are affected with a combined syndrome of HHT and another autosomal dominant disorder, juvenile polyposis (JP-HT; MIM 175050) (Fig. 3.1). These patients have polyps in the gastrointestinal tract [25].

The underlying pathogenic mechanism for HHT remains controversial. It appears that the bone morphogenetic pathway (BMP) is likely perturbed. It is evidenced that the ligands that bind ACVRL1 are BMP9 and BMP10 [26]. This is supported by the finding that three patients exhibiting HHT-like symptoms harbor mutations in the gene coding for BMP9/GDF2 (MIM 605120) (HHT5; MIM 615506) [27]. Several drugs currently used to treat other diseases are able to alleviate the life-impeding symptoms of HHT, for example, thalidomide, tranexamic acid, and bevacizumab [28–32]. However, how these drugs act in HHT has not been fully explored.

As in the VMs, the severity of symptoms unpredictably varies among HHT patients, even for those in the same family and mutation. Though a somatic second hit has not been confirmed in patients, mouse models have suggested the combination of three hits to contribute to lesion progression. Conditional knockout of *Acvrl* and *Eng* in adult mice reliably formed AVMs when given a pro-angiogenic stressor, such as wounding or treatment with LPS or VEGF [33–38]. The mouse models suggest that in addition to the predisposing germline mutation and complete localized loss of the gene function, a pro-angiogenic environmental element strongly contributes to lesion formation.

Germline mutations also occur in CM-AVM, either in the RASA1 or the EPHB4 gene, and result in loss of function. The affected gene for CM-AVM1, RASA1 (MIM 139150), encodes the GTPase-activating protein p120-RasGAP [39–41] (Fig. 3.1). The loss of RASA1 causes hyperactivation of the RAS/MAPK signaling pathway, resulting in altered cell proliferation, differentiation, and growth. Mice homozygous for p120rasGap loss die during embryogenesis, whereas embryos mosaic for wild-type and p120RasGap-null cells generate abnormal cutaneous vessels [42]. Additionally, a somatic second hit has been identified in lesional tissue from three CM-AVM1 patients, (1) in a Parkes-Weber syndrome, (2) in a capillary malformation, and (3) in an arteriovenous malformation, underscoring the necessity of complete localized loss of function of p120rasGap for lesions to develop [40, 43, 44].

CM-AVM2 is caused by alterations in the EPH receptor B4 (EPHB4) (MIM 600011), which, along with its ligand Ephrin B2 (EFNB2), plays a major role in arteriovenous differentiation [45, 46]. EPHB4 mutations were also found in sporadic Vein of Galen aneurysmal malformations, which are a subtype of cerebral AVMs [47, 48]. In zebrafish, RASA1 functions downstream of EPHB4, and knocking down either led to enlarged vessels and arrested blood flow [49].

In sporadically occurring AVMs, activating mutations in the KRAS (MIM 190070), NRAS (MIM 164790), BRAF (MIM 164757), and MAP2K1 (MIM 176872) have been found [50–52], further implicating the MAPK signaling in the development of AVMs. The majority of the discovered hotspot mutations are the same as those commonly seen in various types of cancers (e.g., KRAS glycine-12-to-aspartic acid (G12D)). Thus, it raises the possibility to repurpose currently used therapeutic cancer drugs for treatment of AVMs. A preclinical model showed promise as blood flow was normalized in zebrafish AVM models treated with a BRAF inhibitor, vemurafenib [51].

Capillary Malformations

Capillary malformations (CM; MIM 16300) are the most common vascular malformations, with a reported incidence of 0.3% [53]. They appear sporadically, except in the CM-AVM described above. CM can be an isolated cutaneous lesion or associated with leptomeningeal vascular anomalies (Sturge-Weber syndrome). In both cases, somatic changes in the guanine nucleotide-binding protein G (GNAQ; MIM 600998) are attributed to the disorder, with the most frequent variant being an arginine183-to-glycine (R183Q) substitution [54–56] (Fig. 3.1). This mutation may cause an overstimulation of the MAPK/ERK pathway, as HEK293 cells transfected with mutant GNAQ expressed an increase in ERK activation, compared to control cells [54]. Although it is unknown whether other signaling pathways are involved, ERK inhibition may thus block development of these lesions.

Cerebral Cavernous Malformations, Hyperkeratotic Cutaneous Capillary-Venous Malformations, and Verrucous Venous Malformations

Cerebral cavernous malformations (CCM) are lesions located within the CNS parenchyma. They can be inherited (commonly multifocal) or occur *de novo*. Familial cases are passed on in an autosomal dominant manner, and CCMs also follow paradominant inheritance [57, 58]. Three causative genes are known: Krev interaction trapped-1 (MIM 604214) (KRIT1/CCM1; MIM 116860), malcavernin (MIM 607929) (CCM2; MIM 607929), and programmed cell death 10 (MIM 609118) (PDCD10/CCM3; MIM 603285) (Fig. 3.1). A fourth locus on chromosome 3 has been suggested, but the gene is unknown.

The three CCM proteins interact with each other among several signaling pathways. KRIT1 is involved in the Delta-Notch signaling pathway and regulates endothelial cell (EC)-cell junctions [59], while the delta-like ligand 4 (DLL4) may be targeted by PDCD10. PDCD10 has also been reported to play a role in apoptosis and in the vascular endothelial growth factor (VEGF) signaling pathway [60]. CCM2 is a scaffolding protein for MEKK3/MAP3K3 [61]. Studies in endothelial directed *Krit1* and *CCM2* knockout mice, and evaluation of CCM lesions, suggests the mitogen-activated kinase (MAPK) signaling pathway is affected as the loss of these genes lead to inappropriately active MEKK3 and Kruppel-like factor(KLF)-2 and KLF-4 [62].

Loss of function of CCM1 (KRIT1) is also associated with cutaneous vascular lesions known as hyperkeratotic cutaneous capillary-venous malformations

(HCCVMs) [63, 64] (Fig. 3.1). These lesions are similar to verrucous venous malformations (VVM), which develop sporadically within the skin without associated CCMs. VVMs are caused by activating mutations in the *MAP3K3* gene (MIM 602539) [65] (Fig. 3.1). Thus, MAP3K3 inhibition may be a way to control the development of CCMs, HCCVMs, and VVMs.

Lymphatic Malformations

Lymphatic malformations (LM) are congenital, isolated macro- or micro-cystic lesions that appear sporadically. Exome sequencing was key in identifying activating somatic mutations in the catalytic domain of PIK3CA in lesional tissue [66–68] (Fig. 3.1). As with the 20% of VMs with a PIK3CA mutation, the change causes overstimulation of the PI3K/AKT signaling pathway. Consequently, mutant lymphatic EC isolated from LMs exhibited increased proliferation and sprouting in collagen. Similar to VMs, sirolimus proved effective in improving the quality of life of LM patients [3]. Thus, a new era of treatment now combines conventional therapies with molecular approaches.

Complex and Combined Syndromes

Occasionally, a vascular malformation is present in conjunction with other defects and symptoms, typically connective tissue or bony overgrowth. There are a variety of clinical presentations of such syndromes. Next generation sequencing has been paramount in discovering somatic mutations in the heterogeneous lesions. Many of the identified affected genes are part of the PI3K/AKT signaling pathway. Interestingly, activating alterations in PIK3CA have been implicated in several syndromes. These include congenital lipomatous overgrowth vascular malformations, epidermal nevi, scoliosis/skeletal and spinal (CLOVES; MIM 612918) syndrome, megalencephaly-CM (MCAP; MIM 602501), fibroadipose overgrowth (FAO), and capillary-lymphatico-venous malformation with overgrowth/Klippel-Trenaunay syndrome (KTS; 149000) [69, 70]. Consequently, these are categorized within the PIK3CA-related overgrowth spectrum (PROS) [69], and they have shared molecular pathophysiology despite phenotypic heterogeneity (Fig. 3.1).

Genes encoding proteins of other members of the PI3K/AKT signaling are responsible for additional syndromes. Missense mutations in the serine threonine protein kinase AKT3 (MIM 611223) in some MCAP patients have been found [71]. Activating somatic mutations in AKT1 (MIM 164730) are seen in Proteus syndrome (PLS; MIM 176920) [72] (Fig. 3.1). The role of AKT1 in skin hyperplasia was confirmed in a mouse model, as hyperactivation of AKT in murine skin led to overgrowth [73]. These syndromes and the PROS spectrum may be amenable to management with PI3K-AKT pathway inhibitors, such as sirolimus and BYL719.

Vascular Tumors: Congenital Hemangiomas

Vascular tumors, which are largely accounted for by hemangiomas, are defects with hyperactive EC proliferation. Infantile hemangiomas (IH; MIM 602089) are the most common benign pediatric tumors (of vascular endothelial cells), found in 5–10% of children. IHs express the cell surface marker glucose transporter-1 (GLUT1). IH has a propensity toward race and sex, as it is found predominantly in the Caucasian population and three times more often in females. However, a genetic cause is unknown, although familial aggregation is sometimes seen [74–76].

Congenital hemangiomas are much less frequent than IH and differ in that the tumors are fully formed at birth and the ECs are negative for GLUT-1. There are three types of congenital hemangiomas. Rapidly involuting congenital hemangiomas (RICH) regress early in life, sometimes completely involuting within 12–14 months. Noninvoluting congenital hemangiomas (NICH) do not regress. Partially involuting congenital hemangiomas (PICH) are phenotypically between RICH and NICH.

Somatic missense mutations that disrupt the glutamine at amino acid position 209 (Glu20) in both GNAQ and GNA11, which have 90% sequence similarity, were discovered in RICH and NICH (Fig. 3.1). The finding that the same change in GNAQ and GNA11 (c.626A > T) can be observed in RICH and in NICH suggests that additional factors (be it environmental, genetic, developmental context, or others) strongly influence lesional phenotype [77]. Furthermore, the association of specific "hot spot" GNAQ mutations with corresponding vascular anomalies with very different characteristics (RICH/NICH vs. SWS and CM) exemplifies how it is crucial to understand the effects the changes have on underlying molecular signaling pathways. Although both alterations lead to moderate hyperactivation of GNAQ, various factors, such as the downstream signaling pathway, frequency of the mutant allele, and cell type affected apparently contribute to the lesion type that arises.

Pyogenic Granuloma

Pyogenic granuloma (PG), also referred to as lobular capillary hemangioma, is a benign vascular tumor. PGs often appear as singular red or blue papular growths that are susceptible to bleeding, though multifocal cases can occur. They are typically found on the surface of the skin or mucosa along the head and neck [78]. PGs have a propensity toward affecting women and children. Proposed causes for PG development include trauma, infection, or other events stimulating angiogenesis [78, 79].

An uncommon form of PG is associated with CM. Recent findings suggest overactivation of RAS as a culprit [80]. In particular, a c.1799T>A change in BRAF within ECs was implied as a major genetic hit in the progression of secondary PG on CM with a GNAQ R183Q change (Fig. 3.1). A mutation in KRAS further suggests the involvement of the MAPK signaling pathway [81].

Concluding Remarks

The knowledge gained from the oftentimes rare, inherited forms of vascular malformations was essential in opening the doors toward understanding the etiopathogenic causes of vascular anomalies. Since it was demonstrated that the reduced penetrance and variable expressivity for inherited vascular anomalies was due to somatic second hits, the focus was directed toward studies on the sporadically occurring forms focusing on involved tissues. However, such work was previously difficult because somatic changes are present at low allelic frequencies, below the detection threshold of traditional genetic tools, such as Sanger sequencing (which is ~10%). This issue is compounded by the fact that tissues are heterogenous cell populations, and the mutant allele is likely restricted to a certain number/population of cells, e.g., vascular EC. With the development of highly-sensitive, massively parallel sequencing and digital PCR (ddPCR), the ability to detect somatic genetic changes has significantly improved.

For the first time in history, we have insight into the pathophysiological bases of a large number of vascular anomalies, which often pinpoint to the disruption of intracellular signaling pathways in ECs (Fig. 3.1). As the same pathways are implicated in various cancers, and several inhibitors have been developed and used in their treatment, preclinical and clinical trials have been initiated for vascular anomalies. These trials need to be rigorously conducted and documented, in order to objectively evaluate the benefits and side effects, which could differ from cancer patients. Improved quality of life for affected patients is an important goal, thus an essential outcome measure in any such study. It is currently unknown how much a developmental vascular anomaly with continued angiogenic potential can be reduced in size with molecular approaches.

References

1. Limaye N, et al. Somatic mutations in angiopoietin receptor gene TEK cause solitary and multiple sporadic venous malformations. Nat Genet. 2009;41(1):118–24.
2. Limaye N, Boon LM, Vikkula M. From germline towards somatic mutations in the pathophysiology of vascular anomalies. Hum Mol Genet. 2009;18(R1):R65–74.
3. Adams DM, et al. Efficacy and safety of sirolimus in the treatment of complicated vascular anomalies. Pediatrics. 2016;137(2):1–10.
4. Boscolo E, et al. Rapamycin improves TIE2-mutated venous malformation in murine model and human subjects. J Clin Invest. 2015;125(9):3491–504.
5. Boon LM, et al. Glomuvenous malformation (glomangioma) and venous malformation: distinct clinicopathologic and genetic entities. Arch Dermatol. 2004;140(8):971–6.
6. Soblet J, et al. Blue Rubber Bleb Nevus (BRBN) syndrome is caused by somatic TEK (TIE2) mutations. J Invest Dermatol. In press.
7. Dompmartin A, et al. Elevated D-dimer level in the differential diagnosis of venous malformations. Arch Dermatol. 2009;145(11):1239–44.
8. Soblet J, et al. Variable somatic TIE2 mutations in half of sporadic venous malformations. Mol Syndromol. 2013;4(4):179–83.
9. Hammer J, et al. Sirolimus is efficacious in treatment for extensive and/or complex slow-flow vascular malformations: a monocentric prospective phase II study. Orphanet J Rare Dis. 2018;13(1):191.

10. Limaye N, et al. Somatic activating PIK3CA mutations cause venous malformation. Am J Hum Genet. 2015;97(6):914–21.
11. Venot Q, et al. Targeted therapy in patients with PIK3CA-related overgrowth syndrome. Nature. 2018;558(7711):540–6.
12. Brouillard P, et al. Mutations in a novel factor, glomulin, are responsible for glomuvenous malformations ("glomangiomas"). Am J Hum Genet. 2002;70(4):866–74.
13. Brouillard P, et al. Genotypes and phenotypes of 162 families with a glomulin mutation. Mol Syndromol. 2013;4(4):157–64.
14. Amyere M, et al. Somatic uniparental isodisomy explains multifocality of glomuvenous malformations. Am J Hum Genet. 2013;92(2):188–96.
15. McIntyre BA, et al. Glomulin is predominantly expressed in vascular smooth muscle cells in the embryonic and adult mouse. Gene Expr Patterns. 2004;4(3):351–8.
16. Chambraud B, et al. FAP48, a new protein that forms specific complexes with both immunophilins FKBP59 and FKBP12. Prevention by the immunosuppressant drugs FK506 and rapamycin. J Biol Chem. 1996;271(51):32923–9.
17. Grisendi S, et al. Ligand-regulated binding of FAP68 to the hepatocyte growth factor receptor. J Biol Chem. 2001;276(49):46632–8.
18. Tron AE, et al. The glomuvenous malformation protein Glomulin binds Rbx1 and regulates cullin RING ligase-mediated turnover of Fbw7. Mol Cell. 2012;46(1):67–78.
19. Faughnan ME, et al. International guidelines for the diagnosis and management of hereditary haemorrhagic telangiectasia. J Med Genet. 2011;48(2):73–87.
20. Cole SG, et al. A new locus for hereditary haemorrhagic telangiectasia (HHT3) maps to chromosome 5. J Med Genet. 2005;42(7):577–82.
21. Bayrak-Toydemir P, et al. A fourth locus for hereditary hemorrhagic telangiectasia maps to chromosome 7. Am J Med Genet A. 2006;140(20):2155–62.
22. McAllister KA, et al. Endoglin, a TGF-beta binding protein of endothelial cells, is the gene for hereditary haemorrhagic telangiectasia type 1. Nat Genet. 1994;8(4):345–51.
23. Johnson DW, et al. Mutations in the activin receptor-like kinase 1 gene in hereditary haemorrhagic telangiectasia type 2. Nat Genet. 1996;13(2):189–95.
24. Desloover J, et al. Autotrophic nitrous oxide removal in bioelectrochemical systems. Commun Agric Appl Biol Sci. 2011;76(2):51–3.
25. Gallione CJ, et al. SMAD4 mutations found in unselected HHT patients. J Med Genet. 2006;43(10):793–7.
26. David L, et al. Identification of BMP9 and BMP10 as functional activators of the orphan activin receptor-like kinase 1 (ALK1) in endothelial cells. Blood. 2007;109(5):1953–61.
27. Wooderchak-Donahue WL, et al. BMP9 mutations cause a vascular-anomaly syndrome with phenotypic overlap with hereditary hemorrhagic telangiectasia. Am J Hum Genet. 2013;93(3):530–7.
28. Lebrin F, et al. Thalidomide stimulates vessel maturation and reduces epistaxis in individuals with hereditary hemorrhagic telangiectasia. Nat Med. 2010;16(4):420–8.
29. Gaillard S, et al. Tranexamic acid for epistaxis in hereditary hemorrhagic telangiectasia patients: a European cross-over controlled trial in a rare disease. J Thromb Haemost. 2014;12(9):1494–502.
30. Geisthoff UW, et al. Treatment of epistaxis in hereditary hemorrhagic telangiectasia with tranexamic acid - a double-blind placebo-controlled cross-over phase IIIB study. Thromb Res. 2014;134(3):565–71.
31. Dupuis-Girod S, et al. Bevacizumab in patients with hereditary hemorrhagic telangiectasia and severe hepatic vascular malformations and high cardiac output. JAMA. 2012;307(9):948–55.
32. Thompson AB, et al. Very low dose bevacizumab for the treatment of epistaxis in patients with hereditary hemorrhagic telangiectasia. Allergy Rhinol (Providence). 2014;5(2):91–5.
33. Park SO, et al. Real-time imaging of de novo arteriovenous malformation in a mouse model of hereditary hemorrhagic telangiectasia. J Clin Invest. 2009;119(11):3487–96.

34. Choi EJ, et al. Minimal homozygous endothelial deletion of Eng with VEGF stimulation is sufficient to cause cerebrovascular dysplasia in the adult mouse. Cerebrovasc Dis. 2012;33(6):540–7.
35. Choi EJ, et al. Novel brain arteriovenous malformation mouse models for type 1 hereditary hemorrhagic telangiectasia. PLoS One. 2014;9(2):e88511.
36. Garrido-Martin EM, et al. Common and distinctive pathogenetic features of arteriovenous malformations in hereditary hemorrhagic telangiectasia 1 and hereditary hemorrhagic telangiectasia 2 animal models--brief report. Arterioscler Thromb Vasc Biol. 2014;34(10):2232–6.
37. Fontalba A, et al. Mutation study of Spanish patients with hereditary hemorrhagic telangiectasia. BMC Med Genet. 2008;9:75.
38. Han C, et al. VEGF neutralization can prevent and normalize arteriovenous malformations in an animal model for hereditary hemorrhagic telangiectasia 2. Angiogenesis. 2014;17(4):823–30.
39. Boon LM, Mulliken JB, Vikkula M. RASA1: variable phenotype with capillary and arteriovenous malformations. Curr Opin Genet Dev. 2005;15(3):265–9.
40. Revencu N, et al. RASA1 mutations and associated phenotypes in 68 families with capillary malformation-arteriovenous malformation. Hum Mutat. 2013;34(12):1632–41.
41. Eerola I, et al. Capillary malformation-arteriovenous malformation, a new clinical and genetic disorder caused by RASA1 mutations. Am J Hum Genet. 2003;73(6):1240–9.
42. Henkemeyer M, et al. Vascular system defects and neuronal apoptosis in mice lacking ras GTPase-activating protein. Nature. 1995;377(6551):695–701.
43. Macmurdo CF, et al. RASA1 somatic mutation and variable expressivity in capillary malformation/arteriovenous malformation (CM/AVM) syndrome. Am J Med Genet A. 2016;170(6):1450.
44. Revencu N, Fastre ERavoet M, Helaers R, Brouillard P, Chung C, Gerard M, Irvine A, Boon L, Vikkula M. RASA1 mosaic mutations in patients with capillary malformation – arteriovenous malformation. Submitted.
45. Amyere M, et al. Germline loss-of-function mutations in EPHB4 cause a second form of capillary malformation-arteriovenous malformation (CM-AVM2) deregulating RAS-MAPK signaling. Circulation. 2017;136(11):1037.
46. Yu J, et al. EPHB4 mutation implicated in capillary malformation-arteriovenous malformation syndrome: a case report. Pediatr Dermatol. 2017;34(5):e227–30.
47. Vivanti A, et al. Loss of function mutations in EPHB4 are responsible for vein of Galen aneurysmal malformation. Brain. 2018;141(4):979–88.
48. Duran D, et al. Mutations in chromatin modifier and ephrin signaling genes in vein of Galen malformation. Neuron. 2018;101(3):429.
49. Kawasaki J, et al. RASA1 functions in EPHB4 signaling pathway to suppress endothelial mTORC1 activity. J Clin Invest. 2014;124(6):2774–84.
50. Nikolaev SI, et al. Somatic activating KRAS mutations in arteriovenous malformations of the brain. N Engl J Med. 2018;378(3):250–61.
51. Al-Olabi L, et al. Mosaic RAS/MAPK variants cause sporadic vascular malformations which respond to targeted therapy. J Clin Invest. 2018;128(4):1496–508.
52. Hong T, Yan Y, Li J, Radovanovic I, Ma X, Shao YW, Yu J, Ma Y, Zhang P, Ling F, Huang S, Zhang H, Wang Y. High prevalence of KRAS/BRAF somatic mutations in brain and spinal cord arteriovenous malformations. Brain. 2019;142(1):23–34.
53. Jacobs AH, Walton RG. The incidence of birthmarks in the neonate. Pediatrics. 1976;58(2):218–22.
54. Shirley MD, et al. Sturge-Weber syndrome and port-wine stains caused by somatic mutation in GNAQ. N Engl J Med. 2013;368(21):1971–9.
55. Couto JA, et al. Endothelial cells from capillary malformations are enriched for somatic GNAQ mutations. Plast Reconstr Surg. 2016;137(1):77e–82e.
56. Tan W, et al. The somatic GNAQ mutation (R183Q) is primarily located within the blood vessels of port wine stains. J Am Acad Dermatol. 2016;74(2):380–3.
57. Akers AL, et al. Biallelic somatic and germline mutations in cerebral cavernous malformations (CCMs): evidence for a two-hit mechanism of CCM pathogenesis. Hum Mol Genet. 2009;18(5):919–30.

58. Pagenstecher A, et al. A two-hit mechanism causes cerebral cavernous malformations: complete inactivation of CCM1, CCM2 or CCM3 in affected endothelial cells. Hum Mol Genet. 2009;18(5):911–8.
59. Wustehube J, et al. Cerebral cavernous malformation protein CCM1 inhibits sprouting angiogenesis by activating DELTA-NOTCH signaling. Proc Natl Acad Sci U S A. 2010;107(28):12640–5.
60. Chen L, et al. Apoptotic functions of PDCD10/CCM3, the gene mutated in cerebral cavernous malformation 3. Stroke. 2009;40(4):1474–81.
61. Uhlik MT, et al. Rac-MEKK3-MKK3 scaffolding for p38 MAPK activation during hyperosmotic shock. Nat Cell Biol. 2003;5(12):1104–10.
62. Zhou Z, et al. Cerebral cavernous malformations arise from endothelial gain of MEKK3-KLF2/4 signalling. Nature. 2016;532(7597):122.
63. Eerola I, et al. KRIT1 is mutated in hyperkeratotic cutaneous capillary-venous malformation associated with cerebral capillary malformation. Hum Mol Genet. 2000;9(9):1351–5.
64. Sirvente J, et al. Frequency and phenotypes of cutaneous vascular malformations in a consecutive series of 417 patients with familial cerebral cavernous malformations. J Eur Acad Dermatol Venereol. 2009;23(9):1066–72.
65. Couto JA, et al. A somatic MAP3K3 mutation is associated with verrucous venous malformation. Am J Hum Genet. 2015;96(3):480–6.
66. Boscolo E, et al. AKT hyper-phosphorylation associated with PI3K mutations in lymphatic endothelial cells from a patient with lymphatic malformation. Angiogenesis. 2015;18(2):151–62.
67. Osborn AJ, et al. Activating PIK3CA alleles and lymphangiogenic phenotype of lymphatic endothelial cells isolated from lymphatic malformations. Hum Mol Genet. 2015;24(4):926–38.
68. Luks VL, et al. Lymphatic and other vascular malformative/overgrowth disorders are caused by somatic mutations in PIK3CA. J Pediatr. 2015;166(4):1048–54 e1-5.
69. Keppler-Noreuil KM, et al. PIK3CA-related overgrowth spectrum (PROS): diagnostic and testing eligibility criteria, differential diagnosis, and evaluation. Am J Med Genet A. 2015;167A(2):287–95.
70. Vahidnezhad H, Youssefian L, Uitto J. Klippel-Trenaunay syndrome belongs to the PIK3CA-related overgrowth spectrum (PROS). Exp Dermatol. 2016;25(1):17–9.
71. Harada A, et al. Sudden death in a case of megalencephaly capillary malformation associated with a de novo mutation in AKT3. Childs Nerv Syst. 2015;31(3):465–71.
72. Lindhurst MJ, et al. A mosaic activating mutation in AKT1 associated with the Proteus syndrome. N Engl J Med. 2011;365(7):611–9.
73. Segrelles C, et al. Constitutively active Akt induces ectodermal defects and impaired bone morphogenetic protein signaling. Mol Biol Cell. 2008;19(1):137–49.
74. Walter JW, et al. Genetic mapping of a novel familial form of infantile hemangioma. Am J Med Genet. 1999;82(1):77–83.
75. Grimmer JF, et al. Familial clustering of hemangiomas. Arch Otolaryngol Head Neck Surg. 2011;137(8):757–60.
76. Castrén E, et al. Inheritance patterns of Infantile Hemangioma. submitted.
77. Ayturk UM, et al. Somatic activating mutations in GNAQ and GNA11 are associated with congenital hemangioma. Am J Hum Genet. 2016;98(4):789–95.
78. Giblin AV, et al. Pyogenic granuloma - the quest for optimum treatment: audit of treatment of 408 cases. J Plast Reconstr Aesthet Surg. 2007;60(9):1030–5.
79. Dastgheib L, Maghami Z, Aslani FS. Infantile multiple large pyogenic granuloma on burned skin. Case report and review of literature. An Bras Dermatol. 2016;91(2):212–4.
80. Lim YH, et al. Somatic activating RAS mutations cause vascular tumors including pyogenic granuloma. J Invest Dermatol. 2015;135(6):1698–700.
81. Groesser L, et al. BRAF and RAS mutations in sporadic and secondary pyogenic granuloma. J Invest Dermatol. 2016;136(2):481–6.

Sirolimus for the Treatment of Vascular Anomalies

4

Joana M. Mack, Denise M. Adams, and Kiersten W. Ricci

Introduction

Sirolimus, also known as rapamycin, is a specific and potent inhibitor of mammalian target of rapamycin (mTOR), a serine/threonine kinase in the phosphoinositide-3-kinase (PI3K)/Akt pathway which regulates numerous cellular processes including cellular catabolism and anabolism, cell motility, angiogenesis, and cell growth [1]. Prior to its use in vascular anomalies, sirolimus was used to treat patients with tuberous sclerosis (TS) and lymphangioleiomyomatosis (LAM), both of which result from mutations of important regulators, tuberous sclerosis complex 1 and 2, of the PI3K/Akt/mTOR pathway [2]. Given its effectiveness in these conditions, sirolimus was first trialed as a treatment for vascular anomalies in an infant with kaposiform hemangioendothelioma (KHE) and severe Kasabach-Merritt phenomenon (KMP), whose disease was refractory to all treatment regimens (steroids, vincristine, cyclophosphamide, bevacizumab, and embolization therapy). The patient not only had complete resolution of coagulopathy within 2 months of sirolimus initiation but also experienced substantial improvements in pain, lesion size, and function [3]. This initial success prompted the prospective phase 2 clinical trial

J. M. Mack
Vascular Anomalies Center, Division of Hematology/Oncology, Cancer and Blood Disorders Program, Arkansas Children's Hospital, Little Rock, AR, USA

D. M. Adams (✉)
Dana-Farber Cancer Institute, Boston Children's Hospital, Boston, MA, USA

Division of Hematology/Oncology, Vascular Anomalies Center, Harvard Medical School, Boston Children's Hospital, Boston, MA, USA
e-mail: Denise.adams@childrens.harvard.edu

K. W. Ricci
Hemangioma and Vascular Malformation Center, Division of Hematology, Cincinnati Children's Hospital Medical Center and University of Cincinnati College of Medicine, Cincinnati, OH, USA

C. C. Trenor III, D. M. Adams (eds.), *Vascular Anomalies*,
https://doi.org/10.1007/978-3-030-25624-1_4

assessing the safety and efficacy of sirolimus in the treatment of complicated vascular anomalies. The phase 2 study demonstrated that sirolimus was a safe treatment option with remarkable responses in the majority of patients with microcystic and complex lymphatic malformations, capillary lymphatic venous malformations (CLVM), PTEN hamartoma tumor syndrome (PHTS), venous lymphatic malformations (VLM), and kaposiform hemangioendothelioma (KHE). Many of these patients experienced improvement in clinical symptoms and quality of life regardless of whether improvement or stable disease was noted radiologically [4]. Since these early successes, the use of sirolimus has rapidly expanded and appears efficacious in a variety of vascular tumors and malformations [5]. Sirolimus has also been safely used in combination with surgery and interventional procedures allowing for improved overall patient outcomes [6–9]. Because of the widespread use of sirolimus, standards of practice are needed and are currently being developed through pediatric hematology/oncology professionals involved in vascular anomalies.

Mechanism of Action

Sirolimus forms a complex with FK506-binding protein (FKBP12), which then binds to several other proteins to produce two distinct complexes, mTOR complex 1 and 2 (mTORC1/2), which differ in protein components, substrate specificity, and regulation. mTOR mainly functions to regulate protein synthesis and cell growth through the downstream molecules, 4E-BP1 and S6K, and is acutely inhibited by rapamycin. While mTORC1 regulates cell growth and metabolism, mTORC2 instead controls proliferation and survival and is acutely insensitive to rapamycin. However, after prolonged exposure to sirolimus, mTORC2 levels have been found to be reduced in some but not all cell types [10]. Although rapamycin is a potent and specific inhibitor of mTOR, the inhibitory effects are partial due to several factors. First, the effects of sirolimus on cellular processes are cytostatic rather than cytotoxic. Several studies have shown that sirolimus can stabilize and decrease the volume of tumors, but once discontinued, the tumors return to their original state [2, 11, 12]. Additionally, multiple negative feedback loops are only temporarily suppressed by sirolimus, and numerous compensatory pathways are upregulated in response to chronic therapy [10]. The exact mechanism of action of sirolimus responsible for its beneficial effects in vascular anomalies is not completely understood, but is likely multifactorial, including inhibition of downstream mTOR signaling in endothelial cells and suppression of lymphocyte function.

Pharmacokinetics

Sirolimus has a relatively narrow therapeutic index and large interpatient pharmacokinetic variability, likely due to genetic differences in the drug metabolizing enzymes (CYP3A4, CYP3A5, CYP2C8) required for hepatic and intestinal metabolism [13]. Oral bioavailability is low (27% in tablet versus 14% in solution form), which has been attributed to a combination of extensive intestinal and hepatic first pass metabolism by cytochrome P450 (CYP) 3A4 and intestinal P-glycoprotein efflux pump. Sirolimus has a large distribution of volume (mean 12 L/kg) and is primarily eliminated through fecal/biliary pathways with a mean half-life of 62 hours in adults [14]. The half-life of sirolimus is extended with hepatic impairment [15]. A phase I clinic trial evaluated 45 healthy adults between the age of 19 and 36 and showed tolerance of single oral dose of sirolimus between 0.3 and 8 mg/m^2 [16]. There were no serious adverse events during the study.

In children, particularly in neonates and infants, close monitoring is essential given differences in drug elimination, at least in part, due to developing organ functions [17]. Based on the phase II clinical trial in children and young adults (ages 0–31 years) with vascular anomalies, sirolimus was administered orally as a tablet or liquid suspension at an initial dose of 0.8 mg/m^2 per dose at 12-hour intervals and titrated to maintain a goal serum trough level of 10–15 ng/mL. This goal drug level was based on the use of sirolimus in pediatric renal transplant patients [4]. However, lower sirolimus doses, corresponding to lower trough levels, have been efficacious in patients with vascular anomalies, so many providers now titrate the dose to desired effect with consideration of side effects. Higher trough levels (8–13 ng/mL) are used in the initial treatment of complicated vascular anomalies such as kaposiform hemangioendotheliomas and Kasabach-Merritt phenomenon (KHE and KMP), lymphatic anomalies (Gorham-Stout disease(GSD), generalized lymphatic anomaly (GLA), kaposiform lymphangiomatosis (KLA), and Klippel-Trenaunay syndrome (KTS). Less complicated patients can be treated with levels ranging from 4 to 8 ng/mL and maintenance dosing can be effective with levels less than 4 ng/mL. Dosing and drug levels are based on severity of disease and therapy goals. For maintenance therapy, the goal of treatment is to provide the lowest dose with the greatest effect. Initial adult dosing is 2 mg a day for uncomplicated patients [18].

Dosing for infants and young children has been studied and recently reported with data from the noted phase II study [19]. Neonates (0–1 month of age) require a lower starting dose of 0.4–0.45 mg/m^2/dose administered twice daily (target concentration levels between 10 and 15 ng/mL) due to the decreased CYP3A enzymes that are found in the liver and intestine compared to older infants, children, and adults.

Effectiveness of Sirolimus

The phase II clinical trial assessing the safety and efficacy of sirolimus in the treatment of complicated vascular anomalies included planned treatment duration of 12 courses with each course being 28 days [4]. Fifty-three patients were evaluable at the end of course 12. Patients who had responsive or stable disease were continued on treatment at the discretion of the treating institution. At the end of course 12, 85% of patients had a partial response to therapy. Complete resolution of disease was not expected for these congenital disorders. Because of significant benefits of sirolimus, 42 out of the 53 patients continued treatment after 12 courses. Six patients discontinued treatment at the end of course 12 but restarted therapy upon recurrence of symptoms. Time to response varies among patients, but maximal effect generally does not occur until months after achieving therapeutic sirolimus trough levels. Duration and timing of treatment are not defined and are determined on an individual basis. Since this initial study, somatic activating mutations have been reported in the PI3K/Akt/mTOR pathway [20]. There have been many publications reinforcing the effectiveness of sirolimus in the literature to date [4–9].

Adverse Effects

Common side effects, which are generally dose-dependent, include headaches, gastrointestinal discomfort, mouth sores, elevated cholesterol levels, and bone marrow suppression. Rare but important and/or life-threatening side effects are listed in Table 4.1. Frequent monitoring (physical exam and blood work) is necessary while on sirolimus therapy to ensure adequate drug levels and to monitor for toxicities. Suggested monitoring evaluations range from every 1 to 3 months depending on the target blood level.

Table 4.1 Adverse effects of sirolimus

Side effects	Rare but important and/or life-threatening
Cardiovascular – chest pain, edema, hypertension, peripheral edema, tachycardia	Ascites Azoospermia Cardiac tamponade
Central nervous system – dizziness, headache	Cytomegalovirus Epstein-Barr infection
Dermatologic – acne vulgaris, skin rash	Exfoliative dermatitis
Endocrine and metabolic – amenorrhea, hyperglycemia, hypercholesterolemia, hypertriglyceridemia	Focal segmental glomerulosclerosis Hemolytic uremic syndrome Hepatic necrosis
Gastrointestinal – abdominal pain, constipation, diarrhea, nausea, mouth sores	Hepatotoxicity Hypersensitivity angiitis
Genitourinary – urinary tract infection	Interstitial pulmonary disease
Hematologic and oncologic – anemia, leukopenia, thrombocytopenia	Pneumonitis Pulmonary fibrosis
Infection – herpes simplex infection, herpes zoster	Bronchiolitis obliterans organizing pneumonia Lymphedema
Neuromuscular and skeletal – arthralgia, myalgia, osteonecrosis	Lymphoma Pericardial effusion
Renal – increased serum creatinine, pyelonephritis	Pleural effusion Pneumonia due to *Pneumocystis jirovecii*
Respiratory – epistaxis, nasopharyngitis, pneumonia	Progressive multifocal leukoencephalopathy Pseudomembranous colitis
Miscellaneous – wound healing impairment	Pulmonary hemorrhage Reversible posterior leukoencephalopathy syndrome Sepsis Skin carcinoma Thrombotic thrombocytopenic purpura

Immunology: Immunosuppression

Critical for immune response, T-cell production and proliferation are heavily regulated through the mTOR signaling pathway through complex cellular signaling interactions. Once the naïve T-cell receptor (TCR) is engaged after antigen exposure (Signal "1") and recognition, a cascade of responses is dependent on the immune microenvironment. In addition to antigen recognition, T-cells are dependent on co-stimulation by "Signal 2" in order to have full activation, production, and proliferation. Waickman et al. propose that mTOR is a central integrator of diverse signals derived from the immune microenvironment that constitute "Signal 2" [21].

Activated T-cells expend a tremendous amount of energy obtained through aerobic glycolysis [22]. The mTOR pathway, specifically mTORC1, regulates several important transcriptions of glycolytic enzymes. Several other metabolic pathways like the pentose phosphate pathway (PPP), the tricarboxylic acid cycle (TCA), and fatty acid oxidation all provide substrates for resting and activated T-cells [23, 24]. Thus, mTOR inhibition decreases expression of the important genes and metabolic substrates involved in providing energy for T-cells [23, 25].

T-cells are generally divided into two main categories, cytotoxic and helper T-cells, although other less prominent types do exist [25, 26]. Cytotoxic T-cells include CD8+ T-cells which function to eliminate pathogen-infected cells by directly delivering cytotoxic granules. Helper T-cells include CD4+ T-cells which function to activate specific cytokines or recruit new immune cells to fight the pathogen-infected cell. T-cell helper (T_h) subsets, which rely on mTOR signaling for metabolism, produce certain cytokines responsible for fighting specific infections [21]. Therefore, in the presence of mTOR inhibition with sirolimus, CD4+ T-cells do not differentiate into specific effector cells leaving the host vulnerable to infections [27].

One of the most concerning side effects of sirolimus is immunosuppression though the drug has been very well tolerated. The degree of immunosuppression caused by sirolimus in the treatment of vascular anomalies is unclear. Vascular anomalies particularly "leaky" lymphatic anomalies such as KLA and central conducting lymphatic anomalies (CCLA) are associated with protein loss and hypogammaglobulinemia. Furthermore, infants with vascular anomalies on sirolimus who already have immature immune systems are presumed to be at higher risk. Formal testing for immune dysfunction is suggested in these high-risk patients.

Pneumocystis jirovecii Prophylaxis

Pneumocystis jirovecii (formerly *Pneumocystis carinii*) pneumonia (PJP) is a potentially life-threatening fungal lung infection that occurs in solid organ transplant recipients, individuals with human immunodeficiency virus (HIV), and immunocompromised patients. PJP has been reported in patients receiving sirolimus after solid organ transplantation and in at least one pediatric patient with a vascular anomaly, an infant on concurrent corticosteroids [28].

Consideration of PJP susceptibility in immunocompromised individuals, including those on sirolimus therapy, is essential due to its serious implications and ability of prophylaxis. Presently it is suggested that those patients at high risk should be placed on PJP prophylaxis with the patient's institutions guidelines. It is less clear if older patients or those with lower goal trough levels need PJP prophylaxis.

Infectious Screening

Sirolimus therapy can potentially reactivate or exacerbate latent or current infections. Specific routine screening has not been established for patients starting sirolimus, but adaption of infectious screening for patients undergoing solid organ transplantation should be a consideration. Pretransplant screening includes HIV, herpes simplex virus, hepatitis B virus, hepatitis C virus, cytomegalovirus (CMV), Epstein-Barr virus (EBV), and varicella-zoster virus (VZV) testing. Further infectious screening is warranted based on a detailed history including exposures, active symptoms, and prior infections [29].

Vaccinations

Vaccine-preventable diseases can lead to significant morbidity and mortality in immunocompromised patients. Vaccination guidelines with sirolimus use are not established, particularly in patients in vascular anomalies. Similarly to infection screening, the most data on vaccination recommendations arise from studies in solid organ transplantation (SOT) and hematopoietic stem cell transplantation (HSCT) recipients pre- and post-transplantation. Transplant guidelines recommend that live vaccines can be administered to SOT recipients at least 4 weeks prior to transplantation if not on immunosuppression [30]. Live vaccinations such as those for varicella and measles, mumps, and rubella (MMR) are not recommended post-transplant due to lifelong immunosuppression to prevent graft rejection. Prior to transplantation in patients who will require significant immunosuppression, antibody titers testing is recommended for tetanus, diphtheria, measles, mumps, and pneumococcal disease.

It is unclear what effect sirolimus has on the waning on immunity induced by vaccines. Therefore, live vaccines should be administered prior to the start of sirolimus, if possible. Non-live or killed vaccines are safe and recommended in patients on sirolimus therapy. However, the need for titer monitoring and booster immunizations is unclear at this time [31].

Future Therapies

Research in vascular anomalies has entered into the genetic era with the identification of several mutations in vascular tumors and malformations, not only allowing for a better understanding of the pathophysiology of these conditions but also directing our field towards additional rational and targeted medical therapies. Activating mutations of the PI3K/AKT/mTOR or the RAS/mitogen-activated protein kinase (MAPK)/MAP-extracellular signal-regulated kinase (MEK) pathway lead to dysregulation of normal cellular functions, resulting in cellular proliferation, survival advantage, and angiogenesis, and are thought to be the driver for the development and/or progression of vascular anomalies.

BYL719 (alpelisib), a PIK3CA inhibitor, was first used in 2015 in a patient with CLOVES (congenital lipomatous overgrowth-vascular malformation-epidermal nevi-scoliosis/skeletal/spinal anomaly syndrome) [32]. This overgrowth syndrome has been found to have somatic genetic mutations involving the *PIK3CA* gene and belongs to the spectrum of PIK3CA-related overgrowth syndromes (PROS). After developing a mouse model with PROS/CLOVES and demonstrating the prevention and improvement of overgrowth with the use of BYL719, Venot et al. treated 19 patients (4 adults and 15 children) with PROS under compassionate care protocol. All patients had symptom improvement and measurable tumor decrease (radiologically and clinically). Venot et al. reported no significant adverse effects, but some patients developed hyperglycemia that was controlled with diet. BYL719 appears to act by decreasing AKT phosphorylation, which results in less inhibition of tuberous sclerosis complex 2

(TSC2), a negative regulator of mTORC1, and thus, decreases mTORC1 activation. Venot and colleagues suggested that the beneficial effect of BYL719 in this patient population was driven by more complete blockage of AKT in comparison to sirolimus, which is less effective in inhibiting phosphorylation of mTORC2, allowing for persistent phosphorylation of AKT [32]. PIK3CA inhibition is a promising treatment for patients with PROS who overall have high morbidity and mortality, particularly those who have suboptimal response to sirolimus therapy.

Components of the PIK3CA/AKT/mTOR and RAS/MAPK/MEK pathways interact and regulate each other via cross-inhibition and cross-activation. Activation of RAS/MAPK leads to a cascade with activation of BRAF and then MEK. Mutations in EPHB4, KRAS, HRAS, NRAS, BRAF, RAF1, PTPN11, and SOS1 have been recently reported in vascular anomalies, which assumingly result from dysregulation of the RAS pathway. These mutations have been found in lymphedema syndromes, KHE, KLA, CCLA, and capillary malformation/arteriovenous malformation 2 (CM-AVM2) [33, 34]. RASA1 is inhibitory regulator of the RAS/MAPK/MEK pathway, and therefore, loss-of-function *RASA1* mutations result in RAS/MAPK over activation. RASA1 mutations have been implicated in several vascular malformations including multiple capillary malformation syndrome, Parkes Weber syndrome, and capillary malformation-arteriovenous malformation (CM-AVM) [35]. BRAF and MEK mutations have also been discovered in arteriovenous malformations. Al-Olabi et al. demonstrated improved blood flow with vemurafenib, a BRAF inhibitor, in a transgenic zebrafish AVM model with a BRAF mutation [36]. Additionally, mutations of the mitogen-activated protein kinase 1 (*MAP2K1*) gene, which encodes for MEK1, were found in 64% of endothelial cells from extracranial AVM in one study [37]. MEK and BRAF inhibitors have been safely used in treatment regimens for certain benign and malignant tumors and may be beneficial in certain complicated vascular anomalies. Barclay et al. recently published a NRAS mutation in patients with KLA, inviting consideration of using MEK inhibitors and other agents for this high-risk lymphatic diagnosis.

Conclusion

The discovery of germline and somatic genetic mutations has led to a better understanding of the correlation between phenotype and genotype in vascular anomalies. Many of these mutations occur in the same cellular signaling pathways, specifically PIK3CA/AKT/mTOR and RAS/MAPK/MEK, that are involved in cancer. Classification of vascular anomalies based on genetic abnormalities, along with continued scientific and clinical research, will potentially reveal novel uses of existing medications or the development of new targeted therapies and, ultimately, expand therapeutic options and improve disease outcomes [5]. Because vascular anomalies are congenital, the need for medication may be lifelong, but the dosage required may be less than in cancer. The identification of medications with a tolerable toxicity profile, both short- and long-term, will be critical to patients with vascular anomalies.

References

1. Huber S, Bruns CJ, Schmid G, et al. Inhibition of the mammalian target of rapamycin impedes lymphangiogenesis. Kidney Int. 2007;71(8):771–7.
2. Bissler JJ, McCormack FX, Young LR, et al. Sirolimus for angiomyolipoma in tuberous sclerosis complex or lymphangioleiomyomatosis. N Engl J Med. 2008;358(2):140–51.
3. Hammill AM, Wentzel M, Gupta A, et al. Sirolimus for the treatment of complicated vascular anomalies in children. Pediatr Blood Cancer. 2011;57(6):1018–24.
4. Adams DM, Trenor CC 3rd, Hammill AM, et al. Efficacy and safety of sirolimus in the treatment of complicated vascular anomalies. Pediatrics. 2016;137(2):e20153257.
5. Adams DM, Ricci KW. Vascular anomalies: diagnosis of complicated anomalies and new medical treatment options. Hematol Oncol Clin North Am. 2019;33(3):455–70.
6. Kim D, Benjamin L, Wysong A, Hovsepian D, Teng J. Treatment of complex periorbital venolymphatic malformation in a neonate with a combination therapy of sirolimus and prednisolone. Dermatol Ther. 2015;28(4):218–21.
7. Akyuz C, Atas E, Varan A. Treatment of a tongue lymphangioma with sirolimus after failure of surgical resection and propranolol. Pediatr Blood Cancer. 2014;61(5):931–2.
8. Vlahovic AM, Vlahovic NS, Haxhija EQ. Sirolimus for the treatment of a massive capillary-lymphatico-venous malformation: a case report. Pediatrics. 2015;136(2):e513–6.
9. Triana P, Dore M, Cerezo VN, et al. Sirolimus in the treatment of vascular anomalies. Eur J Pediatr Surg. 2017;27(1):86–90.
10. Sarbassov DD, Ali SM, Sengupta S, et al. Prolonged rapamycin treatment inhibits mTORC2 assembly and Akt/PKB. Mol Cell. 2006;22(2):159–68.
11. Li J, Kim SG, Blenis J. Rapamycin: one drug, many effects. Cell Metab. 2014;19(3):373–9.
12. Marsh DJ, Trahair TN, Martin JL, et al. Rapamycin treatment for a child with germline PTEN mutation. Nat Clin Pract Oncol. 2008;5(6):357–61.
13. Jacobsen W, Serkova N, Hausen B, Morris RE, Benet LZ, Christians U. Comparison of the in vitro metabolism of the macrolide immunosuppressants sirolimus and RAD. Transplant Proc. 2001;33(1–2):514–5.
14. Stenton SB, Partovi N, Ensom MH. Sirolimus: the evidence for clinical pharmacokinetic monitoring. Clin Pharmacokinet. 2005;44(8):769–86.

15. Emoto C, Fukuda T, Cox S, Christians U, Vinks AA. Development of a physiologically-based pharmacokinetic model for sirolimus: predicting bioavailability based on intestinal CYP3A content. CPT Pharmacometrics Syst Pharmacol. 2013;2(7):e59.
16. Brattstrom C, Sawe J, Jansson B, et al. Pharmacokinetics and safety of single oral doses of sirolimus (rapamycin) in healthy male volunteers. Ther Drug Monit. 2000;22(5):537–44.
17. Kearns GL, Abdel-Rahman SM, Alander SW, Blowey DL, Leeder JS, Kauffman RE. Developmental pharmacology--drug disposition, action, and therapy in infants and children. N Engl J Med. 2003;349(12):1157–67.
18. McCormack FX, Inoue Y, Moss J, et al. Efficacy and saferty of sirolimus in lymphangioleiomyomatosis. N Engl J Med. 2011;364(17):1595–606.
19. Mizuno T, Fukuda T, Emoto C, et al. Developmental pharmacokinetics of sirolimus: implications for precision dosing in neonates and infants with complicated vascular anomalies. Pediatr Blood Cancer. 2017;64(8):e26470.
20. Kurek KC, Liks VL, Ayturk UM, et al. Somatic mosaic activating mutations in PIK3CA cause CLOVES syndrome. Am J Hum Genet. 2012;90(6):1108–15.
21. Waickman AT, Powell JD. mTOR, metabolism, and the regulation of T-cell differentiation and function. Immunol Rev. 2012;249(1):43–58.
22. Fox CJ, Hammerman PS, Thompson CB. Fuel feeds function: energy metabolism and the T-cell response. Nat Rev Immunol. 2005;5(11):844–52.
23. Duvel K, Yecies JL, Menon S, et al. Activation of a metabolic gene regulatory network downstream of mTOR complex 1. Mol Cell. 2010;39(2):171–83.
24. Sipula IJ, Brown NF, Perdomo G. Rapamycin-mediated inhibition of mammalian target of rapamycin in skeletal muscle cells reduces glucose utilization and increases fatty acid oxidation. Metabolism. 2006;55(12):1637–44.
25. Michalek RD, Gerriets VA, Jacobs SR, et al. Cutting edge: distinct glycolytic and lipid oxidative metabolic programs are essential for effector and regulatory CD4+ T cell subsets. J Immunol. 2011;186(6):3299–303.
26. Pennock ND, White JT, Cross EW, Cheney EE, Tamburini BA, Kedl RM. T cell responses: naive to memory and everything in between. Adv Physiol Educ. 2013;37(4):273–83.
27. Delgoffe GM, Kole TP, Zheng Y, et al. The mTOR kinase differentially regulates effector and regulatory T cell lineage commitment. Immunity. 2009;30(6):832–44.
28. Russell TB, Rinker EK, Dillingham CS, Givner LB, McLean TW. *Pneumocystis jirovecii* pneumonia during sirolimus therapy for Kaposiform hemangioendothelioma. Pediatrics. 2018;141(5):S421–S4.
29. Fischer SA, Lu K, Practice ASTIDCo. Screening of donor and recipient in solid organ transplantation. Am J Transplant. 2013;13(S4):9–21.
30. Chong PP, Avery RK. A comprehensive review of immunization practices in solid organ transplant and hematopoietic stem cell transplant recipients. Clin Ther. 2017;39(8):1581–98.
31. Miyairi I, Funaki T, Saitoh A. Immunization practices in solid organ transplant recipients. Vaccine. 2016;34(16):1958–64.
32. Venot Q, Blanc T, Rabia SH, et al. Targeted therapy in patients with PIK3CA-related overgrowth syndrome. Nature. 2018;558(7711):540–6.
33. Amyere M, Revencu N, Helaers R, et al. Germline loss-of-function mutations in EPHB4 cause a second form of capillary malformation-arteriovenous malformation (CM-AVM2) deregulating RAS-MAPK signaling. Circulation. 2017;136(11):1037–48.
34. Barclay SF, Inman KW, Luks VL, et al. A somatic activating NRAS variant associated with kaposiform lymphangiomatosis. Genet Med. 2018; https://doi.org/10.1038/s41436-018-0390-0. [Epub ahead of print].
35. Nguyen HL, Boon LM, Vikkula M. Vascular anomalies caused by abnormal signaling within endothelial cells: targets for novel therapies. Semin Intervent Radiol. 2017;34(3):233–8.
36. Al-Olabi L, Polubothu S, Dowsett K, et al. Mosaic RAS/MAPK variants cause sporadic vascular malformations which respond to targeted therapy. J Clin Invest. 2018;128(4):1496–508.
37. Couto JA, Huang AY, Konczyk DJ, et al. Somatic MAP2K1 mutations are associated with extracranial arteriovenous malformation. Am J Hum Genet. 2017;100(3):546–54.

Infantile and Congenital Hemangiomas: Natural History, Complications, and When and How to Treat

5

Margaret T. Lee and Sheilagh Maguiness

Infantile Hemangioma

Natural History and Growth Characteristics

Infantile hemangiomas occur in about 4% of newborns [1]. They are more common in fair-skinned, preterm, low birth weight infants and females. Though lesions are not generally present at birth, it is not uncommon for a precursor lesion to be present, such as a bruise-like patch or an area of pallor/vasoconstriction. Hemangiomas then mark out their borders early, with the most rapid period of growth (at least in the superficial component) occurring between 5 and 7 weeks of age [2]. Following this, there can be a deeper component, which tends to grow more in volume than area over the ensuing 3–6 months. Finally, growth stabilizes and a slow regression of the lesion occurs over years. In the case of superficial infantile hemangiomas or large, bulky lesions, natural involution does not necessarily predict the ultimate presence of normal-appearing skin. In many cases, the skin becomes stretched "anetodermatous," and the texture appears scar-like. In other cases residual fibrofatty tissue may be left behind post-involution, and patients and parents may desire intervention to prevent or treat these changes.

M. T. Lee (✉)
Division of Pediatric Hematology/Oncology/Stem Cell Transplantation, Columbia University Medical Center, New York, NY, USA
e-mail: ml653@cumc.columbia.edu

S. Maguiness
Dermatology, University of Minnesota, Minneapolis, MN, USA
e-mail: smaguine@umn.edu

C. C. Trenor III, D. M. Adams (eds.), *Vascular Anomalies*,
https://doi.org/10.1007/978-3-030-25624-1_5

Types and Morphology

Hemangiomas have four distinct clinical variants: superficial, deep, mixed, and arrested/minimal growth. Superficial infantile hemangiomas are the classic, bright red plaques which are minimally elevated and often do resemble a strawberry (Fig. 5.1a Superficial IH). There are deep infantile hemangiomas, which are not usually noted in the first few weeks of life, but enlarge around 3–6 months of life, presenting as soft, rubbery, blue-hued subcutaneous nodules (Fig. 5.1b Deep IH). Mixed hemangiomas can have both a superficial and a deep component (Fig. 5.1c Mixed IH). Finally, some infantile hemangiomas remain quite flat and don't seem to proliferate much if at all; these are termed "infantile hemangiomas with minimal or arrested growth" [3] (Fig. 5.1d IH-MAG). All types of infantile hemangiomas share similar histopathology and express the immunohistochemical marker GLUT-1, which is unique to infantile hemangioma tissue and helpful in confirming the diagnosis if there is any clinical confusion.

Infantile hemangiomas can occur in different morphologic patterns including solitary, segmental/regional, or multifocal. Solitary infantile hemangiomas are the most common, and the majority are uncomplicated, occurring in non-cosmetically

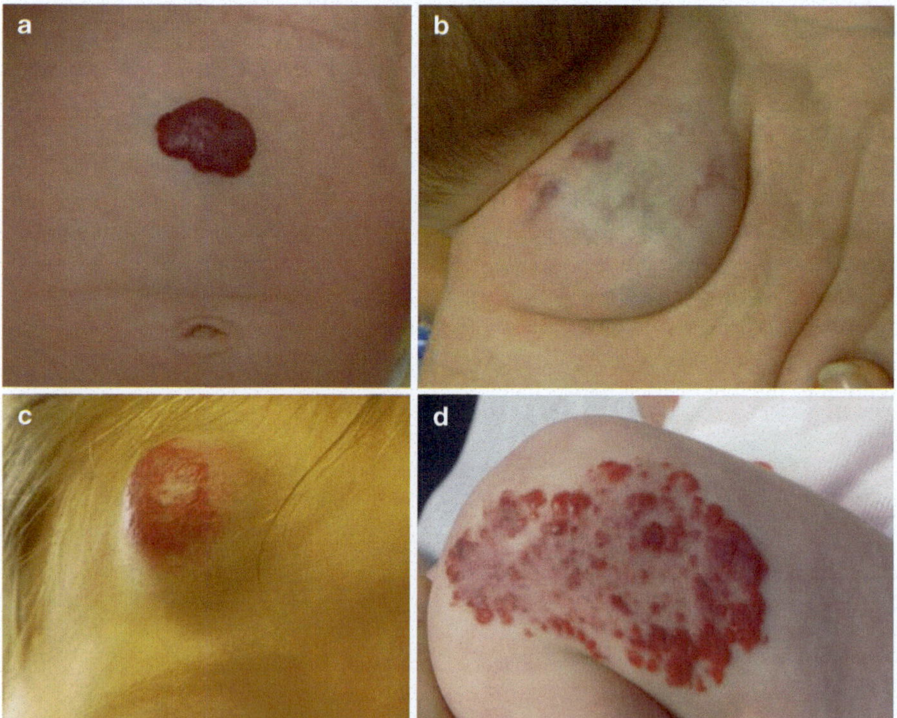

Fig. 5.1 (**a**) Superficial infantile hemangioma. (**b**) Deep infantile hemangioma. (**c**) Mixed, superficial, and deep infantile hemangioma. (**d**) Minimal or arrested growth (IH-MAG)

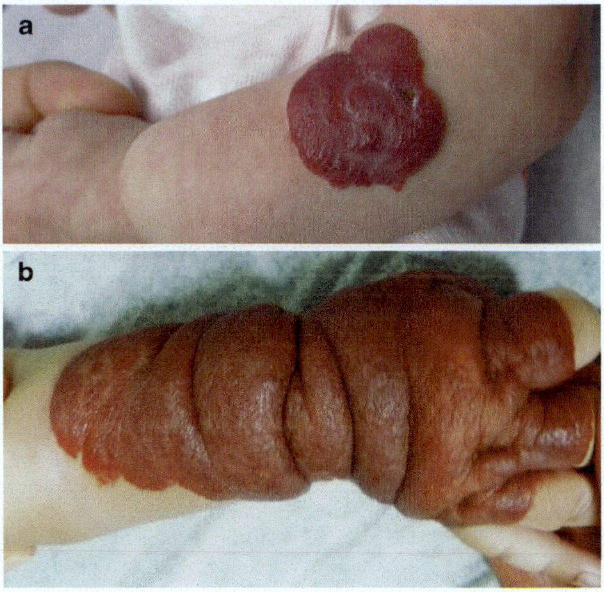

Fig. 5.2 (**a**) Localized superficial hemangioma of the forearm with small ulceration. (**b**) Segmental/ regional, superficial infantile hemangioma of the forearm

sensitive areas that do not require intervention. Alternatively, infantile hemangiomas may appear to cover an entire region or segment of the body. This is particularly concerning when located on the head and neck or lumbosacral areas. Regional/ segmental infantile hemangiomas are associated with more potential complications than localized infantile hemangiomas (Fig. 5.2a, b Localized versus segmental). For example, segmental infantile hemangiomas tend to be larger and more prone to ulceration. In addition, segmental distribution can herald underlying structural anomalies or syndromic associations. Finally, infantile hemangiomas can occur in a multifocal presentation when numerous lesions are randomly scattered over the body. In cases where there are five or more cutaneous hemangiomas, there are also specific potential complications to keep in mind including possible hepatic involvement (see Table 5.1 and Hepatic Hemangioma below).

Complications

Infantile hemangiomas are extremely heterogeneous and can occur anywhere on the body. As such, the range of potential complications ranges from life- or function-threatening to disfigurement and aesthetic concerns. Hemangiomas can also be unpredictable, so while complications may be anticipated based on subtype and anatomic location, close follow-up is recommended during the early proliferative phase between 5 and 7 weeks of age [2]. Knowledge and understanding of the growth characteristics and potential complications of infantile hemangiomas are critical to the decision on when and how to treat each unique patient. With the advent of propranolol as a safe and effective treatment, early intervention around

Table 5.1 Infantile hemangiomas: location, potential complications, and suggested workup

Anatomic distribution	Potential complications	Suggested workup
Periorbital: upper, lower eyelid, and intraocular	Visual obstruction, amblyopia, astigmatism	Ophthalmology examination, baseline, and monthly
Mandibular "Beard distribution"	Airway involvement, respiratory compromise	Prompt/urgent referral to pediatric otolaryngology. Laryngoscopy for direct evaluation of the airway
Lumbosacral area > 2.5 cm	Potential spinal dysraphism/ tethered cord	Ultrasound prior to age 3 months, MRI after age 6 months
Multifocal	Hepatic involvement, hypothyroidism, high-output cardiac failure	Abdominal US. If hepatic hemangiomas present, consider thyroid function studies and cardiac evaluation
Large facial	Hemangioma ≥5 cm on the face may herald PHACE association	MRI/MRA of the head and neck, eye examination, echocardiogram
[a]Nasal tip	Destruction of cartilage, ulceration, nasal deformity	Imaging not usually needed unless in the setting of suspected PHACE
[a]Auricular	Destruction of cartilage, ulceration, distortion of helices	Further workup not usually needed unless in the setting of suspected PHACE

[a]Locations at high risk for aesthetic complication

2–3 months of life may have the most impact in preventing complications over the long term. Thus, for high-risk hemangiomas where complications are anticipated, treatment should be started as early as possible around the time of rapid proliferation, ideally prior to 3 months of age.

A summary of anticipated complications based on anatomic site is outlined in Table 5.1, and the necessary workup is suggested. High-risk anatomic sites include the following: periorbital location, mandibular or beard distribution, nasal tip, auricular, lumbosacral, large facial lesions, and multifocal presentation. In all of these cases, early intervention is likely to be beneficial and may prevent complications and/or obviate the need for surgical correction in the future.

Complex Regional Infantile Hemangiomas

In specific cases, infantile hemangiomas can be associated with underlying structural anomalies. This typically occurs in the setting of large hemangiomas overlying a high-risk anatomic site such as the face or lumbosacral area. The underlying anomalies are structural or developmental in nature, and thus, further workup is warranted when assessing an infant with segmental/regional infantile hemangiomas in these areas.

PHACE Association

PHACE (posterior fossa brain malformations, hemangiomas, arterial anomalies, coarctation of the aorta and cardiac defects, eye abnormalities) is the association of large facial infantile hemangioma with other structural or developmental anomalies. It was first recognized in 1996 and over the years has become better characterized. The etiology for this condition is still unknown. In infants with large facial

Table 5.2 Clinical features of PHACE association (adapted from Metry's diagnostic criteria for PHACE 2009) [5]

Organ	Developmental anomalies
Skin	Large facial hemangioma (>5 cm) Frontotemporal location or multiple facial segments are higher risk for PHACE Midline or ventral scarring defects
Brain	Cerebrovascular anomalies including: dysplasia, stenosis/occlusion, hypoplasia/aplasia, aberrant origin, persistent trigeminal artery, saccular aneurysm Persistent embryonic arteries Cerebellar anomalies (Dandy-Walker malformation)
Heart	Aortic arch anomalies including coarctation of the aorta, aortic dysplasia, aberrant subclavian artery, right-sided aortic arch
Eye	Posterior segment abnormalities, morning glory malformation

hemangioma >5 cm, concern should be raised for PHACE association, in particular if the lesion is located on the frontotemporal area of the face. In one prospective study, about 30% of infants with large facial hemangioma measuring >22cm^2 had underlying anomalies in keeping with PHACE association [4]. Diagnostic criteria for PHACE association have previously been published [5]. The most common extracutaneous manifestations of PHACE association are cerebrovascular anomalies followed by congenital heart disease, ocular abnormalities, and midline defects. Importantly, the cerebrovascular and cardiac/aortic arch anomalies often occur in the same patient, compounding the risk for ischemic events and stroke [6]. See Table 5.2 for summary of the clinical features of PHACE association.

Hematologists/oncologists are often called upon to help in the multidisciplinary management of these complex patients who, due to their underlying structural anomalies of vessels in the brain and heart, are at increased risk for cerebral ischemia. Patients with PHACE association and large facial infantile hemangiomas often require systemic therapy for their hemangiomas. In this case, special consideration must be given to the possibility of underlying cerebrovascular disease and pre-treatment workup including MRI/MRA of the head and neck, and cardiac evaluation is generally recommended prior to initiation of therapy.

LUMBAR Association

LUMBAR (lower body congenital infantile hemangiomas and other skin defects, urogenital anomalies and ulceration, myelopathy, bony deformities, anorectal malformations and arterial anomalies, and rectal anomalies) is the association of a large infantile hemangioma of the lumbosacral area with other underlying structural or developmental anomalies [7]. Different acronyms have been published to describe the same constellation of findings [8, 9]. LUMBAR is considered the lower body counterpart for PHACE association, and infantile hemangioma in this location deserves further workup and close monitoring for possible complications. In one prospective study, hemangiomas >2.5 cm located on the lumbosacral area had a high risk for associated spinal dysraphism with 50% of patients demonstrating spinal anomalies. Ultrasonography was not specific in the diagnosis of underlying spinal cord abnormalities; thus, MRI of the lumbosacral spine is recommended.

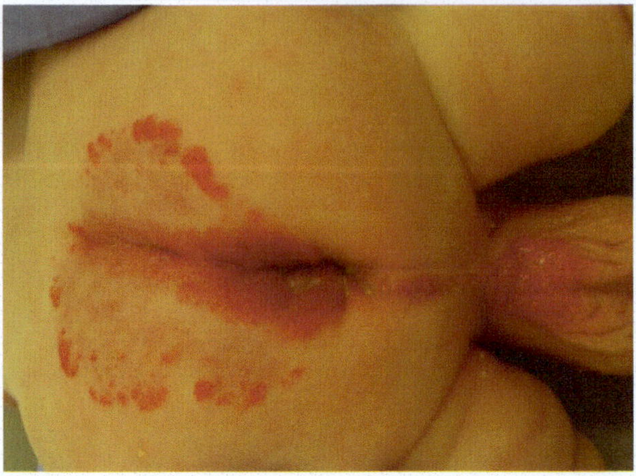

Fig. 5.3 Lumbosacral infantile hemangioma (IH-MAG type) at risk for spinal dysraphism small perianal ulceration

Segmental infantile hemangiomas in the lumbosacral and gluteal areas are also at very high risk for ulceration (Fig. 5.3). In some cases, ulceration is the primary presenting sign of a sacral infantile hemangioma. Thus treatment is often warranted in large hemangiomas in this location, arguably as a preventive measure against the likelihood of painful ulceration.

When and How to Treat

The majority of uncomplicated infantile hemangiomas do not require intervention. Watchful observation and anticipatory guidance is the most common treatment. Complicated hemangiomas and those in high-risk anatomic sites as summarized in Table 5.1 require active intervention. In the next section, current treatment for infantile hemangiomas will be discussed. All available therapies including systemic, topical, intralesional, and laser modalities will be outlined. In addition, treatment for ulceration will be reviewed including appropriate wound care and topical therapies specific to this clinical setting. Though hematologists/oncologists may not regularly prescribe topical or perform intralesional treatments for infantile hemangiomas, a working knowledge of the range of available therapies is important as interdisciplinary management of complicated infantile hemangioma is increasingly common.

Ulceration

Ulceration is the most frequent and urgent complication for infantile hemangiomas. Risk factors for ulceration include large size, a predominant superficial component, mucosal sites (lip, anogenital), upper back, chest, lumbosacral, and gluteal areas. Ulceration tends to occur early in the course of proliferation, prior to 4 months of age [10]. Early white/gray discoloration of the surface of a superficial hemangioma may herald ulceration [11]. As ulceration leads to pain and scarring, treatment is recommended in this setting. Treatment of ulceration depends on the clinical situation but most commonly includes basic wound care, and topical or systemic therapies, of which oral propranolol is the treatment of choice.

For hemangiomas in which painful ulceration has already occurred, treatment consists of several aims: (1) appropriate wound care, (2) pain control, and (3) halting progressive ulceration.

Appropriate wound care with topical modalities such as thick ointments (e.g., Aquaphor® or white petrolatum) can help to reduce crusting and decrease friction. They also provide an important barrier in anogenital or other mucosal sites. The use of non-adherent dressings, such as thin hydrocolloid dressings or petrolatum impregnated gauze, to provide occlusion can also be helpful. When crusting is present, it must be debrided with dilute hydrogen peroxide or saline soaks 2–3 times daily, as crusting impedes reepithelialization and can lead to superinfection. To help with pain control, topical lidocaine 5% ointment can be applied directly to the ulcer in small (pea-sized) amounts up to 3–4 times daily and is extremely helpful prior to cleansing or diaper changes. Other topical treatments used in the setting of ulceration include topical antibiotics such as metronidazole cream and mupirocin ointment. Another physical modality used with some success in the treatment of ulcerated hemangiomas is pulsed dye laser, which has been reported to be effective in both pain relief and expediting healing [12].

To halt progression of ulceration, systemic therapy with propranolol is the treatment of choice (Fig. 5.4). However there is some evidence that topical timolol maleate gel may be helpful. Timolol has been reported safe and effective in the treatment of ulcerated hemangiomas in all locations, with shorter time to healing and pain control than untreated hemangiomas [13]. In the authors' experience, systemic corticosteroids are of minimal benefit for ulceration. Prevention of ulceration is obviously ideal. Identifying hemangiomas at high risk for ulceration and initiating early systemic therapy with propranolol may be helpful in preventing the ulceration from occurring. In smaller lesions or when propranolol is contraindicated, topical timolol and/or pulsed dye laser treatment may also be helpful.

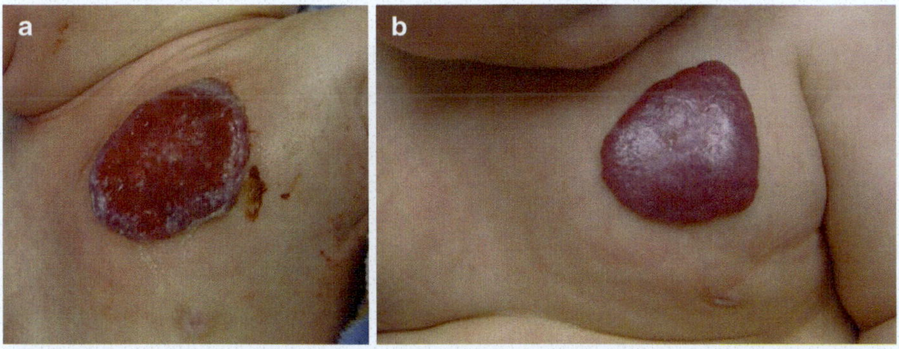

Fig. 5.4 Ulcerated superficial hemangioma of the chest (**a**) Infantile hemangioma of the upper chest with extensive ulceration. (**b**) Complete healing of the ulceration with oral propranolol in 2.5 weeks

Systemic Therapy

Historically, prior to 2008, oral corticosteroids were the mainstay of treatment for infantile hemangiomas, and no FDA-approved therapy existed. Oral corticosteroids were effective at halting proliferation of infantile hemangiomas; however, adverse events typical for chronic use of oral corticosteroids such as weight gain, growth delay, sleep disturbance, irritability, Cushingoid facies, and hypertension were common. Thus, this treatment was used only in life- or function-threatening lesions. Similarly, chemotherapeutic agents such as alpha interferon and vincristine were also used in severe complicated infantile hemangiomas requiring aggressive management, both with undesirable side effect profiles. Interferon was found to be associated with development of spastic diplegia when used in infants <1 year of age, while vincristine almost always requires administration through a central venous line and causes other adverse effects.

The advent of propranolol as a safe and effective therapy and its recent FDA approval for this indication have resulted in a paradigm shift in the management of complicated infantile hemangiomas in a relatively short time. With improved results and excellent safety profile, oral propranolol is the first-line therapy for infantile hemangiomas requiring treatment.

Propranolol

Since the serendipitous observation by Leaute-Labreze and colleagues that children receiving oral beta-blockade for other indications had improvement in their cutaneous infantile hemangiomas, there have been many case reports, series, and two randomized controlled trials (RCT) demonstrating its safety and efficacy [14]. There have been numerous publications which support propranolol as first-line therapy in most clinical situations, with a very high clinical response rate and low side effect profile [15] (see Fig. 5.5 for treatment examples). In the largest RCT comparing oral propranolol to placebo in 401 treated infants versus 55 in the placebo group, 60% of patients in the treatment arm had complete or near complete resolution of the hemangioma at 24 weeks compared to 5% of placebo [16]. A dose of 3 mg/kg/d divided BID was found to be superior to 1 mg/kg/day for a duration of 6 months. Rebound growth of about 10% was observed. The most common side effects included sleep disturbance, diarrhea, cool extremities, and bronchial hyper-reactivity. Symptomatic hypoglycemia has been reported in the literature as a potential serious side effect, but this is rare. Due to the potential for crossing the blood-brain barrier, propranolol has theoretic risk for late neurodevelopmental effects; however, this has not been reported. In one study, infants treated with propranolol had a higher incidence for delayed walking, but this risk was not sustained with all four children walking unassisted by 20 months [17]. There is one RCT comparing efficacy of oral propranolol with oral prednisolone. This study showed similar efficacy between the two modalities but fewer serious adverse effects with propranolol; however, results are limited due to small size [18]. The mechanism of action for oral propranolol is unknown. Recent studies and literature reviews indicate that a variety of possible mechanisms may be at play. These include the promotion of pericyte-mediated vasoconstriction, inhibition of vasculogenesis/angiogenesis, disruption of hemodynamic force-induced cell survival, and the inactivation of the renin-angiotensin system [19].

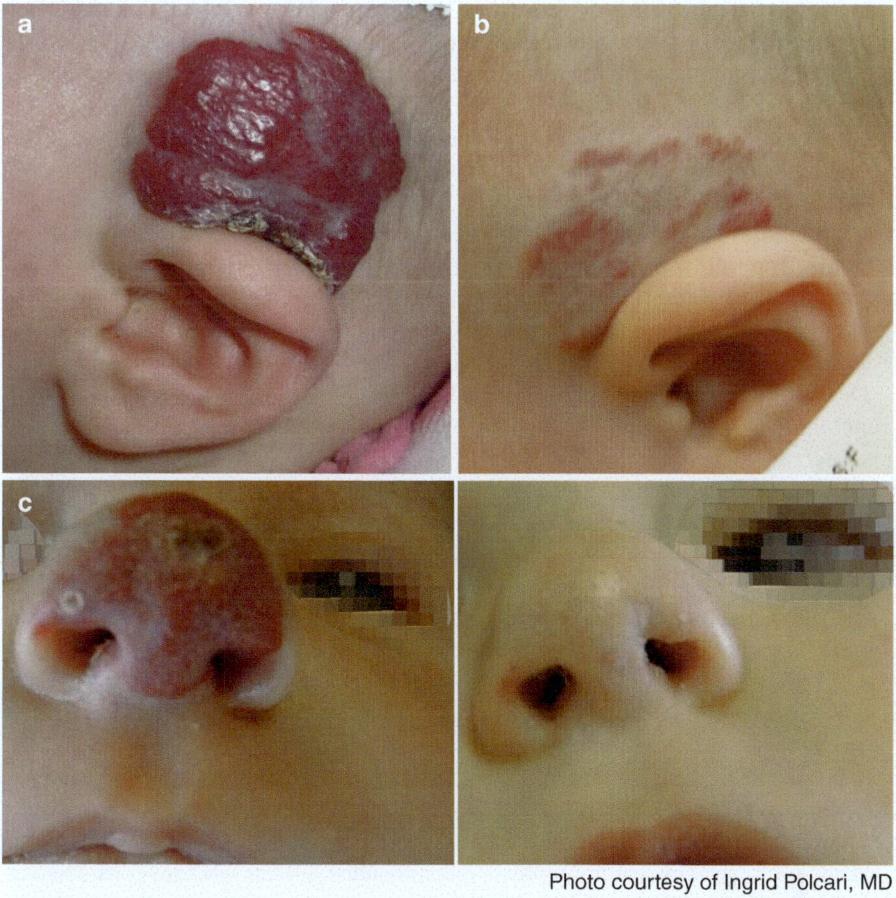

Fig. 5.5 (**a, b**) Periauricular ulcerated infantile hemangioma (**a**) before and (**b**) after 3 months of treatment with propranolol. (**c**) Infantile hemangioma of the nasal tip at age 6 weeks before and after treatment with propranolol. (Photo courtesy of Dr. Ingrid Polcari)

Propranolol is indicated in infants with complicated or high-risk infantile hemangiomas (see Table 5.1). Propranolol is usually administered in an outpatient setting, with dose escalation over days to weeks. Doses of between 1 and 3 mg/kg/day divided BID or TID are the most widely used. Contraindications to propranolol include weight < 2 kg, sinus bradycardia, hypotension, cardiogenic shock, heart block, congestive heart failure, reactive airway disease, potential for hypoglycemia, and known hypersensitivity.

Initiation and use of oral propranolol for infantile hemangiomas has been discussed in two consensus guideline statements from both the USA and Canada [20] and an expert group from Europe [21]. In general, outpatient initiation of propranolol is recommended for most healthy infants in the absence of any contraindications. A pre-treatment history and full physical examination are recommended. A baseline EKG is recommended specifically when the history or physical examination reveals concern for heart rhythm abnormalities. Inpatient initiation is recommended for infants <2 months of age (corrected for prematurity) and/or those <3.5 kg. Other indications for inpatient admission include life-threatening hemangioma (subglottic or diffuse hepatic), inadequate social support, or significant comorbidities, cardiac or otherwise. During an inpatient admission, close monitoring allows for rapid dose escalation, and many infants can be discharged on a full dose of the medication. An initial dose of 0.33 mg/kg/dose every 8 hours with monitoring of heart rate and blood pressure 1–2 hours following each dose is recommended during the first 24 hours. The following 24 hours 0.66 mg/kg/dose every 8 hours is given with the same monitoring. If this is tolerated, the infant can be discharged after 48 hours with stable vital signs. Due to the elevated risk for hypoglycemia in very young infants, propranolol is given after feeds and held if the infant has poor oral intake.

Despite the consensus statement in 2013 regarding outpatient initiation of propranolol, there remains some variability in the recommended dose and dose escalation intervals. A baseline history and physical examination +/– pre-treatment EKG are recommended. Infants >3 months of age with weight > 3.5 kg may be started on propranolol on an outpatient basis at doses of 1 mg/kg/day divided BID or TID with 0.5–1 mg/kg/day dose escalations every 3–7 days until goal dose is achieved (2–3 mg/kg/day). Families should be counseled to always feed the infant prior to giving the medication and hold the dose as discussed above, with poor oral intake, vomiting, prolonged diarrhea, or evidence of reactive airway disease.

Special Considerations

In infants with large facial infantile hemangioma at risk for PHACE association, care must be taken with administration of propranolol due to the high incidence of cerebrovascular disease and predisposition to stroke in these patients. Propranolol may be used safely in this setting; however, pre-treatment workup including EKG, MRI/MRA of the head and neck, and echocardiography is recommended. Infants who are considered at high risk for stroke include those with cardiac or aortic arch anomalies, significant narrowing of multiple major cerebral vessels without adequate collateral circulation, severe stenosis of one major cerebral vessel without collateral circulation, concurrent moyamoya disease, and variations of these changes [20]. In these cases, consultation with cardiology and neurology is recommended prior to initiation of propranolol, as use of beta-blocker in this setting would theoretically compound the risk for stroke.

Topical Therapy

Superficial localized hemangiomas may benefit from topical therapy depending on location. On the head and neck, and in particular on the central face, topical therapies have been demonstrated to successfully hasten resolution. In some cases, even deep or ulcerated lesions have responded to topical therapies. Historically, potent topical steroids were sometimes used in attempt to hasten involution for hemangiomas in prominent locations. However, concern regarding side effects (thinning of the skin and dyspigmentation) limited the use of this treatment. More recently, however, there is growing data supporting topical beta-blockers, such as timolol maleate gel, as a safe and effective topical modality. Most pediatric dermatologists use topical timolol maleate gel to treat superficial or even deep infantile hemangiomas on the face, and occasionally periorbital ones, if complications are anticipated. In one recent randomized trial, timolol was effective in reducing the color and predicted volume of superficial infantile hemangiomas without any major side effects [22]. Though there is excellent safety with use of topical beta-blockers, care must be taken as timolol maleate is more concentrated than oral propranolol; thus, there is risk for systemic absorption via the conjunctiva or on large ulcerated or mucosal sites.

Intralesional Therapy

The use of intralesional corticosteroids for infantile hemangiomas, in particular those in the periorbital, nasal tip or lip locations has been used for several decades. A recent review of intralesional triamcinolone acetonide at doses of no more than 3 mg/kg/dose demonstrated good safety and response for this intervention. Most hemangiomas responded to treatment with 67% improving and 33% stabilizing in size. However rebound growth was common (40%) and repeated injections are necessary [23]. Safety concerns with intralesional injection in the periorbital location include retinal artery occlusion with embolization of injected steroid. Though reported, this is rare. Other side effects of intralesional therapy include atrophy of the injected area and systemic absorption. Though many physicians and pediatric dermatologists regularly perform intralesional treatment for infantile hemangiomas, appropriate training is necessary for optimal utilization of this modality, and it is generally reserved for smaller lesions when there are contraindications for systemic therapy. In a recent European expert consensus statement on treatments for infantile hemangiomas, intralesional corticosteroid injection was not considered a recommended or first-line therapy.

Laser Modalities

The pulsed dye laser (PDL) has been used in the past to treat infantile hemangiomas. Its main use is in the treatment of residual lesions and telangiectasias post-involution and can be a helpful tool to decrease redness in this setting. However use of PDL during the proliferative phase of infantile hemangioma growth is no more effective than natural involution and is associated with increased risk for ulceration, scarring, and atrophy [24]. Thus with the advent of propranolol, use of PDL has been limited to post-involution and residual lesions. Similarly, other lasers such as neodymium-doped yttrium aluminum garnet (Nd:YAG) or ablative fractional resurfacing may be helpful post-involution for residual lesions. However, more studies are needed to assess the long-term outcomes. In addition, the efficacy of oral propranolol may obviate the need for these and/or surgical modalities in the future.

Congenital Hemangioma

Natural History and Growth Characteristics

Congenital hemangiomas (CH) can be differentiated from classic infantile hemangiomas by their unique histopathology and growth characteristics. Congenital hemangiomas are fully formed at birth, having completed the majority of their proliferation in utero. They can be detected on prenatal ultrasonography as early as the late first trimester. Although the incidence of congenital hemangiomas is not exactly known, one report documented the presence of congenital hemangiomas in 0.3% of newborns [1]. Congenital hemangiomas lack expression of GLUT-1, a histochemical marker present in all classic infantile hemangiomas, which is helpful in distinguishing between these two distinct vascular tumors. The genetic basis for CH has recently been elucidated; both subtypes described below have been found to be associated with mutations in GNAQ [46]. Congenital hemangiomas have two major clinical subtypes, rapidly involuting congenital hemangiomas (RICH) and non-involuting congenital hemangioma (NICH). Some wonder if the two exist along a spectrum or continuum given their genetic, clinical, and histopathologic similarities [25]. Indeed, other morphologic variants also support this relationship as other variants have recently been reported including those that only partially involute with time (PICH) and RICH with presumed prenatal involution [26, 27].

Types and Morphology

Rapidly Involuting Congenital Hemangioma (RICH)

RICH occur fully formed at birth and are often observed on prenatal ultrasonography. They usually present as large, exophytic, violaceous vascular tumors with surrounding pale halo (Fig. 5.6). Boon's original 1996 paper described three morphologic types: raised violaceous tumor with ectatic veins, raised grayish tumor with multiple tiny telangiectasias surrounded by a pale halo, and flat infiltrative tumor with violaceous overlying skin. RICH are high-flow vascular lesions, and handheld Doppler evaluation will reveal fast blood flow. Similarly, formal ultrasonographic studies demonstrate heterogeneous lesions limited to the skin and subcutaneous fat, with diffuse vascularity and multiple arteries and veins with high-velocity blood flow and occasional calcifications [28]. Larger lesions may

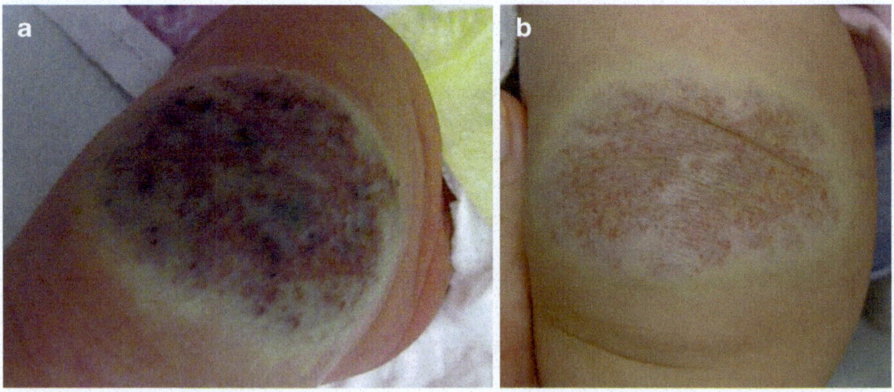

Fig. 5.6 Rapidly involuting congenital hemangioma at (**a**) 4 weeks and (**b**)11 weeks with significant flattening, lightening of color over time. Note the surrounding pale halo characteristic of these lesions

ulcerate leading to pain and bleeding. Their antenatal course is that of rapid involution over weeks to months, with resultant flattening of the lesions leaving characteristic atrophic skin behind.

Non-involuting Congenital Hemangioma (NICH)

NICH are also noted fully formed at birth. They tend to persist unchanged through life and do not regress. Usually lesions are asymptomatic; however, sometimes pain or other symptoms are reported depending on location. Symptoms may be exacerbated during times of growth or increased hormonal activity during puberty. NICH can have two clinical subtypes: patch or plaque/nodular [29]. Compared to RICH, NICH lesions are typically more flat and are usually not exophytic. NICH are most commonly located on the trunk and extremities (Fig. 5.7). In the largest series to date, there is a slight female predominance (57%) [29]. Similar to RICH, NICH are high-flow lesions on ultrasonography and handheld Doppler, and this elevated blood flow persists over time.

Complications

Similar to common infantile hemangiomas, ulceration is a possible complication seen in cutaneous congenital hemangiomas, most commonly with RICH. Ulceration in congenital hemangiomas is particularly worrisome since it can result in life-threatening hemorrhage, due to their underlying high blood flow [30]. Transient thrombocytopenia and mild hypofibrinogenemia have been described [31], but the degree of thrombocytopenia is not as profound and sustained as that seen in Kasabach-Merritt phenomenon seen with other vascular tumors such as tufted angioma or kaposiform hemangioendothelioma. Rarely, congenital hemangiomas can manifest with high-output cardiac failure [32, 33], and hydrops fetalis had been reported to occur with large hemangiomas [34, 35]. Persistent pain is a symptom

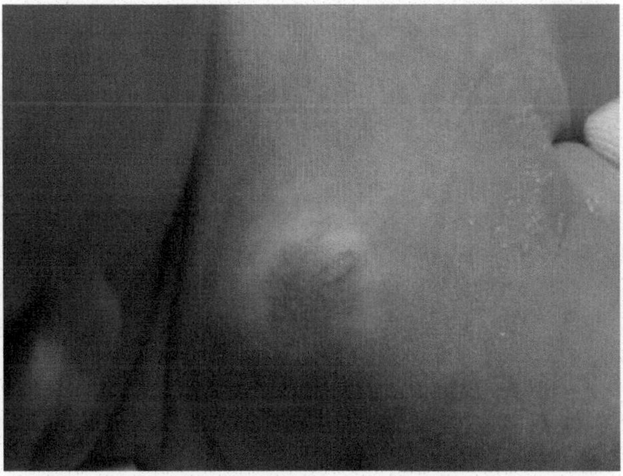

Fig. 5.7 Small NICH on the shoulder of a neonate

reported particularly in NICH, potentially due to vasoconstriction causing local tissue ischemia [29]. Disfigurement from residual skin changes can occur after involution is complete in RICH.

When and How to Treat

Most congenital hemangiomas do not require treatment. For RICH, serial observation during the rapid involution phase is considered the best approach. Treatment is indicated when complications such as ulceration, bleeding, hemodynamic compromise, or significant thrombocytopenia are observed. Unlike infantile hemangiomas, no medical therapy has proven to be effective for these lesions. Appropriate wound care, pain control, and treatment of secondary infections are necessary when ulceration occurs. (see previous section on *Ulceration*). Surgical excision is indicated when medical therapy fails to control ulceration, cardiac failure, or bleeding. Surgery may also be performed to excise residual anetodermatous skin or other disfigurement after involution is complete. For NICH, surgical excision is the recommended treatment for lesions that cause disfigurement or problematic pain when it is discrete and in a location that is surgically amenable. Preoperative embolization may need to be performed prior to excision of larger lesions that are highly vascular because of their potential for bleeding. Pulsed dye laser and/or sclerotherapy is sometimes used to reduce appearance of superficial telangiectasia or prominent veins in residual RICH or sometimes for NICH.

Hepatic Hemangioma

Natural History and Clinical Subtypes

The liver is the most common extracutaneous site of hemangioma. The presence of cutaneous hemangiomas usually lead to the diagnosis of hepatic hemangiomas, although in rare cases, hepatic hemangiomas can present as symptomatic liver disease without associated skin lesions or diagnosed prenatally on routine perinatal ultrasounds [36, 37]. Diagnosis can usually be made by their characteristic appearance on magnetic resonance imaging (MRI) of hypointensity on T1-weighted images and hyperintensity on T2-weighted imaging. Biopsy is oftentimes not necessary and may be contraindicated due to risk of bleeding. Hematologist/oncologists may be called upon to aid in the diagnosis and workup of hepatic hemangiomas as they may mimic other tumors in the liver requiring further imaging or biopsy. Hepatic hemangiomas are the most common benign liver tumors in early infancy. They share the same growth characteristic and involution as their more common cutaneous counterparts. Similar to cutaneous hemangiomas, hepatic hemangiomas occur as true infantile hemangiomas as well as congenital hemangiomas. They are subclassified into three distinct types: focal, multifocal, and diffuse. *Focal* hepatic hemangiomas appear as discrete, solitary, often large hypervascular tumor in the liver, fully grown at birth (Fig. 5.8). They are not classic infantile hemangiomas but

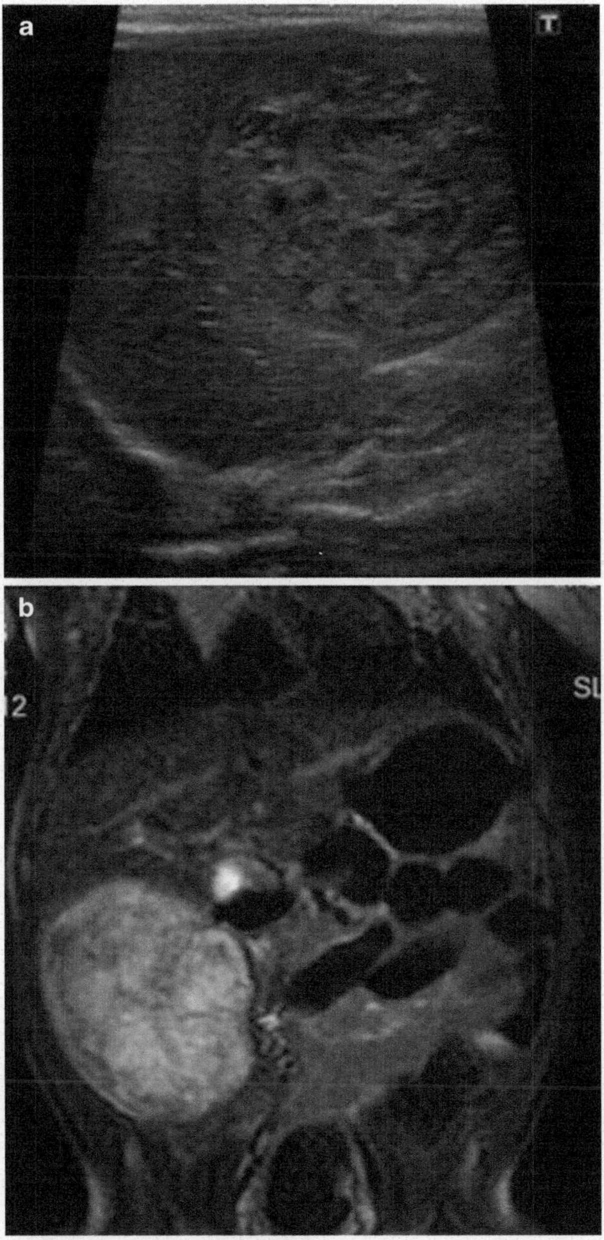

Fig. 5.8 (**a**, **b**) Focal hepatic hemangioma on (**a**) ultrasound and (**b**) MRI. (Reprinted from His Dickie et al. [38]. Copyright (2014), with permission from Elsevier)

are most commonly rapidly involuting congenital hemangiomas. Hepatic RICH are often diagnosed on prenatal ultrasonography and are high-flow vascular lesions that do not express GLUT-1 on histopathologic examination. By contrast, multifocal and diffuse hepatic hemangiomas are true infantile hemangiomas, expressing GLUT-1, and undergo the typical natural history of proliferation over the first few weeks to months of life after birth, followed by slow involution. *Multifocal* hepatic hemangiomas are characterized by multiple lesions with intervening normal hepatic parenchyma (Fig. 5.9), whereas *diffuse* hepatic hemangiomas have far more extensive hepatic involvement with near-total replacement of the liver parenchyma (Fig. 5.10). Focal hepatic hemangiomas must be differentiated from hepatoblastoma, mesenchymal hamartoma, and angiosarcoma, while multifocal and diffuse lesions may be confused for metastatic tumors such as neuroblastoma [38]. Because of intense hypervascularity, hepatic hemangiomas can also be mistaken for hepatic arteriovenous malformations [39].

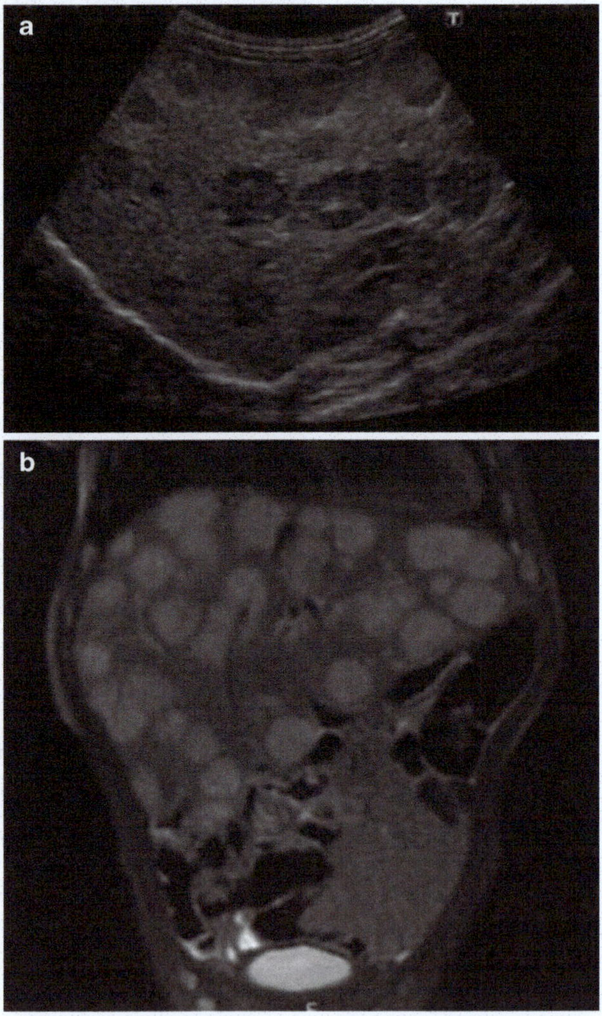

Fig. 5.9 (**a, b**) Multifocal hepatic hemangioma on (**a**) ultrasound and (**b**) MRI. (Reprinted from His Dickie et al. [38]. Copyright (2014), with permission from Elsevier)

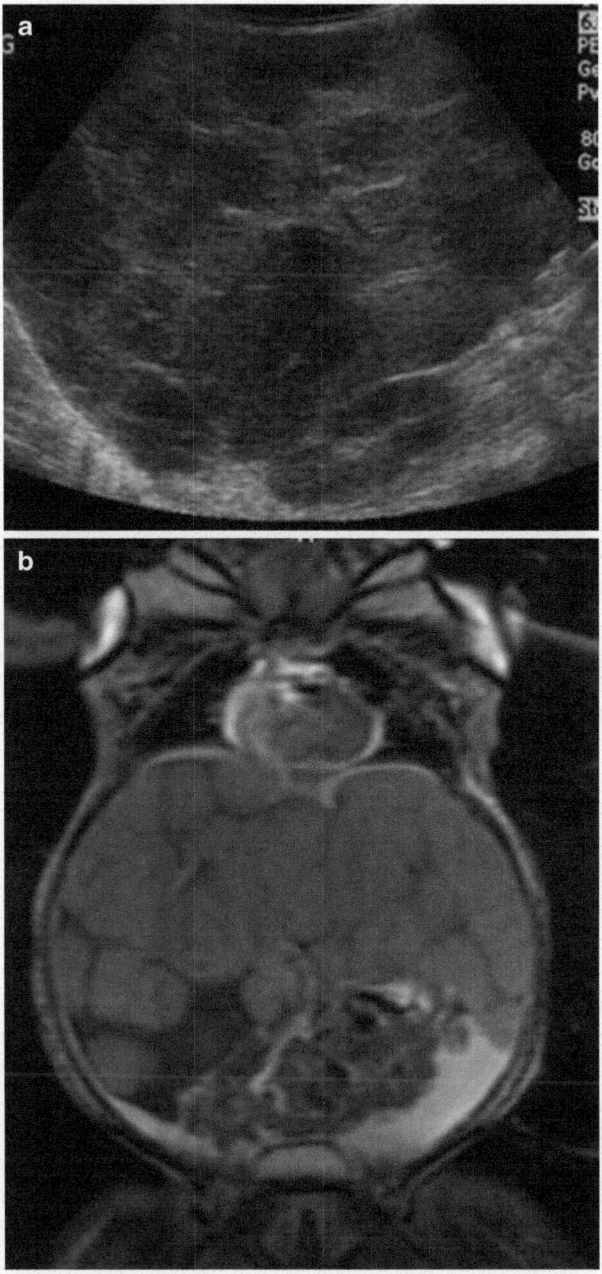

Fig. 5.10 (**a**, **b**) Diffuse hepatic hemangioma on (**a**) ultrasound and (**b**) MRI. (Reprinted from His Dickie et al. [38]. Copyright (2014), with permission from Elsevier)

Complications

The clinical presentations of hepatic hemangiomas vary from being asymptomatic to having life-threatening complications. Focal hepatic hemangiomas can present in the newborn with hepatomegaly, hyperbilirubinemia, thrombocytopenia and anemia from intralesional bleeding and/or thrombosis, and congestive heart failure from arteriovenous shunting. Multifocal and, in particular, diffuse hepatic hemangiomas have been described to cause massive hepatomegaly that can lead to abdominal compartment syndrome with severe cardiorespiratory compromise and fulminant liver failure. Severe acquired hypothyroidism is a well-known association found in almost all diffuse and in some multifocal hepatic hemangiomas. Liver infantile hemangioma tissue produces type 3 iodothyronine deiodinase enzyme that inactivates thyroid hormone causing clinical hypothyroidism. If undetected and left untreated, hypothyroidism can result in neurological impairment and low cardiac output congestive heart failure [40]. Clinically significant ascites during involution have been recently reported in hepatic RICH [41].

When and How to Treat

The majority of patients with hepatic involvement of hemangiomas do well with lesions undergoing regression in a similar manner to their cutaneous counterparts. However, in certain subtypes, there can be a significant risk of mortality. Rialon et al. have reported a mortality rate of 16% in 123 affected patients with diffuse and multifocal hepatic hemangiomas [42]. Risk factors for poor prognosis include diffuse pattern and associated congestive heart failure. Screening for hepatic hemangiomas in infants with five or more multiple cutaneous hemangiomas allows for earlier detection and treatment of affected patients before life-threatening progression ensues, resulting in improved outcomes with reduced mortality [43]. Algorithms have been developed to guide surveillance and management of hepatic hemangiomas [36, 37]. Baseline studies recommended include imaging with abdominal ultrasound and MRI, liver function tests, CBC, coagulation studies, thyroid function test, and alpha-fetoprotein. Cardiac evaluation is also recommended to assess and monitor for cardiac failure. Follow-up requires serial ultrasounds to monitor for progression of lesions, with frequency determined by phase of proliferation and involution. Early and aggressive treatment is imperative when any of the aforementioned complications are detected, particularly congestive heart failure and hypothyroidism. Conventional systemic therapies for infantile hemangioma, mainly oral propranolol or corticosteroids, are used to hasten involution of hepatic hemangiomas [44, 45]. In diffuse or multifocal hepatic hemangiomas with acquired hypothyroidism, very high doses of hormone replacement are usually required to achieve euthyroid status. Embolization to decrease arteriovenous and porto-hepatic venous shunting can be initiated as a temporizing measure until medical therapies take effect in patients with high-output heart failure. Selective hepatic arterial ligation is sometimes still used if embolization is not feasible. In rare cases, surgical resection may be necessary in patients who continue to be symptomatic despite medical therapy. In extreme cases of diffuse hepatic hemangiomas with abdominal compartment syndrome, liver transplantation may be considered as last resort when all other options of treatment have failed.

References

1. Kanada KN, Merin MR, Munden A, Friedlander SF. A prospective study of cutaneous findings in newborns in the United States: correlation with race, ethnicity, and gestational status using updated classification and nomenclature. J Pediatr. 2012;161(2):240–5.
2. Tollefson MM, Frieden IJ. Early growth of infantile hemangiomas: what parents' photographs tell us. Pediatrics. 2012;130(2):e314–20.
3. Suh KY, Frieden IJ. Infantile hemangiomas with minimal or arrested growth: a retrospective case series. Arch Dermatol. 2010;146(9):971–6.
4. Haggstrom AN, Garzon MC, Baselga E, Chamlin SL, Frieden IJ, Holland K, et al. Risk for PHACE syndrome in infants with large facial hemangiomas. Pediatrics. 2010;126(2):e418–26.
5. Metry D, Heyer G, Hess C, Garzon M, Haggstrom A, Frommelt P, et al. Consensus statement on diagnostic criteria for PHACE syndrome. Pediatrics. 2009;124(5):1447–56.
6. Bayer ML, Frommelt PC, Blei F, Breur JM, Cordisco MR, Frieden IJ, et al. Congenital cardiac, aortic arch, and vascular bed anomalies in PHACE syndrome (from the international PHACE syndrome registry). Am J Cardiol. 2013;112(12):1948–52.
7. Iacobas I, Burrows PE, Frieden IJ, Liang MG, Mulliken JB, Mancini AJ, et al. LUMBAR: association between cutaneous infantile hemangiomas of the lower body and regional congenital anomalies. J Pediatr. 2010;157(5):795–801 e1-7.
8. Frade F, Kadlub N, Soupre V, Cassier S, Audry G, Vazquez MP, et al. PELVIS or LUMBAR syndrome: the same entity. Two case reports. Arch Pediatr. 2012;19(1):55–8.
9. Yadav DK, Panda SS, Teckchandani N, Bagga D. SACRAL syndrome. BMJ Case Rep. 2013;2013.
10. Chamlin SL, Haggstrom AN, Drolet BA, Baselga E, Frieden IJ, Garzon MC, et al. Multicenter prospective study of ulcerated hemangiomas. J Pediatr. 2007;151(6):684–9, 9 e1.
11. Maguiness SM, Hoffman WY, McCalmont TH, Frieden IJ. Early white discoloration of infantile hemangioma: a sign of impending ulceration. Arch Dermatol. 2010;146(11):1235–9.
12. Di Maio L, Baldi A, Dimaio V, Barzi A. Use of flashlamp-pumped pulsed dye laser in the treatment of superficial vascular malformations and ulcerated hemangiomas. In Vivo. 2011;25(1):117–23.
13. Oranje AP, Janmohamed SR, Madern GC, de Laat PC. Treatment of small superficial haemangioma with timolol 0.5% ophthalmic solution: a series of 20 cases. Dermatology. 2011;223(4):330–4.
14. Leaute-Labreze C, Dumas de la Roque E, Hubiche T, Boralevi F, Thambo JB, Taieb A. Propranolol for severe hemangiomas of infancy. N Engl J Med. 2008;358(24):2649–51.
15. Hogeling M, Adams S, Wargon O. A randomized controlled trial of propranolol for infantile hemangiomas. Pediatrics. 2011;128(2):e259–66.
16. Leaute-Labreze C, Hoeger P, Mazereeuw-Hautier J, Guibaud L, Baselga E, Posiunas G, et al. A randomized, controlled trial of oral propranolol in infantile hemangioma. N Engl J Med. 2015;372(8):735–46.
17. Gonski K, Wargon O. Retrospective follow up of gross motor development in children using propranolol for treatment of infantile haemangioma at Sydney Children's Hospital. Australas J Dermatol. 2014;55(3):209–11.
18. Bauman NM, McCarter RJ, Guzzetta PC, Shin JJ, Oh AK, Preciado DA, et al. Propranolol vs prednisolone for symptomatic proliferating infantile hemangiomas: a randomized clinical trial. JAMA Otolaryngol Head Neck Surg. 2014;140(4):323–30.

19. Ji Y, Chen S, Xu C, Li L, Xiang B. The use of propranolol in the treatment of infantile haemangiomas: an update on potential mechanisms of action. Br J Dermatol. 2015;172(1):24–32.
20. Drolet BA, Frommelt PC, Chamlin SL, Haggstrom A, Bauman NM, Chiu YE, et al. Initiation and use of propranolol for infantile hemangioma: report of a consensus conference. Pediatrics. 2013;131(1):128–40.
21. Hoeger PH, Harper JI, Baselga E, Bonnet D, Boon LM, Atti MC, et al. Treatment of infantile haemangiomas: recommendations of a European expert group. Eur J Pediatr. 2015;174(7):855–65.
22. Chan H, McKay C, Adams S, Wargon O. RCT of timolol maleate gel for superficial infantile hemangiomas in 5- to 24-week-olds. Pediatrics. 2013;131(6):e1739–47.
23. Couto JA, Greene AK. Management of problematic infantile hemangioma using intralesional triamcinolone: efficacy and safety in 100 infants. J Plast Reconstr Aesthet Surg. 2014;67(11):1469–74.
24. Batta K, Goodyear HM, Moss C, Williams HC, Hiller L, Waters R. Randomised controlled study of early pulsed dye laser treatment of uncomplicated childhood haemangiomas: results of a 1-year analysis. Lancet. 2002;360(9332):521–7.
25. Mulliken JB, Enjolras O. Congenital hemangiomas and infantile hemangioma: missing links. J Am Acad Dermatol. 2004;50(6):875–82.
26. Nasseri E, Piram M, McCuaig CC, Kokta V, Dubois J, Powell J. Partially involuting congenital hemangiomas: a report of 8 cases and review of the literature. J Am Acad Dermatol. 2014;70(1):75–9.
27. Maguiness S, Uihlein LC, Liang MG, Kozakewich H, Mulliken JB. Rapidly involuting congenital hemangioma with fetal involution. Pediatr Dermatol. 2015;32(3):321–6.
28. Gorincour G, Kokta V, Rypens F, Garel L, Powell J, Dubois J. Imaging characteristics of two subtypes of congenital hemangiomas: rapidly involuting congenital hemangiomas and non-involuting congenital hemangiomas. Pediatr Radiol. 2005;35(12):1178–85.
29. Lee PW, Frieden IJ, Streicher JL, McCalmont T, Haggstrom AN. Characteristics of noninvoluting congenital hemangioma: a retrospective review. J Am Acad Dermatol. 2014;70(5):899–903.
30. Liang MG, Frieden IJ. Infantile and congenital hemangiomas. Semin Pediatr Surg. 2014;23(4):162–7.
31. Boon LM, Enjolras O, Mulliken JB. Congenital hemangioma: evidence of accelerated involution. J Pediatr. 1996;128(3):329–35.
32. Cole P, Kaufman Y, Metry D, Hollier L. Non-involuting congenital haemangioma associated with high-output cardiomyopathy. J Plast Reconstr Aesthet Surg. 2009;62(10):e379–82.
33. Weitz NA, Lauren CT, Starc TJ, Kandel JJ, Bateman DA, Morel KD, et al. Congenital cutaneous hemangioma causing cardiac failure: a case report and review of the literature. Pediatr Dermatol. 2013;30(6):e180–90.
34. Daniel SJ, Cassady G. Non-immunologic hydrops fetalis associated with a large hemangioendothelioma. Pediatrics. 1968;42(5):828–33.
35. McGahan JP, Schneider JM. Fetal neck hemangioendothelioma with secondary hydrops fetalis: sonographic diagnosis. J Clin Ultrasound. 1986;14(5):384–8.
36. Dickie B, Dasgupta R, Nair R, Alonso MH, Ryckman FC, Tiao GM, et al. Spectrum of hepatic hemangiomas: management and outcome. J Pediatr Surg. 2009;44(1):125–33.
37. Christison-Lagay ER, Burrows PE, Alomari A, Dubois J, Kozakewich HP, Lane TS, et al. Hepatic hemangiomas: subtype classification and development of a clinical practice algorithm and registry. J Pediatr Surg. 2007;42(1):62–7; discussion 7-8.
38. Hsi Dickie B, Fishman SJ, Azizkhan RG. Hepatic vascular tumors. Semin Pediatr Surg. 2014;23(4):168–72.
39. Alomari AI. Hepatic arteriovenous malformation or rapidly involuting congenital hemangioma? Tex Heart Inst J. 2015;42(4):408.
40. Huang SA, Tu HM, Harney JW, Venihaki M, Butte AJ, Kozakewich HP, et al. Severe hypothyroidism caused by type 3 iodothyronine deiodinase in infantile hemangiomas. N Engl J Med. 2000;343(3):185–9.

41. Klein M, Chang AK, Vasudevan SA, Blatt J, Iacobas I, Lee S. Clinically significant ascites as an indication for resection of rapidly involuting congenital hepatic hemangiomas. Pediatr Blood Cancer. 2018;65(8):e27222.
42. Rialon KL, Murillo R, Fevurly RD, Kulungowski AM, Christison-Lagay ER, Zurakowski D, et al. Risk factors for mortality in patients with multifocal and diffuse hepatic hemangiomas. J Pediatr Surg. 2015;50(5):837–41.
43. Rialon KL, Murillo R, Fevurly RD, Kulungowski AM, Zurakowski D, Liang M, et al. Impact of screening for hepatic hemangiomas in patients with multiple cutaneous infantile hemangiomas. Pediatr Dermatol. 2015;32(6):808–12.
44. Mhanna A, Franklin WH, Mancini AJ. Hepatic infantile hemangiomas treated with oral propranolol--a case series. Pediatr Dermatol. 2011;28(1):39–45.
45. Marsciani A, Pericoli R, Alaggio R, Brisigotti M, Vergine G. Massive response of severe infantile hepatic hemangioma to propranolol. Pediatr Blood Cancer. 2010;54(1):176.
46. Ayturk UM, Couto JA, Hann S, Mulliken JB, Williams KL, Huang AY, Fishman SJ, Boyd TK, Kozakewich HP, Bischoff J, Greene AK. Somatic activating mutations in GNAQ and GNA11 are associated with congenital hemangioma. Am J Human Genet. 2016;98(4):789–95.

Kaposiform Hemangioendothelioma and Kasabach-Merritt Phenomenon: Management of Coagulopathy and Treatment Options

6

Taizo A. Nakano and Ilona J. Frieden

Abbreviations

HHV-8	Human herpesvirus-8
ISSVA	International Society for the Study of Vascular Anomalies
KHE	Kaposiform hemangioendothelioma
KLA	Kaposiform lymphangiomatosis
KMP	Kasabach-Merritt phenomenon
MRI	Magnetic resonance imaging
mTOR	Mammalian target of rapamycin
NICH	Non-involuting congenital hemangioma
rFVIIa	Recombinant activated factor VII
RICH	Rapidly involuting congenital hemangioma
TA	Tufted angioma
VEGFR-3	Vascular endothelial growth factor receptor-3

Introduction

Kaposiform hemangioendothelioma (KHE) is a rare and locally aggressive vascular tumor of infancy and childhood. Accurate classification and diagnosis of this vascular lesion remains challenging; however, great progress has been made to better

T. A. Nakano (✉)
Center for Cancer and Blood Disorders, Children's Hospital Colorado, University of Colorado School of Medicine, Aurora, CO, USA
e-mail: taizo.nakano@childrenscolorado.org

I. J. Frieden
Departments of Dermatology and Pediatrics, University of California, San Francisco, San Francisco, CA, USA
e-mail: Ilona.Frieden@ucsf.edu

C. C. Trenor III, D. M. Adams (eds.), *Vascular Anomalies*,
https://doi.org/10.1007/978-3-030-25624-1_6

characterize the tumor and standardize our diagnostic and therapeutic approach. Rapid recognition and intervention is vital to the management of this lesion as its complications are associated with considerable morbidity and mortality.

Historically, KHE was often lumped together with other "hemangiomas" of infancy [1]. However, a subset of these lesions were recognized as substantially more aggressive, locally invasive, and occasionally associated with a life-threatening consumptive coagulopathy. The gross histology of this subgroup revealed an architecture of sheets and lobules of round- and spindle-shaped endothelial cells reminiscent of Kaposi sarcoma, the aggressive malignancy triggered by infection with human herpesvirus-8 (HHV-8) associated with immunocompromised adults [2]. Recognizing this pathologic similarity, but aware of the substantial difference in pathophysiology of disease, clinical investigators used a variety of names to refer to a lesion of this nature including congenital hemangioendothelioma, Kaposi-like infantile hemangioendothelioma, Kaposi-like hemangioma, and hemangioma with Kaposi-like features [3, 4].

In 1993, Zukerberg et al. coined the term kaposiform hemangioendothelioma that provided this aggressive vascular tumor with a unified identity [5]. In 1996, the International Society for the Study of Vascular Anomalies (ISSVA) adopted a classification of vascular anomalies that recognized KHE as a rare and distinct vascular tumor of infancy and childhood [6]. This classification schema, updated in 2014, categorizes a KHE as a locally aggressive vascular tumor associated with profound thrombocytopenia, hypofibrinogenemia, and/or consumptive coagulopathy, otherwise referred to as the Kasabach-Merritt phenomenon (KMP). Originally described in 1940, the Kasabach-Merritt phenomenon continues to be inappropriately associated with a variety of clinical coagulopathies found in both vascular malformations and tumors. However, we now recognize that KMP is a hallmark of KHE and tufted angioma (TA), a tumor which is now viewed as likely part of the KHE histopathologic spectrum.

The pediatric hematologist oncologist has key roles in the multidisciplinary evaluation and treatment of patients with suspected KHE. Although, historically, surgical and interventional therapies played a first-line role in the treatment of these lesions, subsequent clinical experience has demonstrated a considerable susceptibility to a number of pharmacotherapeutic and chemotherapeutic interventions. The pediatric hematologist oncologist will be called upon to coordinate drug administration and provide careful clinical monitoring. In the case of a KHE associated with life-threatening KMP (which occurs in the majority of cases of large KHE in infancy), the practitioner will be called upon to maintain adequate hemostasis and manage hemorrhagic complications. To facilitate rapid diagnosis and decision making, additional cross-disciplinary involvement should be encouraged from pediatric dermatology, diagnostic and interventional radiology, and general surgery. The goal of this chapter is to outline current approaches to the diagnosis and treatment of KHE with the additional complication of KMP.

Kaposiform Hemangioendothelioma

Kaposiform hemangioendothelioma (KHE) is a vascular neoplasm of infancy and childhood that consists of an abnormal and aggressive proliferation of endothelial and lymphatic cells. Given its infiltrative growth yet low-grade histomorphological features, the World Health Organization and ISSVA classify KHE as a neoplasm of intermediate malignancy. Although there are occasional reports of local spread and regional lymph node involvement, it is not considered a tumor with metastatic potential [2]. Unlike classic infantile hemangiomas (IH), this locally invasive lesion does not spontaneously involute and, importantly, can demonstrate episodes of rapid growth associated with an acquired sequestration of platelets and consumption of clotting factors. Although the mechanism of tumorigenesis has not been fully defined, somatic activating *GNA14* mutations have been identified in some KHE and found to induce changes in cellular morphology and increase cell growth via MAPK activation [7].

Epidemiology

Limited studies have been completed to accurately calculate the incidence of KHE in infants and children. In 2013, Croteau et al. published a single-center cohort retrospective study of KHE and reported an estimated incidence of 0.07 cases per 100,000 children per year [8]. They reported that symptomatic KHE manifested before 1 month of age in 60% of cases and less than 1 year of age in 93% of cases. It is estimated that approximately 50–70% of cases of KHE develop the Kasabach-Merritt phenomenon [2, 9]. No clear gender or ethnic preponderance has been identified.

Clinical Presentation

Most infants and children with KHE display evidence of the vascular anomaly at birth or during early childhood. Although in some cases KHE is fully formed at birth, more often it is mistaken for a "birthmark" or bruise. Initial findings can be either a intradermal and subcutaneous mass with ill-defined borders and violaceous discoloration or as a brown-red vascular stain with a variable degree of induration [5, 10, 11] (Fig. 6.1a, b). Cutaneous lesions are occasionally associated with hypertrichosis and/or hyperhidrosis [12]. Although relatively benign in this quiescent state, a KHE can quickly evolve with rapid growth and development of full-blown coagulopathy, often after exposure to an inflammatory trigger such as trauma or infection [1]. This abrupt exacerbation may occur early from the trauma associated with delivery or be delayed for multiple months. Occasionally, it occurs in utero presenting with premature delivery and features of hydrops fetalis.

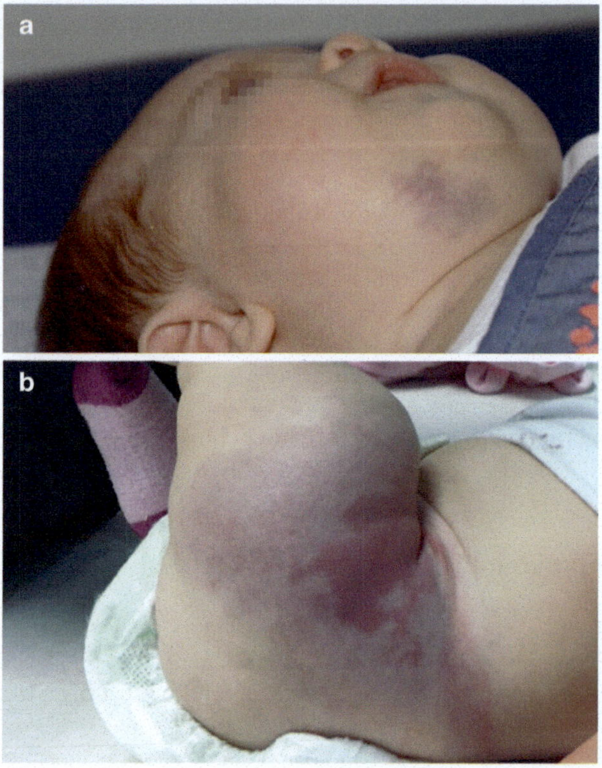

Fig. 6.1 Clinical presentation of KHE. (**a**) 1-month-old with KHE involving the skin of the right lower mandible as an ecchymotic, poorly demarcated soft tissue mass. (**b**) 2-month-old infant with large KHE of the left leg extending onto the torso who progressed to develop KMP

When KHE is complicated by KMP, the tumors typically enlarge dramatically, becoming deeper red to violaceous in color with more edema or leathery quality to their surface (Fig. 6.2a, b). Surrounding purpura extending beyond the border of the apparent tumor is often noted [9]. The tumors are often quite tender, particularly when associated with KMP. The rapid expansion of a KHE typically presents in the first year of life in the following locations: extremities and trunk (75% of cases), retroperitoneal (18% of cases), cervicofacial, visceral, and bone [13]. Although a few case reports of multifocal KHE have been reported, the great majority of lesions are localized without evidence of multifocality or metastatic potential [14, 15].

As a KHE expands, it may negatively impact surrounding structures and function. The tumor may impair muscle and joint function and cause musculoskeletal pain or compress nerves, resulting in acquired nerve palsy or impaired sensation. Depending on the site of presentation, it can additionally disrupt venous return or compress the airway. The cutaneous component may appear inflamed, developing into superficial edema, erosions, or frank ulceration. Over time KHE may continue to demonstrate additional exacerbations of aggravated growth and inflammation in response to subsequent traumatic or infectious stimuli, even after severe coagulopathy has subsided.

Although most KHE lesions present in the skin and subcutaneous tissues with classic cutaneous findings, isolated visceral, retroperitoneal, intrathoracic/mediastinal, and bone lesions have been reported [8, 16]. Isolated bone and visceral KHE

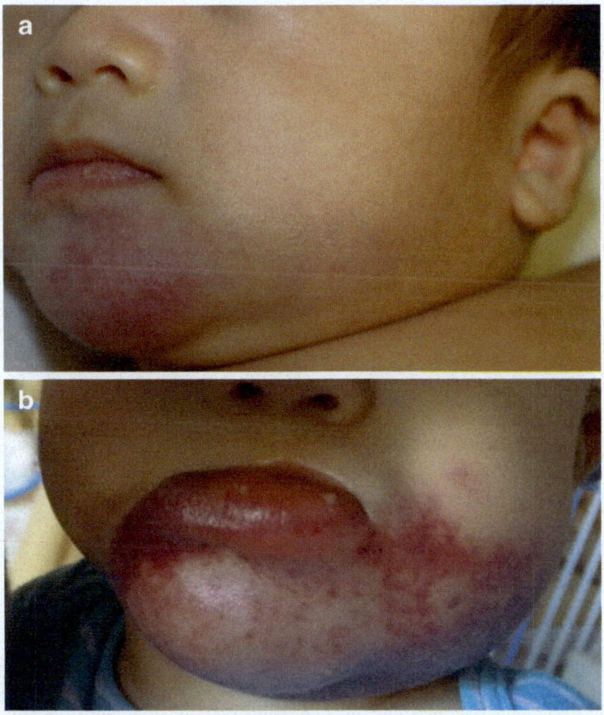

Fig. 6.2 Acute progression to KMP. (**a**) Infant with biopsy-proven tufted angioma at age 2 months. His D-dimers were initially mildly elevated (1100 ng/mL), but platelets remained normal. (**b**) At 9 months of age, the lesion demonstrated acute increase in soft tissue swelling, tenderness, purpura, and severe thrombocytopenia

tend to present without KMP, whereas lesions of the retroperitoneum or mediastinum have a high risk for KMP. Reports of bone KHE emphasize presentation radiographically as lytic lesions without periosteal reaction, commonly mistaken for chondroblastoma [16] (Fig. 6.3a, b). Some have hypothesized that isolated bone lesions are physically constrained from expansion, which limits the tumor's ability to infiltrate the surrounding tissue [8].

Although the most severe and symptomatic signs and symptoms of KHE are typically during infancy, residual tumor can result in long-term effects with both functional and aesthetic impacts. KHE can result in fibrosis or lymphedema which in themselves may be painful or impair function, including long-term impacts on the musculoskeletal system, skin, and nerve [17]. The possibility of these long-term comorbidities justifies the need for long-term clinical surveillance of patients with KHE [18].

Histopathology

The pathologic presentation of KHE is distinctly infiltrative, which can help to differentiate it from other vascular malformations and tumors of infancy and childhood. While the cutaneous component of the lesion demonstrates local inflammation and color change with tumor expansion, the subcutaneous and deep tissue infiltration

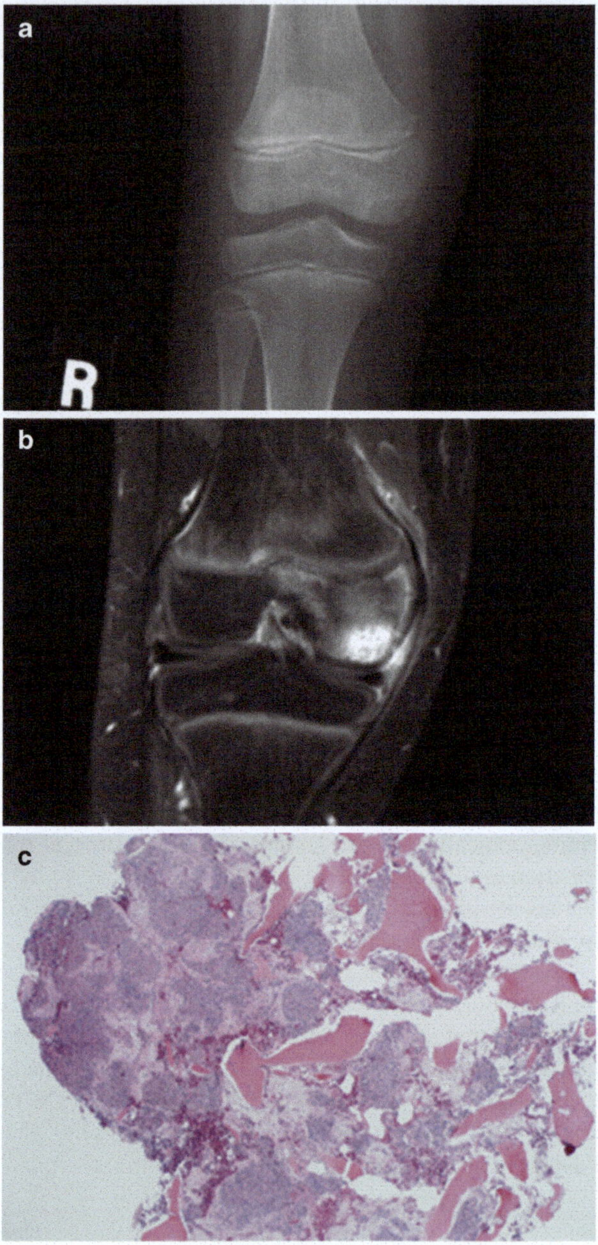

Fig. 6.3 Isolated bone KHE. (**a**) X-ray of right knee demonstrating lytic lesion of distal femur. Lesion was initially mistaken for a chondroblastoma but biopsy demonstrated histology consistent with KHE. (**b**) Right knee coronal T1 MRI after gadolinium contrast demonstrating enhancing epiphyseal lesion of medial femoral condyle with surrounding bone marrow edema. (**c**) H&E 4× demonstrating infiltration of tumor nodules into the marrow space between bony spicules in this case

shows an invasive pattern with possible extension across tissue planes from the dermis, subdermis, subcutaneous fat, muscle, and bone [8] (Fig. 6.4a, d). Although case reports have demonstrated possible regional lymph node involvement, KHE does not demonstrate metastatic potential [2]. Additionally, KHE does not undergo spontaneous involution, differentiating it from a classic infantile hemangioma [9].

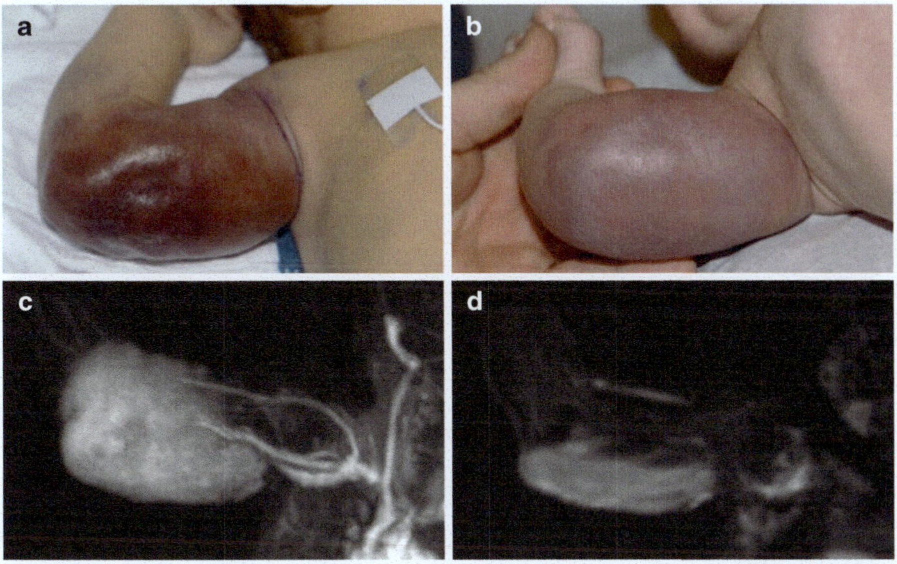

Fig. 6.4 Right arm KHE with KMP. (**a**) Newborn male with rapidly enlarging, circumferential right upper arm KHE with KMP. (**b**) 1 month later, there was marked improvement after initial treatment with oral prednisone and sirolimus followed by sirolimus as monotherapy. (**c**) Coronal MRA of right arm obtained at initial presentation demonstrating abrupt transition from large feeding vessels to tortuous intralesional vessels. (**d**) Coronal T1 MRI of right arm after gadolinium contrast obtained at initial presentation that demonstrated tumor infiltration of the subdermis and muscle

Visualized with hematoxylin and eosin staining, KHE histology demonstrates a pattern of sheets and lobules of round and tightly packed spindle-shaped endothelial cells that infiltrate areas of progressively fibrotic tissue [5, 9] (Figs. 6.3c and 6.5a). The spindled endothelial cells align to form slit-like lumina openings that entrap erythrocytes similar to a Kaposi sarcoma-like histologic pattern [19, 20]. However, there is no association between KHE and the HHV-8 virus, which is the known trigger of Kaposi sarcoma [2]. Throughout the lesion there are infiltrating irregular nodules associated with thin-walled lymphatic vessels, historically referred to as "lymphangiomatosis." [5] Extensive lymphatic involvement is thought to be an intrinsic component of the KHE rather than the result of mass effect or tumor obstruction [1, 2]. Similar to Kaposi sarcoma, the tumor likely arises from lymphatic endothelium and expresses lymphatic markers such as D2-40 and vascular endothelial growth factor receptor-3 (VEGFR-3) [2]. Epithelioid or "glomeruloid" islands within the nodules represent areas of increased platelet trapping and blood destruction (Fig. 6.5b). Histologic evidence of fibrin, microthrombi, and hemosiderin granules can be identified within these areas [5, 9, 21] (Fig. 6.6a). Lymphocytes and macrophages can additionally be identified in these glomeruloid islands [20].

With immunohistochemical staining, KHE tumors stain diffusely positive for the vascular endothelial markers CD31 and CD34 and the endothelial nuclear marker FLI1, which can be identified in most vascular neoplasms (Fig. 6.5c, Table 6.1).

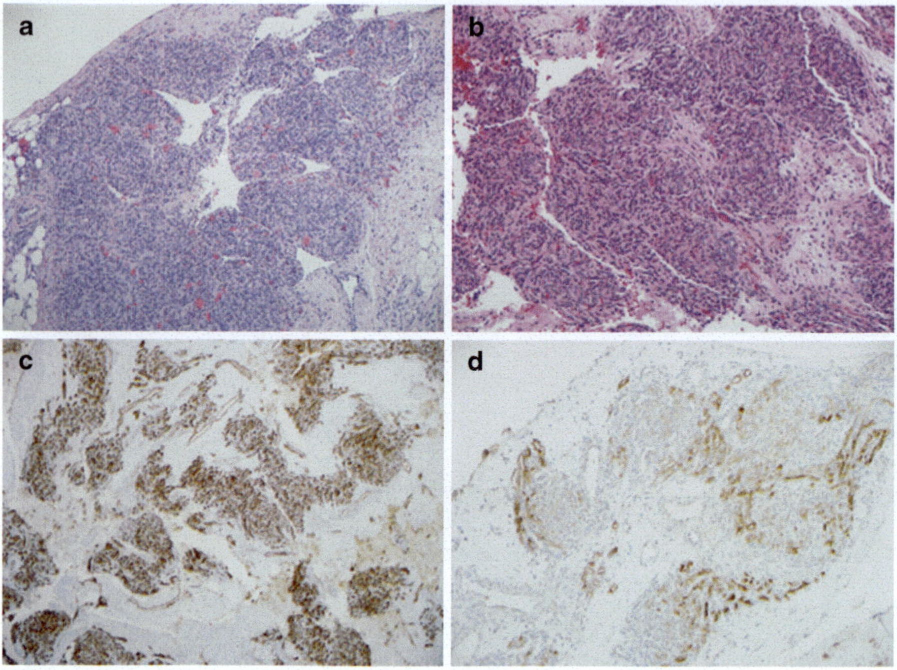

Fig. 6.5 KHE histology and immunohistochemistry. (**a**) H&E 10× view demonstrating infiltrative tumor nodules focally outlined by larger, thin-walled lymphatic spaces. (**b**) H&E 20× view demonstrating characteristic glomeruloid structures composed of whirled nests of epithelioid endothelial cells and pericytes rimmed by small slit-like vascular spaces. (**c**) CD34 immunohistochemical stain 10× view highlighting the nodular architecture of the lesion, with small round and slit-like vascular spaces in the nodules and larger, thin-walled vascular spaces between nodules. (**d**) D2-40 immunohistochemical stain 20× view highlights slit-like lymphatic channels, predominantly at the edges of the nodules and glomeruloid structures

KHE also typically has positive staining for the lymphatic endothelial markers D2-40 and VEGFR-3, a marker of lymphangiogenesis [22, 23] (Fig. 6.5d). Neoplastic spindle cells within KHE stain positively for the lymphatic endothelial markers LYVE-1 and Prox1 (nuclear expression) [19]. Glomeruloid islands stain positively for CD61, otherwise known as platelet glycoprotein IIIa, which is expressed by platelets and megakaryocytes (Fig. 6.6b). Of note, KHE has negative staining for GLUT1 (a specific marker for infantile hemangioma), negative for HHV-8, and negative for LeY [2, 9].

Tufted Angioma

When considering a differential diagnosis of KHE with KMP, it is important to briefly mention a related vascular neoplasm known as the tufted angioma (TA). Thought to be in the same spectrum of disease as KHE, TA is a slower-growing

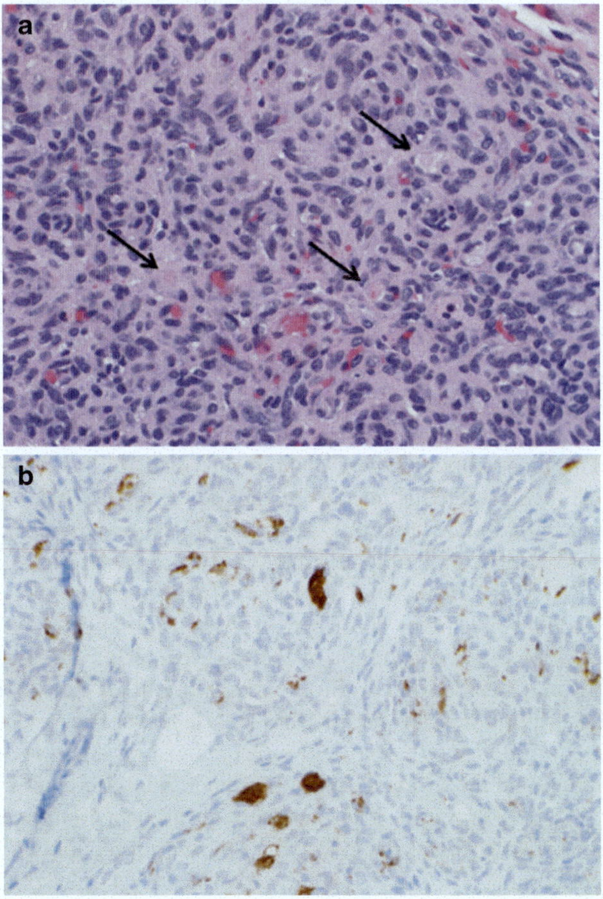

Fig. 6.6 KHE platelet sequestration. (**a**) High-power 40× view of a larger nodule showing multiple vascular spaces containing pink microthrombi (arrows), consistent with red blood cell and platelet breakdown. (**b**) Microthrombi highlighted by a CD61 immunohistochemical stain, 40× view

Table 6.1 Immunohistochemical pattern for KHE

Marker	Staining	Function
CD34	Positive	A marker of early hematopoietic and vascular cells, facilitates cell migration
CD31	Positive	Platelet endothelial cell adhesion molecule (PECAM-1), present on endothelial intercellular junctions
D2-40	Positive	A marker of lymphatic endothelium
VEGFR-3	Positive	Vascular endothelial growth factor 3 mediates lymphangiogenesis, a lymphatic endothelial marker
FLI1	Positive	Friend leukemia integration 1 transcription factor, a proto-oncogene and a broad IHC marker of vascular neoplasm
CD61	Positive	Integrin beta-3, found on thrombocytes, utilized as a marker of platelets and megakaryocytes
GLUT1	Negative	An erythrocyte-type glucose transport protein that is a sensitive marker for infantile hemangioma and placental tissue
LeY	Negative	Lewis Y antigen, of the Lewis human blood group system, a known marker for infantile hemangioma

vascular neoplasm that is more typically confined to the superficial skin [24]. Histologically, TA demonstrate discrete nodules of capillary vessels, circumscribed in groups or "tufts" in a "cannonball" pattern, primarily located in the dermis and hypodermis [1, 25]. Lymphatic channels are often present similar to a KHE, and the two lesions share an identical immunophenotype [9, 19]. Additionally, at least one case report has demonstrated TA progressing to KHE over time [26]. These features further reinforce the concept that KHE and TA fall on a continuum of the same disease process [27]. Distinct from KHE, TA may present in an older age group and have a lower tendency to present associated with thrombocytopenia and consumptive coagulopathy (KMP). TA may also resolve spontaneously in some cases.

Kasabach-Merritt Phenomenon

The most important complication of KHE is the Kasabach-Merritt phenomenon, which is present in the majority of cases of KHE. This is a potentially life-threatening constellation of findings including thrombocytopenia, hypofibrinogenemia, and consumptive coagulopathy that was first described by Kasabach and Merritt in 1940 as "extensive purpura" secondary to a "giant capillary hemangioma" [28]. The 2-month-old infant described in their original case report demonstrated a rapidly enlarging vascular tumor of the leg, severe thrombocytopenia, and severe hemorrhage. Considering current nomenclature, their case most likely represents the first description of KHE with KMP [1, 29]. The development of KMP carries an associated mortality risk of 10–30% [10]. Cause of death is often related to hemorrhage, functional impairment, high-output cardiac failure, and shock.

After this report, KMP was thought to be a complication of infantile hemangiomas (IH); this was disproven in 1997 with the publication of two case series differentiating KHE and IH [1, 29]. Even very large IH fail to demonstrate platelet sequestration and consumptive coagulopathy. Multiple investigators have written about the pathophysiological mechanisms of KHE that lead to KMP and which are lacking in IH. The vascular architecture of a KHE greatly differs from that of IH. The vessels that feed into a KHE demonstrate an abrupt transition from larger vessels to small convoluted capillaries, which results in more turbulent blood flow, increased blood stasis, and activation of primary hemostasis [5, 30] (Fig 6.4c). Additionally, a number of well-characterized lymphoepithelial neoplasms demonstrate dysregulated consumption of hemostatic factors and fibrinolysis including Kaposi sarcoma and kaposiform lymphangiomatosis [31]. In KHE, the rapid expansion of abnormal lymphatic endothelial cells likely creates a pro-thrombotic intravascular environment that manifests as KMP.

Taken together, an intravascular environment of turbulent flow and blood stasis, abnormal lymphatic endothelial dysfunction, and hypercoagulability resembles the pro-thrombotic triad of Virchow. The notable difference between conditions surrounding classic thrombosis formation and the environment of KHE with KMP, however, is concurrent hyperfibrinolysis that promotes a continuous cycle of sequestration and consumption [30]. Eventually, the systemic vasculature becomes depleted of platelets (thrombocytopenia often <20,000/microL), fibrinogen (often <100 mg/dL), and, over time, clotting factors as well (PT/aPTT often normal to minimally elevated). The systemic bleeding risk is substantial, and intralesional hemorrhage is common. The shear stress on red cells passing through this overactive system can result in microangiopathic hemolysis, which may be visualized on a patient's peripheral blood smear and result in mild or severe anemia [32].

KHE is exquisitely sensitive to inflammation and injury, and in response to one of these triggers, the lesion will demonstrate episodic exacerbations of sequestration, consumption, hyperfibrinolysis, and hemorrhage. Although the mechanism for this is incompletely understood, the interspersed presence of lymphatic endothelial cells through the KHE tumor may represent cells with an increased sensitivity to systemic or localized immune or inflammatory changes. The clinical result is a vascular lesion that can rapidly increase in size and induce considerable pain (Figs. 6.4a and 6.7a). The anatomic location of a KHE per se is not predictive of KMP, but size

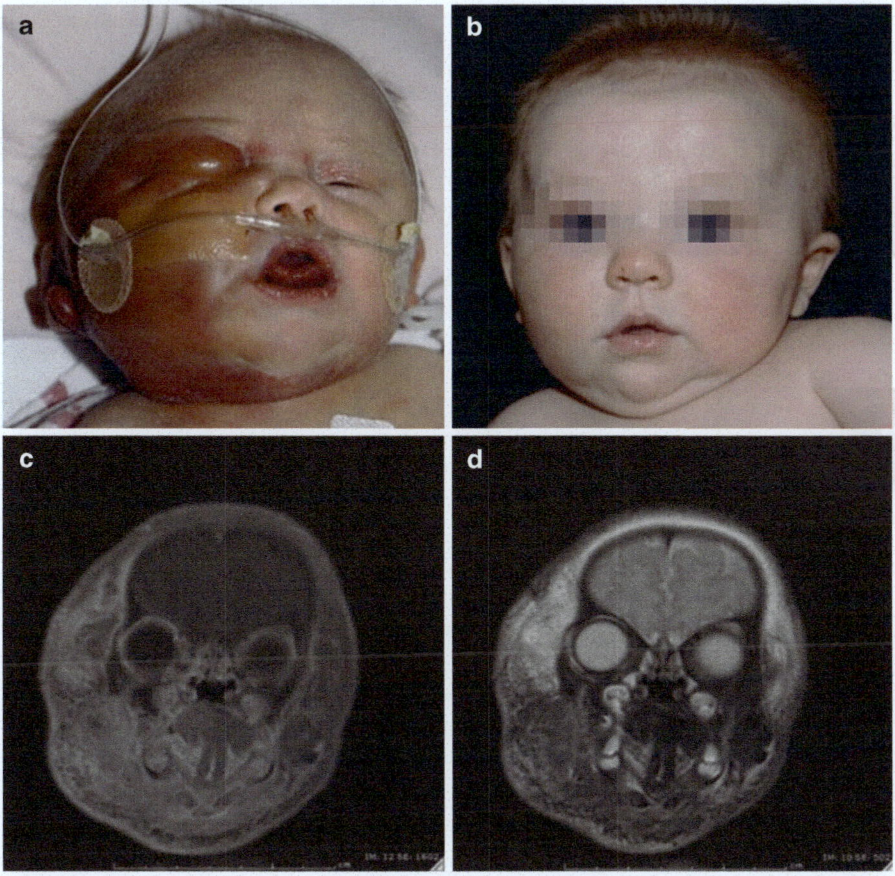

Fig. 6.7 Facial KHE patient with KMP. (**a**) Newborn female with rapidly enlarging facial KHE with KMP. (**b**) Follow-up exam at 4 months of age after multi-agent therapy. Initially received daily prednisone, weekly vincristine, and daily sirolimus. Transitioned to sirolimus monotherapy at 8 weeks of age. (**c**) Coronal T1 MRI obtained at initial presentation demonstrating diffuse enhancement of tumor infiltrating subdermis and muscle of right face, head, and neck. (**d**) Coronal T2 MRI obtained at initial presentation demonstrating diffuse lesion enhancement

is. In particular larger lesions, those invading deeper tissues and muscle, and those presenting in younger infants anecdotally, have increased risk of KMP.

Of note, certain vascular malformations, in particular venous malformations and combined venous-lymphatic malformations, have associated coagulopathy that is distinct in several respects from KMP. These malformations often demonstrate a localized or disseminated intravascular coagulopathy (LIC/DIC) characterized by markedly elevated D-dimer, but minimal thrombocytopenia [33]. Intravascular blood stasis and an abnormally activated endothelium appear to be the primary causes of consumptive coagulopathy in venous malformations, potentially leading to thrombophilia, chronic phlebolith formation, and pain [30, 33]. The chronic slow and intralesional consumption of fibrinogen, factor V, factor VIII, and factor XIII over time increases the periprocedural (surgical or interventional) risk of severe hemorrhage for these patients. In KHE with KMP, platelet trapping is a primary event, and severe thrombocytopenia and hypofibrinogenemia are the hallmark of the disease. It is important to correctly differentiate between these abnormalities of hemostasis as they require different approaches to management [6].

Diagnostic Evaluation

KHE must be considered in the differential diagnosis of any localized or regionally distributed vascular growth with onset during infancy or childhood. Rapid recognition is important because it can result in earlier intervention to help prevent complications and improve outcome. The clinical diagnosis of KHE should be suspected based on history, exam, laboratory studies, imaging, and, if available, histologic and immunohistochemical biopsy evaluation (Table 6.2; see also "Clinical Presentation"). The most common presentation is during the first year of life, as a subcutaneous mass with an ecchymotic, macular cutaneous component with an ill-defined border. The lesion can aggressively expand and infiltrate deeper tissue layers with potential to involve an entire anatomic region (e.g., an extremity).

When the diagnosis of KHE is suspected, the practitioner should rapidly obtain screening laboratory studies to rule out the complication of KMP. Primary laboratory studies should include a CBC with platelets and differential, D-dimer, fibrinogen, and PT/INR/aPTT. Peripheral blood smear should be reviewed to verify thrombocytopenia and document red and white cell morphology. Evidence of red cell fragmentation often secondary to microangiopathic hemolysis has been reported in up to 60% of cases [30, 32]. Interpretation of laboratory results should allow for quick risk stratification assigning those lesions that demonstrate marked platelet consumption and early evidence of consumptive coagulopathy to a higher-risk group. Secondary laboratory studies may include an LDH and fractionated bilirubin to evaluate degree of red cell hemolysis and baseline renal and hepatic function studies in anticipation of initiating pharmacotherapy.

Although multiple imaging modalities can be used to assist in the diagnosis of KHE, magnetic resonance imaging (MRI) remains the diagnostic imaging modality of choice. With T1-weighted imaging, a KHE presents as a soft tissue mass with

Table 6.2 Diagnostic evaluation of KHE

Diagnostic study	Description/rationale
Clinical history	Locally aggressive vascular tumor of infancy and childhood. Often of the extremity, trunk, cervicofacial, or retroperitoneum. Demonstrates exacerbations of growth that impacts surrounding structures and function
Clinical exam	Cutaneous or subcutaneous firm light pink, rusty red, or purpuric soft tissue tumor or plaque with ill-defined borders. With growth or platelet trapping, localized tenderness may be evident
Laboratory evaluation	
CBC with differential	Evaluate the degree of thrombocytopenia and anemia
Peripheral blood smear review	Evaluate for presence of thrombocytopenia, microangiopathic hemolytic anemia
D-dimer	An elevated D-dimer correlates to the degree of increased thrombotic and fibrinolytic activity
Fibrinogen	Evaluate the degree of consumption of fibrinogen, which is required for secondary hemostasis
PT/INR/aPTT	Prolonged values reflect deficiencies of clotting factors, which are required for secondary hemostasis
Renal function panel[a]	Evaluate for evidence of renal dysfunction
Liver function panel[a]	Evaluate for evidence of hepatic dysfunction
Total bilirubin[a]	Evaluate for evidence of microangiopathic hemolytic anemia and/or hepatic dysfunction
LDH[a]	Evaluate for evidence of microangiopathic hemolytic anemia
Imaging	*MRI remains modality of choice*
Ultrasound	Poorly defined highly vascular subcutaneous lesion
MRI	Imaging modality of choice. KHE diffusely enhances on T1 MRI post gadolinium (isointense) and T2 MRI studies (hyperintense)
Biopsy evaluation	*Decision to biopsy based on clinical bleeding risk and need to clarify diagnosis prior to initiation of therapy*
Histology	Sheets and lobules of round and tightly packed spindle shaped endothelial cells that infiltrate areas of tissue
Immunohistochemistry	CD34 +, CD31 +, D2-40 +, PROX1 +, CD61 +, GLUT1 – (see Table 6.1)

[a]Secondary laboratory studies

ill-defined margins, often involving multiple tissue plains that diffusely enhance with gadolinium (Figs. 6.4d and 6.7c). The lesion is T2 hyperintense with stranding of the subcutaneous fat and further demonstrates the presence of hemosiderin deposits and small dilated feeding and draining vessels [9, 11, 13] (Fig. 6.7d). If available, magnetic resonance angiogram (MRA) can be helpful to demonstrate the tortuous vascular architecture of feeding, draining, and intralesional vessels (Fig. 6.4c).

If the clinical diagnosis of KHE remains uncertain after consideration of clinical history, exam, laboratory studies, and imaging, the practitioner should consider pursuing surgical biopsy for histologic and immunohistochemical evaluation. Although pathologic evaluation often provides a more clear diagnosis of KHE, the risk of bleeding complications in the setting of severe KMP may preclude this as an initial diagnostic tool. Multidisciplinary coordination between the surgeon, anesthesiologist, hematologist, and pathologist is required to carry out a safe and informative incisional biopsy. The hematologist/oncologist should aim to maintain hemostatic stability perioperatively through the possible transfusion of cryoprecipitate, fresh frozen plasma (FFP), packed red blood cells, and even platelets in this critical setting. In general, platelet transfusions lead to enlargement of KHE and worsened KMP. If needed for periprocedural hemostasis, slowed administration of platelets may possibly lessen this complication, but platelet transfusions should be avoided as a way to normalize the platelet count outside of the setting of surgery or active bleeding. The histologic and immunohistochemical features of KHE were described previously in this chapter in the section titled "Pathology/Histology" of KHE. Briefly, histology should demonstrate sheets and lobules of round and tightly packed spindle-shaped endothelial cells infiltrating the dermis, subdermis, and muscle. IHC staining pattern should demonstrate CD34+, CD31+, D2-40 +, PROX1 +, and GLUT1 – (Table 6.1).

Differential Diagnosis

Kaposiform hemangioendotheliomas share a number of similar characteristics with more common vascular malformations and tumors of infancy and childhood as well as features of several malignant tumors [34, 35]. It is, therefore, important to consider an appropriate differential diagnosis prior to initiating therapy.

Infantile hemangioma – Infantile hemangiomas (IH) are benign vascular tumors of infancy that demonstrate growth after birth and spontaneous regression over time. They have well-defined borders and are not associated with a coagulopathy. Histologically, they demonstrate lobulated masses of proliferating endothelial cells and are immunohistochemically positive for GLUT1. They are usually softer and non-tender and often have a brighter red color than KHE. They involute spontaneously, and most IH have completed involution by age 4 to 5 years.

Congenital hemangioma – Congenital hemangiomas (CH) are benign vascular tumors of infancy that are fully formed at birth and may (rapidly involuting congenital hemangioma, RICH) or may not (non-involuting congenital hemangioma, NICH) spontaneously regress. Histologically, they demonstrate lobules of capillary proliferations embedded in a fibrous stroma. At birth RICH may demonstrate a transient thrombocytopenia and transient mild consumptive coagulopathy which can cause confusion with KHE. The transient coagulopathy of a RICH is typically less severe, is at low risk for hemorrhage, and resolves within a few days to weeks as the tumor undergoes rapid autoinfarction. In such cases, close serial follow-up and consideration of imaging or biopsy may be needed to differentiate these entities [36]. Somatic activating mutations in *GNAQ* and *GNA11* have now been associated with both RICH and NICH and may become a useful genetic screen to help diagnose lesions with atypical presentations [37].

Kaposiform lymphangiomatosis – Kaposiform lymphangiomatosis (KLA) is a newly described entity which has many similarities for KHE but with a notable difference – its multifocal nature. Unlike most KHE, patients with KLA have multiple areas of tumor and of lymphatic anomalies [38]. Patients with KLA often present with intrathoracic disease and demonstrate symptomatic hemorrhagic or chylous effusions. The diagnosis of KLA should further be considered in any presumed KHE patient found to have or develop other sites of disease involvement (e.g., incidentally found or symptomatic bony lytic lesions).

Infantile fibrosarcoma – Infantile fibrosarcoma is a malignant tumor of infancy that presents as a rounded, firm, deep tissue lesion. They are red to blue in color with surface telangiectasias [35]. The tumor can be associated with thrombocytopenia and consumptive coagulopathy.

Venous malformation – Venous malformations are slow-flow vascular malformations that present at birth as soft, compressible blue lesions. As mentioned previously, a localized intravascular coagulopathy can occur with venous malformation that greatly differs from features and complications of KMP.

Kaposi sarcoma – Kaposi sarcoma is a vascular tumor of the dermis triggered by the viral genome of human herpesvirus-8 (HHV-8). It is extremely rare to see in the pediatric age group in developed countries.

Rhabdomyosarcoma – Rhabdomyosarcoma is the most common soft tissue sarcoma of the head and neck in infants and children. The diagnosis is made through MRI imaging and tissue biopsy demonstrating differentiation toward skeletal muscle cells. Early recognition and aggressive intervention with possible chemotherapy, radiation therapy, and surgery are necessary for best possible outcome.

Infantile hemangiopericytoma – Infantile hemangiopericytoma is a highly vascularized malignant soft tissue tumor of infancy now considered part of the infantile myofibromatosis spectrum of lesions. Infantile hemangiopericytomas may mimic the consumptive coagulopathy and bleeding complications of KMP. Histologically, the tumor demonstrates well-circumscribed nodules of round-shaped and spindle-shaped cells and thin-walled branching "staghorn" vessels. Chemoresponsiveness and spontaneous regression have been reported [39].

Therapeutic Options

While there is tremendous disease heterogeneity in KHE, similar therapeutic goals can guide clinical management. These goals include reducing the risk of severe Kasabach-Merritt phenomenon (including potential mortality); reducing functional and structural morbidity from the invasive, infiltrating tumor; and reducing long-term morbidity from a variety of less critical factors including pain and aesthetics. Upfront risk stratification should differentiate KHE patients with KMP, requiring more rapid and aggressive intervention, from those who do not demonstrate KMP and have a lower risk of life-threatening complications. The prioritized goal, to resolve KMP, is measured by the recovery of hemostatic parameters where minimal adequate response is defined as platelets >20,000/microL and fibrinogen >100 mg/dL [32]. Reduction in functional and structural morbidity is often measured by clinical exam findings including reduction in tumor size and improved surrounding organ and musculoskeletal function. A multidisciplinary approach should be utilized to develop a personalized treatment plan. Although KMP can and usually does resolve, unless small and surgically resectable, KHE will not completely resolve with pharmacotherapy alone. Therapeutic recommendations are also evolving with sirolimus taking on a more important role in recent years, emphasizing the need to review the most current literature and updated consensus recommendations, in deciding on best approaches to management. Patients and families should be made aware that even if they achieve all therapeutic goals, a residual cutaneous and subcutaneous lesion often remains.

KHE Patients with Kasabach-Merritt Phenomenon

Supportive Hemostatic Care

Maintenance of hemodynamic stability should be a prioritized target in KHE patients with KMP to prevent hemorrhagic complications. In addition to reducing unnecessary patient manipulation and procedures, blood counts and coagulation parameters should be monitored closely. Interventions to correct hemostatic abnormalities should be carried out under the following guidelines:

Platelet Transfusions: As stated previously, a KHE with KMP will rapidly sequester and consume platelets and substantially increase the systemic bleeding risk. Despite alarmingly low platelet counts (often <10,000/microL), *the transfusion of platelets should be avoided unless the patient is actively bleeding or is in immediate preparation for invasive surgical intervention* [30]. Essentially "fueling the fire," transfused platelets demonstrate a shortened half-life as they are immediately sequestered into the lesion [32, 40]. This often results in amplified intralesional clotting and aggressive lesion expansion [41]. The multidisciplinary team should treat "the patient" not "the number." [32] When platelets are indicated, a slower infusion or drip may be better tolerated.

Cryoprecipitate: The rapid consumption of fibrinogen in KMP substantially contributes to the overall bleeding risk. Although fresh frozen plasma (FFP) contains both fibrinogen and clotting factors, the larger volume may not be tolerated in infants, especially if they present with evidence of heart failure [32]. The utility of FFP is better directed to the patient with disseminated intravascular coagulation, who demonstrate prolonged PT and aPTT and require the replacement of all clotting factors. Alternatively, cryoprecipitate offers a highly concentrated source of fibrinogen in a relatively small volume. Transfusion with cryoprecipitate should be considered in the patient with KMP at times of active bleeding, in preparation for invasive surgical procedure and, prophylactically, to maintain a serum fibrinogen >100 mg/dl.

Packed Red Blood Cells: The combination of microangiopathic intralesional hemolysis and the potential for active bleeding contribute to the presentation of mild to moderate anemia. Symptomatic anemia should be corrected to support appropriate cardiovascular function.

Recombinant Human Factor VIIa: Currently, recombinant activated human factor VII (rFVIIa) is FDA approved to treat hemophilia patients with high titer inhibitors and patients with Glanzmann's thrombasthenia. An isolated case report demonstrated the use of rFVIIa (at a dose of 90 mcg/kg/dose) to control active hemorrhage during surgical procedures in a KHE patient with KMP [42]. With minimal data to support the use of rFVIIa in KMP, no current recommendation can be made to support its use in the management of the disorder.

Surgical Excision

Complete surgical resection of a KHE with wide margins has shown historic efficacy to rapidly normalize hematologic parameters [43, 44]. Surgical excision is – when possible – a first-line therapy for KHE; however, larger and more infiltrative lesions of KHE are often not amenable to surgical excision. Additionally, surgical intervention takes on considerable bleeding risk in the setting of KMP. Incomplete resection can result in recurrence of tumor growth. For small, early, and localized KHE lesions, surgical excision remains a viable therapeutic option [43, 45, 46]. However, in the setting of KMP, more commonly, pharmacologic agents are used as first-line treatment with surgical excision reserved as a salvage therapy for refractory disease that presents an imminent threat to the patient. Surgical excision may also be considered for residual lesions that no longer demonstrate KMP but impart a negative functional impact on surrounding structures (e.g., a joint).

Systemic Corticosteroids

Corticosteroids have historically been a first-line agent for the treatment of KHE with KMP [32]. Many experts still initiate therapy with either oral prednisone (2–4 mg/kg body weight per day) or intravenous methylprednisolone (1.6 mg/kg body weight per day). However, as few as 10% of patients may see therapeutic goals met with corticosteroid monotherapy, and up to 30% of patients may be completely unresponsive to corticosteroids [47]. Bolus methylprednisolone at extreme dosing (30 mg/kg per day for 3 days) has been reported in refractory cases with inconclusive efficacy [48]. The majority of patients responding to corticosteroids will demonstrate some degree of response within the first week and should be considered a failure of therapy if no response is noted by 2 weeks [32].

Prolonged use of steroids in infants and children risks a number of important side effects including hypertension, impaired growth, osteopenia, and opportunistic infection. If an increase in platelet count is noted within the first 2 weeks of therapy, corticosteroids should be slowly tapered off over the following 4 weeks to reduce cumulative toxicity. Recent consensus-derived therapeutic guidelines suggest the concurrent use of corticosteroids and vincristine as first-line pharmacotherapy for KHE with KMP [43].

Vincristine

Vincristine is a potent first-line or early second-line agent for the treatment of KHE with KMP [49]. A naturally occurring vinca alkaloid isolated from the leaves of the periwinkle plant *Catharanthus roseus*, vincristine is an antimitotic chemotherapeutic agent that interferes with mitotic spindle microtubules. When utilized to treat KHE, it acts to reduce endothelial expansion, induce endothelial apoptosis, and inhibit angiogenesis [50]. Typically dosed at 0.05 mg/kg body weight weekly in infants <10 kg, vincristine can induce a correction in hematologic parameters, specifically the normalization of platelet counts and fibrinogen levels, and decrease the overall size of and soften a KHE lesion [47, 49] (Fig. 6.7b). Treatment is often continued until there is sustained improvement in platelet count [51]. If a response is demonstrated, it is reasonable to decrease the frequency of administration to every 2 weeks for 2 months and then to every 3 weeks for two additional months.

If dosed and monitored appropriately, weekly vincristine is well tolerated in infants and children. Common side effects include peripheral polyneuropathy, loss of tendon reflexes, autonomic neuropathy (constipation, ileus), and myelosuppression with prolonged use. Physical exam should be completed prior to each administration. Blood counts should be monitored for acquired cytopenias and electrolytes, and liver functions should be monitored to ensure appropriate drug clearance. Antibiotic prophylaxis to cover pneumocystis is recommended. As vincristine is a potent vesicant, administration requires the use of a central venous catheter. There is considerable bleeding risk to the placement of a central venous catheter in a patient with KMP, and the decision to use vincristine may be impaired because of this.

Sirolimus

Sirolimus, also known as rapamycin, is emerging as an important therapeutic option for KHE and has been reported in several studies as a first-line therapy [52, 53]. Sirolimus is an FDA-approved inhibitor of the mammalian target of rapamycin (mTOR) and acts in KHE to prevent downstream protein synthesis, angiogenesis, and subsequent cell proliferation. Preliminary reports of using sirolimus for KMP demonstrate rapid normalization of platelet counts and softening of the tumor (Fig. 6.4b) within days, whereas with combination corticosteroids and vincristine, it can take several weeks for hematologic parameters to normalize [54–56]. The majority of these studies have proposed a starting dose of 0.8 mg/m^2 per dose in infants <1 year of age, administered twice daily at 12-hour intervals [55]. The dose is titrated to obtain a goal serum trough level of 10–15 ng/ml. Of note, it can take up to 2–4 weeks to achieve a consistent therapeutic serum level of sirolimus. Caution should be taken to further dose reduce sirolimus in newborn and premature infants that demonstrate immature drug clearance [57, 58]. Concurrent pneumocystis prophylaxis is recommended.

Adams et al. recently published a phase II clinical trial evaluating the efficacy and safety of sirolimus in the treatment of complicated vascular anomalies [59]. Additionally, the safety profile for sirolimus is well established as it is widely used in renal transplant patients to prevent kidney allograft rejection. Although it is well tolerated when serum levels remain therapeutic, toxicity has been demonstrated to induce neutropenia, mucositis, peripheral edema, hypertension, hypertriglyceridemia, hypercholesterolemia, poor wound healing, headache, and elevation of liver transaminases. Antibiotic prophylaxis to cover pneumocystis should be considered while receiving sirolimus therapy, particularly in children less than 2 years of age [60].

The basis for its efficacy is not entirely known, but mTOR is an important activator/regulator of cell growth and angiogenesis. Conditions involving mutations that upregulate mTOR activity, like tuberous sclerosis and lymphangioleiomyomatosis, have demonstrated safe and efficacious response to sirolimus [61]. mTOR is overexpressed in a number of vascular anomalies, and sirolimus has been suggested as a treatment option for a number of pediatric vascular malformations and tumors [55, 62]. Other rapamycin analogs (temsirolimus, everolimus, and deforolimus) continue to demonstrate clinical efficacy in the treatment of advanced adult neoplasms including renal cell carcinoma and other refractory solid tumors [63].

Multi-agent Chemotherapy

Other chemotherapeutic agents including cyclophosphamide and actinomycin have been administered in combination with vincristine in a handful of case reports [64–66]. It is difficult to extrapolate outcome data from such few patients and literature that report inconsistent response rates from protocols that vary greatly.

Antifibrinolytic Agents

The antifibrinolitic agents, aminocaproic acid and tranexamic acid, are analogs of the amino acid lysine. They act to inhibit plasmin breakdown of thrombosis and are widely utilized to manage minor bleeding in patients with known bleeding disorders. As previously stated, KHE lesions with KMP demonstrate hyperfibrinolytic activity, and an antifibrinolytic agent could be considered as an adjuvant to more definitive therapy in the setting of worsening disease and active bleeding [40, 67].

Antiplatelet Agents

As platelets are sequestered into the tortuous vasculature of a KHE, they adhere, aggregate, and activate as part of an uncontrolled cycle of primary hemostasis. Antiplatelet agents such as aspirin and ticlopidine have been utilized to reduce platelet adhesion, aggregation, and activation [51]. Aspirin decreases synthesis of thromboxane A2 and prostacyclin by inhibiting prostaglandin endoperoxide synthase. Use of aspirin as adjuvant therapy has demonstrated reduction of bulk disease, improved color, and improved perilesional function [68, 69]. Ticlopidine decreases platelet adhesion by inhibiting the adenosine diphosphate binding of fibrinogen with platelet membranes. Multiple case reports have described the use of ticlopidine as an adjuvant to vincristine therapy or used concurrently with aspirin as adjuvants to vincristine [70]. It has yet to be studied if the addition of any antiplatelet agent could worsen the bleeding risk in KHE patients with KMP. While initiation of antiplatelet therapy for KHE is no longer considered first-line therapy, their use is a treatment option for long-term maintenance management and in cases of KHE or tufted angioma without KMP.

Interferon Alpha

In early studies, interferon alpha-2a demonstrated efficacy to correct coagulopathy and reduce tumor size in life-threatening "giant" or "alarming" hemangiomas that were unresponsive to corticosteroids [71]. Based on their description, these vascular tumors were likely KHE with KMP. However, cases of irreversible spastic diplegia were reported in a significant minority of those treated. Side effects also included lethargy and flu-like symptoms. Because of potential neurotoxicity (especially in younger infants) [30, 72], interferon alpha should only be considered in life-threatening lesions refractory to first-line agents.

Propranolol

Propranolol has demonstrated impressive efficacy to induce a more rapid regression of classic infantile hemangiomas. Although many have trialed propranolol for the treatment of KHE with KMP, it has not demonstrated a consistent response pattern and, at best, could be considered a second-line intervention if a lesion is refractory to first-line agents [73, 74].

Interventional Embolization

Large vessel embolization may be considered as a therapeutic option in cases of bulky KHE with radiologic evidence of larger feeding vessels [75]. The procedure often results in a temporary inhibition of KMP and often requires multiple sequential procedures to sustain efficacy [32]. Vessel embolization should be considered as an adjunctive therapy to first-line pharmacotherapy in life-threatening lesions on a case-by-case basis. The interventional procedure is technically challenging, especially when only small feeder vessels are present, and may result in a number of complications including unintended thrombosis and long-term structural and functional defects [32].

Radiation

Although low-dose radiation therapy may disrupt KMP and reduce KHE tumor expansion, well-established risks of secondary malignancy, neuroendocrine dysfunction, and growth delay contraindicate its use as standard therapy in infants and children. Its use should only be considered in refractory, life-threatening KHE with KMP [76, 77].

Clinical Care Summary (KHE with KMP)

Astute recognition of a KHE lesion is required to quickly evaluate and diagnose life-threatening KMP. Upon first suspicion of the diagnosis, it is appropriate to recommend initiating therapy with systemic corticosteroids. As additional laboratory studies, patient history, and more thorough physical exam are obtained, the medical team should decide to either place a central venous catheter and initiate weekly vincristine or initiate oral sirolimus as first-line therapy [43]. The choice between agents should be individualized based on the patient's clinical condition, specifically their risk for catastrophic hemorrhage and family preferences.

When corticosteroids are used, they should be weaned relatively quickly once the patient demonstrates a good clinical response or after 2 weeks if there is not a demonstrable clinical response. Additional vincristine is often administered past hematologic recovery (typically for a total of 20–24 weeks), so long as the patient continues to demonstrate marked improvement on therapy and minimal therapy-related toxicity. Additional sirolimus is also often administered past hematology recovery (potentially for 1–2 years), so long as the patient continues to demonstrate marked improvement on therapy and minimal therapy-related toxicity. Long-term follow-up studies have demonstrated a significant number of children who remain on sirolimus therapy at 4–5 years of age and have identified a risk of recurrence when therapy is weaned off early [78].

Lesions that are refractory to first-line therapy and continue to demonstrate life-threatening features should proceed to second-line interventions including additional pharmacotherapy and consultation for possible surgical or interventional procedures. If dual or multi-agent pharmacotherapy fails to correct hematologic parameters, surgical excision and/or embolization of feeder vessels may provide additional time for pharmacotherapy to be effective. Close multidisciplinary collaboration, specifically between the hematologist/oncologist, dermatologist, general surgeon, and interventional radiologist, is essential to providing comprehensive and efficient therapy for a KHE with KMP.

KHE Patients Without Kasabach-Merritt Phenomenon

The diagnosis of KHE without Kasabach-Merritt phenomenon is often challenging given the broad differential diagnosis for localized vascular anomalies of infancy and childhood. Tissue biopsy is recommended to confirm histologic and immunohistologic diagnosis and, more specifically, to exclude malignant neoplasms such as fibrosarcoma. It remains difficult to propose a standardized treatment approach as current literature on these lesions is limited to small case series and case reports. However, generalized guidelines that outline the therapeutic approach can be proposed based on available clinical experience and recently published expert consensus opinion [43].

Close clinical observation without intervention remains an option for small, localized lesions that neither impair surrounding structure or function. However, if the lesion negatively influences its surroundings, intervention is often necessary. If the KHE is well demarcated and located in an area with an easy surgical approach, complete excisional biopsy may be a more reasonable therapeutic option in the patient without KMP. If the lesion is more invasive crossing tissue planes, surgical excision is less feasible, and pharmacotherapy can be initiated with either corticosteroid monotherapy (oral prednisone 2 mg/kg per day) or sirolimus monotherapy [43, 79, 80]. The use of aspirin (5 to 10 mg/kg/day) or other antiplatelet agents may be considered as adjunctive therapy. The duration of pharmacotherapy should be individualized, and the goals of therapy remain to reduce functional and structural morbidity from the invasive, infiltrating tumor and to reduce long-term morbidity from a variety of less critical factors including pain and aesthetics.

Conclusion

The diagnosis and treatment of KHE patients with KMP has improved dramatically, thanks to a better-defined classification of vascular anomalies, better understanding of the pathophysiology of disease, and the expanded use of novel pharmacotherapeutic agents. Treatment options continue to evolve, making it imperative that treating physicians keep abreast of new and recent developments. Few studies have documented long-term outcome data though it is logical that early recognition of KHE and intervention could minimize long-term sequelae. The mortality rate for KMP is still reported as 10–30% based on limited epidemiologic studies carried out over a decade ago, but with current treatment modalities and multidisciplinary care, it is far lower [81]. The majority of patients demonstrate benefit from multimodal therapy and have long-term remission from their coagulopathy, as well as improved tumor size and appearance. However, evidence of persistent tumor is a likely outcome in larger lesions [17]. Those that infiltrate muscle, bone, and joints can impact long-term musculoskeletal mobility and result in chronic pain and lymphedema. There is a need for multi-institutional collaborative studies to improve clinical outcomes and better investigate the basic pathophysiology of KHE [82].

References

1. Enjolras O, Wassef M, Mazoyer E, Frieden IJ, Rieu PN, Drouet L, et al. Infants with Kasabach-Merritt syndrome do not have "true" hemangiomas. J Pediatr. 1997;130(4):631–40.
2. Lyons LL, North PE, Mac-Moune Lai F, Stoler MH, Folpe AL, Weiss SW. Kaposiform hemangioendothelioma: a study of 33 cases emphasizing its pathologic, immunophenotypic, and biologic uniqueness from juvenile hemangioma. Am J Surg Pathol. 2004;28(5):559–68.
3. Niedt GW, Greco MA, Wieczorek R, Blanc WA, Knowles DM 2nd. Hemangioma with Kaposi's sarcoma-like features: report of two cases. Pediatr Pathol. 1989;9(5):567–75.
4. Tsang WY, Chan JK. Kaposi-like infantile hemangioendothelioma. A distinctive vascular neoplasm of the retroperitoneum. Am J Surg Pathol. 1991;15(10):982–9.
5. Zukerberg LR, Nickoloff BJ, Weiss SW. Kaposiform hemangioendothelioma of infancy and childhood. An aggressive neoplasm associated with Kasabach-Merritt syndrome and lymphangiomatosis. Am J Surg Pathol. 1993;17(4):321–8.
6. Akbayrak T, Orhan C, Baran E, Kaya S, Coskun G, Varan A. Effects of physiotherapy combined with sirolimus in a patient with vascular malformation: a case report. Turk J Pediatr. 2016;58(2):203–7.
7. Lim YH, Bacchiocchi A, Qiu J, Straub R, Bruckner A, Bercovitch L, et al. GNA14 somatic mutation causes congenital and sporadic vascular tumors by MAPK activation. Am J Hum Genet. 2016;99(2):443–50.
8. Croteau SE, Liang MG, Kozakewich HP, Alomari AI, Fishman SJ, Mulliken JB, et al. Kaposiform hemangioendothelioma: atypical features and risks of Kasabach-Merritt phenomenon in 107 referrals. J Pediatr. 2013;162(1):142–7.
9. Kelly M. Kasabach-Merritt phenomenon. Pediatr Clin N Am. 2010;57(5):1085–9.
10. Mulliken JB, Anupindi S, Ezekowitz RA, Mihm MC Jr. Case records of the Massachusetts General Hospital. Weekly clinicopathological exercises. Case 13-2004. A newborn girl with a large cutaneous lesion, thrombocytopenia, and anemia. N Engl J Med. 2004;350(17):1764–75.

11. Gruman A, Liang MG, Mulliken JB, Fishman SJ, Burrows PE, Kozakewich HP, et al. Kaposiform hemangioendothelioma without Kasabach-Merritt phenomenon. J Am Acad Dermatol. 2005;52(4):616–22.
12. Adams D, Frieden IJ. Tufted angioma, kaposiform hemangioendothelioma, and the Kasabach-Merritt phenomenon. Up ToDate, Post TW (Ed), Up ToDate, Waltham, MA (Accessed on December 3, 2015). 2015.
13. Fernandez Y, Bernabeu-Wittel M, Garcia-Morillo JS. Kaposiform hemangioendothelioma. Eur J Intern Med. 2009;20(2):106–13.
14. Veening MA, Verbeke JI, Witbreuk MM, Kaspers GJ. Kaposiform (spindle cell) hemangioendothelioma in a child with an unusual presentation. J Pediatr Hematol Oncol. 2010;32(3):240–2.
15. Deraedt K, Vander Poorten V, Van Geet C, Renard M, De Wever I, Sciot R. Multifocal kaposiform hemangioendothelioma. Virchows Arch. 2006;448(6):843–6.
16. Ma J, Shi QL, Jiang SJ, Zhou HB, Zhou XJ. Primary kaposiform hemangioendothelioma of a long bone: two cases in unusual locations with long-term follow up. Pathol Int. 2011;61(6):382–6.
17. Enjolras O, Mulliken JB, Wassef M, Frieden IJ, Rieu PN, Burrows PE, et al. Residual lesions after Kasabach-Merritt phenomenon in 41 patients. J Am Acad Dermatol. 2000;42(2 Pt 1):225–35.
18. Schaefer BA, Wang D, Merrow AC, Dickie BH, Adams DM. Long-term outcome for kaposiform hemangioendothelioma: a report of two cases. Pediatr Blood Cancer. 2017;64(2):284–6.
19. Le Huu AR, Jokinen CH, Rubin BP, Mihm MC, Weiss SW, North PE, et al. Expression of prox1, lymphatic endothelial nuclear transcription factor, in Kaposiform hemangioendothelioma and tufted angioma. Am J Surg Pathol. 2010;34(11):1563–73.
20. Yuan SM, Hong ZJ, Chen HN, Shen WM, Zhou XJ. Kaposiform hemangioendothelioma complicated by Kasabach-Merritt phenomenon: ultrastructural observation and immunohistochemistry staining reveal the trapping of blood components. Ultrastruct Pathol. 2013;37(6):452–5.
21. Seo SK, Suh JC, Na GY, Kim IS, Sohn KR. Kasabach-Merritt syndrome: identification of platelet trapping in a tufted angioma by immunohistochemistry technique using monoclonal antibody to CD61. Pediatr Dermatol. 1999;16(5):392–4.
22. Saito M, Gunji Y, Kashii Y, Odaka J, Yamauchi T, Kanai N, et al. Refractory kaposiform hemangioendothelioma that expressed vascular endothelial growth factor receptor (VEGFR)-2 and VEGFR-3: a case report. J Pediatr Hematol Oncol. 2009;31(3):194–7.
23. Debelenko LV, Perez-Atayde AR, Mulliken JB, Liang MG, Archibald TH, Kozakewich HP. D2-40 immunohistochemical analysis of pediatric vascular tumors reveals positivity in kaposiform hemangioendothelioma. Mod Pathol. 2005;18(11):1454–60.
24. Arai E, Kuramochi A, Tsuchida T, Tsuneyoshi M, Kage M, Fukunaga M, et al. Usefulness of D2-40 immunohistochemistry for differentiation between kaposiform hemangioendothelioma and tufted angioma. J Cutan Pathol. 2006;33(7):492–7.
25. Jones EW, Orkin M. Tufted angioma (angioblastoma). A benign progressive angioma, not to be confused with Kaposi's sarcoma or low-grade angiosarcoma. J Am Acad Dermatol. 1989;20(2 Pt 1):214–25.
26. Chu CY, Hsiao CH, Chiu HC. Transformation between Kaposiform hemangioendothelioma and tufted angioma. Dermatology. 2003;206(4):334–7.
27. Croteau SE, Gupta D. The clinical spectrum of kaposiform hemangioendothelioma and tufted angioma. Semin Cutan Med Surg. 2016;35(3):147–52.
28. Kasabach HHMK. Capillary hemangioma with extensive purpura: report of a case. Am J Dis Child. 1940;59:1063.
29. Sarkar M, Mulliken JB, Kozakewich HP, Robertson RL, Burrows PE. Thrombocytopenic coagulopathy (Kasabach-Merritt phenomenon) is associated with Kaposiform hemangioendothelioma and not with common infantile hemangioma. Plast Reconstr Surg. 1997;100(6):1377–86.
30. Rodriguez V, Lee A, Witman PM, Anderson PA. Kasabach-Merritt phenomenon: case series and retrospective review of the mayo clinic experience. J Pediatr Hematol Oncol. 2009;31(7):522–6.

31. Sondel PM, Ritter MW, Wilson DG, Lieberman LM. Use of 111In platelet scans in the detection and treatment of Kasabach-Merritt syndrome. J Pediatr. 1984;104(1):87–9.
32. Ryan C, Price V, John P, Mahant S, Baruchel S, Brandao L, et al. Kasabach-Merritt phenomenon: a single centre experience. Eur J Haematol. 2010;84(2):97–104.
33. Dompmartin A, Acher A, Thibon P, Tourbach S, Hermans C, Deneys V, et al. Association of localized intravascular coagulopathy with venous malformations. Arch Dermatol. 2008;144(7):873–7.
34. Frieden IJ, Rogers M, Garzon MC. Conditions masquerading as infantile haemangioma: part 1. Australas J Dermatol. 2009;50(2):77–97.. quiz 8
35. Frieden IJ, Rogers M, Garzon MC. Conditions masquerading as infantile haemangioma: part 2. Australas J Dermatol. 2009;50(3):153–68.. quiz 69-70
36. Rangwala S, Wysong A, Tollefson MM, Khuu P, Benjamin LT, Bruckner AL. Rapidly involuting congenital hemangioma associated with profound, transient thrombocytopenia. Pediatr Dermatol. 2014;31(3):402–4.
37. Ayturk UM, Couto JA, Hann S, Mulliken JB, Williams KL, Huang AY, et al. Somatic activating mutations in GNAQ and GNA11 are associated with congenital hemangioma. Am J Hum Genet. 2016;98(6):1271.
38. Croteau SE, Kozakewich HP, Perez-Atayde AR, Fishman SJ, Alomari AI, Chaudry G, et al. Kaposiform lymphangiomatosis: a distinct aggressive lymphatic anomaly. J Pediatr. 2014;164(2):383–8.
39. Fernandez-Pineda I, Parida L, Jenkins JJ, Davidoff AM, Rao BN, Rodriguez-Galindo C. Childhood hemangiopericytoma: review of St Jude Children's Research Hospital. J Pediatr Hematol Oncol. 2011;33(5):356–9.
40. Shulkin BL, Argenta LC, Cho KJ, Castle VP. Kasabach-Merritt syndrome: treatment with epsilon-aminocaproic acid and assessment by indium 111 platelet scintigraphy. J Pediatr. 1990;117(5):746–9.
41. Phillips WG, Marsden JR. Kasabach-Merritt syndrome exacerbated by platelet transfusion. J R Soc Med. 1993;86(4):231–2.
42. Janic D, Brasanac D, Krstovski N, Dokmanovic L, Lazic J, Krstic Z. The use of recombinant activated factor VII during major surgery in a child with Kasabach-Merritt syndrome. Paediatr Anaesth. 2009;19(2):177–9.
43. Drolet BA, Trenor CC 3rd, Brandao LR, Chiu YE, Chun RH, Dasgupta R, et al. Consensus-derived practice standards plan for complicated Kaposiform hemangioendothelioma. J Pediatr. 2013;163(1):285–91.
44. Guo X, Gong Y, Dong C. Surgical treatment of a huge kaposiform hemangioendothelioma in the chest wall: A case study. SAGE Open Med Case Rep. 2016;4:2050313X16684742.
45. Drolet BA, Scott LA, Esterly NB, Gosain AK. Early surgical intervention in a patient with Kasabach-Merritt phenomenon. J Pediatr. 2001;138(5):756–8.
46. Schmid I, Klenk AK, Sparber-Sauer M, Koscielniak E, Maxwell R, Haberle B. Kaposiform hemangioendothelioma in children: a benign vascular tumor with multiple treatment options. World J Pediatr. 2018;14:322.
47. Wang Z, Li K, Yao W, Dong K, Xiao X, Zheng S. Steroid-resistant kaposiform hemangioendothelioma: a retrospective study of 37 patients treated with vincristine and long-term follow-up. Pediatr Blood Cancer. 2015;62(4):577–80.
48. Ozsoylu S. Megadose methylprednisolone for Kasabach-Merritt syndrome. Eur J Pediatr. 2003;162(7–8):562.. author reply 3–4
49. Haisley-Royster C, Enjolras O, Frieden IJ, Garzon M, Lee M, Oranje A, et al. Kasabach-Merritt phenomenon: a retrospective study of treatment with vincristine. J Pediatr Hematol Oncol. 2002;24(6):459–62.
50. Fahrtash F, McCahon E, Arbuckle S. Successful treatment of kaposiform hemangioendothelioma and tufted angioma with vincristine. J Pediatr Hematol Oncol. 2010;32(6):506–10.
51. Fernandez-Pineda I, Lopez-Gutierrez JC, Ramirez G, Marquez C. Vincristine-ticlopidine-aspirin: an effective therapy in children with Kasabach-Merritt phenomenon associated with vascular tumors. Pediatr Hematol Oncol. 2010;27(8):641–5.

52. Kai L, Wang Z, Yao W, Dong K, Xiao X. Sirolimus, a promising treatment for refractory Kaposiform hemangioendothelioma. J Cancer Res Clin Oncol. 2014;140(3):471–6.
53. Jahnel J, Lackner H, Reiterer F, Urlesberger B, Urban C. Kaposiform hemangioendothelioma with Kasabach-Merritt phenomenon: from vincristine to sirolimus. Klin Padiatr. 2012;224(6):395–7.
54. Wang H, Guo X, Duan Y, Zheng B, Gao Y. Sirolimus as initial therapy for kaposiform hemangioendothelioma and tufted angioma. Pediatr Dermatol. 2018;35(5):635–8.
55. Hammill AM, Wentzel M, Gupta A, Nelson S, Lucky A, Elluru R, et al. Sirolimus for the treatment of complicated vascular anomalies in children. Pediatr Blood Cancer. 2011;57(6):1018–24.
56. Ji Y, Chen S, Xiang B, Li K, Xu Z, Yao W, et al. Sirolimus for the treatment of progressive kaposiform hemangioendothelioma: a multicenter retrospective study. Int J Cancer. 2017;141(4):848–55.
57. Emoto C, Fukuda T, Mizuno T, Schniedewind B, Christians U, Adams DM, et al. Characterizing the developmental trajectory of Sirolimus clearance in neonates and infants. CPT Pharmacometrics Syst Pharmacol. 2016;5(8):411–7.
58. Czechowicz JA, Long-Boyle JR, Rosbe KW, Mathes EF, Frieden IJ, Shimano KA. Sirolimus for management of complex vascular anomalies – a proposed dosing regimen for very young infants. Int J Pediatr Otorhinolaryngol. 2018;105:48–51.
59. Adams DM, Trenor CC 3rd, Hammill AM, Vinks AA, Patel MN, Chaudry G, et al. Efficacy and safety of Sirolimus in the treatment of complicated vascular anomalies. Pediatrics. 2016;137(2):e20153257.
60. Russell TB, Rinker EK, Dillingham CS, Givner LB, McLean TW. *Pneumocystis Jirovecii* pneumonia during Sirolimus therapy for Kaposiform Hemangioendothelioma. Pediatrics. 2018;141(Suppl 5):S421–S4.
61. McCormack FX, Inoue Y, Moss J, Singer LG, Strange C, Nakata K, et al. Efficacy and safety of sirolimus in lymphangioleiomyomatosis. N Engl J Med. 2011;364(17):1595–606.
62. Blatt J, Stavas J, Moats-Staats B, Woosley J, Morrell DS. Treatment of childhood kaposiform hemangioendothelioma with sirolimus. Pediatr Blood Cancer. 2010;55(7):1396–8.
63. Wong MK, Yang H, Signorovitch JE, Wang X, Liu Z, Liu NS, et al. Comparative outcomes of everolimus, temsirolimus and sorafenib as second targeted therapies for metastatic renal cell carcinoma: a US medical record review. Curr Med Res Opin. 2014;30(4):537–45.
64. Hauer J, Graubner U, Konstantopoulos N, Schmidt S, Pfluger T, Schmid I. Effective treatment of kaposiform hemangioendotheliomas associated with Kasabach-Merritt phenomenon using four-drug regimen. Pediatr Blood Cancer. 2007;49(6):852–4.
65. Blei F, Karp N, Rofsky N, Rosen R, Greco MA. Successful multimodal therapy for kaposiform hemangioendothelioma complicated by Kasabach-Merritt phenomenon: case report and review of the literature. Pediatr Hematol Oncol. 1998;15(4):295–305.
66. Fuchimoto Y, Morikawa N, Kuroda T, Hirobe S, Kamagata S, Kumagai M, et al. Vincristine, actinomycin D, cyclophosphamide chemotherapy resolves Kasabach-Merritt syndrome resistant to conventional therapies. Pediatr Int. 2012;54(2):285–7.
67. Ortel TL, Onorato JJ, Bedrosian CL, Kaufman RE. Antifibrinolytic therapy in the management of the Kasabach Merritt syndrome. Am J Hematol. 1988;29(1):44–8.
68. Javvaji S, Frieden IJ. Response of tufted angiomas to low-dose aspirin. Pediatr Dermatol. 2013;30(1):124–7.
69. MacFarland SP, Sullivan LM, States LJ, Bailey LC, Balamuth NJ, Womer RB, et al. Management of refractory pediatric Kaposiform Hemangioendothelioma with Sirolimus and aspirin. J Pediatr Hematol Oncol. 2018;40(4):e239–e42.
70. Fernandez-Pineda I, Lopez-Gutierrez JC, Chocarro G, Bernabeu-Wittel J, Ramirez-Villar GL. Long-term outcome of vincristine-aspirin-ticlopidine (VAT) therapy for vascular tumors associated with Kasabach-Merritt phenomenon. Pediatr Blood Cancer. 2013;60(9):1478–81.
71. Ezekowitz RA, Mulliken JB, Folkman J. Interferon alfa-2a therapy for life-threatening hemangiomas of infancy. N Engl J Med. 1992;326(22):1456–63.

72. Barlow CF, Priebe CJ, Mulliken JB, Barnes PD, Mac Donald D, Folkman J, et al. Spastic diplegia as a complication of interferon alfa-2a treatment of hemangiomas of infancy. J Pediatr. 1998;132(3 Pt 1):527–30.
73. Chiu YE, Drolet BA, Blei F, Carcao M, Fangusaro J, Kelly ME, et al. Variable response to propranolol treatment of kaposiform hemangioendothelioma, tufted angioma, and Kasabach-Merritt phenomenon. Pediatr Blood Cancer. 2012;59(5):934–8.
74. Wang Z, Li K, Dong K, Xiao X, Zheng S. Variable response to propranolol treatment of kaposiform hemangioendothelioma, tufted angioma, and Kasabach-Merritt phenomenon. Pediatr Blood Cancer. 2014;61(8):1518–9.
75. Zhou SY, Li HB, Mao YM, Liu PY, Zhang J. Successful treatment of Kasabach-Merritt syndrome with transarterial embolization and corticosteroids. J Pediatr Surg. 2013;48(3):673–6.
76. Leong E, Bydder S. Use of radiotherapy to treat life-threatening Kasabach-Merritt syndrome. J Med Imaging Radiat Oncol. 2009;53(1):87–91.
77. Kwok-Williams M, Perez Z, Squire R, Glaser A, Bew S, Taylor R. Radiotherapy for life-threatening mediastinal hemangioma with Kasabach-Merritt syndrome. Pediatr Blood Cancer. 2007;49(5):739–44.
78. Adams DM, Trenor III C, Ricci K, Patel M, Chaudry G, Mobberley-Schuman P, Klajn J, Gupta A, Chute C, Merrow A, Dasgupta R, Dickie B, Hammill AM. Phase II Study of Sirolimus and complicated vascular Anomalies: Long term outcomes in Kaposiform Hemangioendothelioma [abstract]. International Society for the Study of vascular anomalies; June 1, 2018; Amsterdam, Netherlands.
79. Patel S, Kamath S, Shillingford NM, Zeinati C, Tolo V, Luu M. Restricted range of motion and a cold upper extremity in a two-year-old boy: Kaposiform Hemangioendothelioma of the bone and the brachial plexus: a case report. JBJS Case Connect. 2017;7(4):e79.
80. Oza VS, Mamlouk MD, Hess CP, Mathes EF, Frieden IJ. Role of Sirolimus in advanced Kaposiform Hemangioendothelioma. Pediatr Dermatol. 2016;33(2):e88–92.
81. Wong BL, Lee VN, Tikka T, Kim D, Dwivedi RC. Kaposiform hemangioendothelioma of the head and neck. Crit Rev Oncol Hematol. 2016;104:156–68.
82. Adams DM, Hammill AM, Mobberley-Schuman PS, Trenor CC 3rd. Comment on: steroid-resistant kaposiform hemangioendothelioma: a retrospective study of 37 patients treated with vincristine and long-term follow-up. Pediatr Blood Cancer. 2015;62(11):2056.

Rare Vascular Tumors

7

Roshni Dasgupta, Ionela Iacobas, and Kristen Snyder

Introduction

Vascular tumors are rare in both children and adults. The relative paucity of cases, diverse phenotypes, and heterogeneous clinical outcomes of these tumors has made their classification difficult. In 2013, The World Health Organization (WHO) updated the classification of soft tissue vascular tumors [1]. Pediatric tumors were not independently classified, but an intermediate category of tumors was created and subsequently further divided into locally aggressive and rarely metastasizing tumors. The International Society for the Study of Vascular Anomalies (ISSVA) created a classification system of vascular anomalies at the 1996 meeting in Rome. This schema divided vascular anomalies into tumors and malformations and provided the framework for great strides in research and treatment in the field. The classification system was expanded at the 2014 ISSVA workshop in Melbourne [2] and updated again in 2018 in Amsterdam (ISSVA Classification of Vascular Anomalies ©2018 International Society for the Study of Vascular Anomalies) is available at "issva.org/classification" accessed [August 21, 2018]).

These revisions were essential to fully encompass further advances in knowledge and understanding in the field. Vascular anomalies continue to be classified as

R. Dasgupta (✉)
Division of Pediatric General and Thoracic Surgery, Cincinnati Children's Hospital Medical Center, Hemangioma and Vascular Malformation Center, Cincinnati, OH, USA
e-mail: roshni.dasgupta@cchmc.org

I. Iacobas
Pediatric Cancer and Hematology Centers, Texas Children's Hospital/Baylor College of Medicine, Houston, TX, USA

K. Snyder
Cancer Center, Children's Hospital of Philadelphia, Philadelphia, PA, USA

C. C. Trenor III, D. M. Adams (eds.), *Vascular Anomalies*,
https://doi.org/10.1007/978-3-030-25624-1_7

tumors and malformations. Vascular tumors are classified into benign, locally aggressive or borderline, and malignant entities.

Benign Tumors

Epithelioid Hemangioma

Epithelioid hemangiomas (EH) were first described by Wells and Whimster in 1969 [3]. EH is a very rare lesion and represents less than 1% of all vascular tumors. EH are benign lesions that usually occur in the skin and subcutaneous tissues. They may also occur in other regions such as bone and can often mimic malignant neoplasms [4, 5]. EH should not be confused with epithelioid hemangioendothelioma or epithelioid angiosarcoma, which are much more aggressive lesions. Clinically, EH appear as erythematous cysts or plaques and can present with local ulceration and pain. They are often mistaken for hemangiomas or pyogenic granulomas. EH may be a reactive process and have been associated with trauma, infections, or hyperestrogen states. They can involve the metaphysis and diaphysis of long bones, may be unifocal or multicentric, and may cause fracture secondary to lytic lesions [4, 6].

Histologically, EH are well-defined proliferations of capillaries surrounding a larger central vessel. The proliferation is generally due to an inflammatory infiltrate of lymphocytes. Solid portions of EH can also be present, which is atypical and may complicate the diagnosis. Tumor cells are positive for endothelial and lymphatic markers including CD31, ERG, and D2–40 and negative for cytokeratin and CAMTA1. However, lesions lack well-formed vascular channels and do not possess any cytologic atypia or mitotic activity [7]. Primary treatment of these lesions is surgical excision. Curettage and sclerotherapy have also been described. EH often recur locally, but do not have a history of distant spread and can be re-resected if necessary [5].

A recent review found that in pediatric cases there was a higher incidence of multifocal disease compared to adults (45%) and a higher recurrence rate (43% compared to 8–24% in adults) [8].

EH can present as focal or multifocal disease. When EH presents as multifocal disease, or in areas where surgical resection is not an option such as multifocal bone or hepatic lesions, medical therapy with anti-angiogenic agents may stabilize the disease and delay the destructive process. Sirolimus and interferon have both been used in patients ineligible for surgical resection with good long-term results [8]. A few patients with EH were noted to have FOS rearrangements, and targeted therapy with FOS inhibitors may bring better solutions for these patients in the near future [9].

Pyogenic Granuloma

Pyogenic granuloma (PG), also known as "lobular capillary hemangioma" is a benign reactive lesion that predominantly affects children and young adults [10]. This tumor is found between 0.5% and 1% of children typically presenting after 4 months of age. These lesions can arise spontaneously or in sites of trauma, eczema, bug bites, and burns or within capillary malformations [11]. Pyogenic granulomas have also been associated with the use of retinoic acid compounds and contraceptives. They are characterized by erythematous vascular papules generally found on the head and neck but can also be found throughout the body.

PG can range in size from 1 millimeter to several centimeters. These lesions appear as small or large, smooth, or lobulated vascular nodules that can grow rapidly, sometimes over weeks to months, and have a tendency to bleed profusely with even minor trauma [12]. The pathophysiology of PG is not completely understood. However, it is thought to be secondary to reactive neovascularization. Microscopically, there is a proliferation of lobules of capillary vessels with fibromyxoid stroma; the surface epithelium is frequently attenuated. Ulceration and neutrophilic infiltration is often seen [13].

Some untreated lesions eventually atrophy, become fibromatous, and slowly regress. However, the vast majority of lesions require medical attention primarily because of recurrent bleeding. Localized treatment for smaller PG (less than 0.5 cm) can include cryotherapy and chemical coagulation such as silver nitrate or laser treatment [14, 15]. For lesions larger than 0.5 cm, full thickness excision to subcutaneous tissue is often required. Unfortunately, recurrences of PG are quite common. [13] Topical imiquimod may help prevent recurrence but prolonged treatment may cause irritation particularly in facial lesions [16]. There is also a report of lesion resolution in over half of patients after use of topical 1% propranolol ointment [17] Somatic activating RAS mutations have been found in Pyogenic granulomas and may lead additional therapies in the future [18].

Locally Aggressive Rare Vascular Tumors

Retiform Hemangioendothelioma

Retiform hemangioendothelioma (RH) was initially reported in 1994 by Calonje who described 15 patients with a type of low-grade angiosarcoma [19]. This tumor has been entered in the WHO reclassification as an intermediate (rarely metastasizing) vascular tumor [20]. These tumors generally have been described in young adults in the upper and lower extremities. Phenotypically they appear as a slow-growing solitary mass with a plaque-like appearance or as a subcutaneous firm nodule [21].

Pathologically, RHE involves the entire thickness of dermis and often extends into the subcutaneous tissue. Hyperchromatic hobnail endothelial cells are a common finding. Mitotic figures are rare. The vessels are elongated and arranged in a pattern which resembles the rete testis. The hobnail cells express endothelial markers including von Willebrand factor, CD31, and CD34 [22]. It is unclear whether these tumors express lymphatic endothelial markers, as conflicting reports have been found for podoplanin and other lymphatic marker expressions [23, 24]. Treatment consists of surgical excision with adequate margins and lymph node sampling (preferably by a sentinel lymph node technique). In the reported cases, local recurrence appears to be common [21]. Reports note two of 15 patients with regional lymph node metastases without any deaths due to distant disease [25]. Long-term monitoring for local recurrence is recommended.

Papillary Intralymphatic Angioendothelioma

Papillary intralymphatic angioendothelioma (PILA) also known as Dabska tumor was first described by Maria Dabska in 1969 when she reported six patients with a locally aggressive hemangioendothelioma [26]. These lesions originate within the dermis and superficial soft tissues of trunk, head and neck, or extremities. They have also been reported to arise from a pre-existing lymphatic or venolymphatic malformation and in patients with lymphedema [27]. Clinically, they appear as violaceous nodules that may be raised. They share a similar appearance to the retiform hemangioendothelioma both clinically and pathologically.

Histologically, under low power they are similar to a lymphatic malformation with large lymphatic channels and aggregates. The vessels are lined by hobnail endothelial cells which are pathognomonic of this tumor [28]. Intravascular endothelial tufts are also noted within the tumor. The endothelial cells also express von Willebrand factor, CD31, and CD34. Lymphatic markers, VEGFR3 and podoplanin, are also expressed with minimal cytologic atypia. As all tumors described showed papillary intravascular proliferation and evidence of lymphatic vessels, they were given the name PILA [29].

Wide surgical excision with lymph node sampling (using a sentinel lymph node technique) is recommended. PILA is known to spread to local regional nodes, and distant spread is uncommon [30]. However, in two cases in the original series it metastasized and caused death. Systemic chemotherapy, if required, should incorporate sarcoma-based therapies [29]. Long-term surveillance for local recurrence and distant spread is recommended.

Composite Hemangioendothelioma

Composite hemangioendothelioma (CHE) was first described in 2000 as a subset of superficial dermal and subcutaneous hemangioendothelioma tumors containing overlapping histologies: epithelioid, retiform, and spindle cell hemangioendotheliomas as well as angiosarcoma-like areas within a single tumor [31] with areas of vacuolated endothelial cells, and other vascular lesions although no lesion contains all subtypes. The definition of composite HE was redefined by the WHO in 2013 as "locally aggressive, rarely metastasizing vascular neoplasm, containing an admixture of histologically distinct components." Importantly, small biopsies of these lesions are unlikely to sample these numerous lesional components and thus may limit accuracy of diagnosis.

To date, less than 40 cases have been reported in the literature [32]. Cases have been reported from infancy to late adulthood and may be associated with other vascular anomalies including arteriovenous malformation, lymphangioma malformaitons, and lymphedema [32]. Based on reviews of the literature, most CHE lesions occur on the extremities but have also occurred in the tongue, mandibular vestibule, cheek, hypopharynx, torso, and inguinal lymph nodes. They appear reddish to bluish-purple and plaque-like to nodular ranging in size from 0.7 to 30 cm; median, 3.2 cm. Lesions are most often associated with normal laboratory findings [32–34].

Treatment with local or wide local excision without chemotherapy or radiation is typically curative. Local recurrence has been documented in 11% to 57% of cases in the literature [32, 35] with rare metastases and without tumor-related deaths. Follow-up imaging surveillance with computed tomography or magnetic resonance imaging is recommended.

Malignant Tumors

Epithelioid Hemangioendothelioma

Epithelioid Hemangioendothelioma (EHE) was first described by Weiss and Enzinger in 1982 as a tumor of intermediate malignancy that was often misdiagnosed as a carcinoma [36]. EHE generally occurs in middle-aged adult patients as a solitary mass in the deep soft tissue, viscera, or bone [37]. The WHO classifies this tumor as a variant of angiosarcoma, a locally aggressive tumor with metastatic potential. [38] The estimated prevalence of EHE is less than one in one million. The majority of patients are female with a mean age at diagnosis of 36 years of age [5]. Some epidemiologic studies have linked chronic *Bartonella* infection with development of EHE [5].

The liver appears to be the most common site of EHE presentation, followed by the lung and bone, but has been reported in numerous sites. Thirty percent of soft tissue cases are associated with metastases and when present, it is often difficult to distinguish the primary tumor from metastatic sites. Cutaneous lesions can be raised and nodular and often pigmented a red-brown color [39].

EHE is often diagnosed incidentally and symptoms are specific to the location of the lesion. Hemolytic anemia and a consumptive coagulopathy have been rarely described as presenting signs. MRI imaging for primary site is important for determining the extent of the tumor and determining surgical resectability. Patients presenting with pleural EHE may have lung nodules often within the lower portion of the lungs with hilar nodal enlargement [40]. Surveillance imaging for staging potential metastatic sites should include the liver, bone, and lung. Bony disease is noted as single or multiple lytic lesions on plain films and cross-sectional imaging. Bone metastases involving more than 50% of cortex represent a high risk of pathologic fractures. There is also some early experience using PET scanning for staging of the lesion, and F-fluorodeoxyglucose (FDG) uptake has been used as a means of assessing response [41, 42].

EHE is characterized by the t(1;3)(p36;q23–25) translocation. This translocation fuses the WWTR1 gene in 3q23–24 with the CAMTA1 in 1p36 [43]. This appears to be a unique translocation and can be very helpful for diagnosis. A fusion protein between the Yes-associated protein 1 (YAP1) gene and the transcription factor E3 (TFE3) gene has been discovered [44]. Lee et al. recently documented the co-expression for some of the patients in the series of both TFE3 and CAMTA. Lesions that were TFE3 positive were noted to be a single larger lesion and to have greater nuclear atypia and hypercellularity compared to those that were TFE3 negative [45].

Microscopically EHE are epithelioid lesions arranged in nests or cord-like patterns. Spindle cells may be present as well. Immunohistochemically, these cells express Fli-1 and CD31, and podoplanin is expressed by lymphatic endothelial cells [38]. Cellular atypia, an increased number of spindled cells, and regions of focal necrosis are thought to be associated with a more aggressive course in adults [46].

Treatment is individualized depending on the type of lesion and metastatic pattern at presentation. Aggressive surgical resection is indicated, with wide margins in soft tissue and bone. Regional lymph nodes should also be evaluated as they are the most frequent sites for metastases [21]. Metastases appear to be more common when cytologic atypia is present. Amputation should be considered particularly in lesions that have an aggressive histological appearance [47]. Liver EHE has been treated with aggressive resection and transplantation with good outcomes. For pleural EHE with multiple nodules, it is often difficult to achieve curative margins and generally requires neoadjuvant therapy prior to resection attempts [48].

Radiotherapy may have a role in localized EHE to prevent local recurrence [49]. Most cases will require adjuvant chemotherapeutic regimens. Multiple medications have been utilized including steroids, bevacizumab, paclitaxel, thalidomide, sorafenib, sunitinib [50], and sirolimus [38]. The choice of sirolimus is based on noted activation of the Ras//PI3K/PTEN /mTOR pathwath in other vascular tumors. Twenty-four patients, age 2–26 years, were evaluated in a multi-institutional case series with epithelioid hemangioendothelioma and 3 patients were treated with sirolimus achieving stable disease or partial response for more than 2.5 years [51], there are limited open clinical trials investigating the effect of targeted therapy on EHE. One includes a MEK inhibitor, trametinib, in patients > than 15 years of age with EHE and progressive disease (NCT 03148275).

Data on survival, response and reoccurence is mostly based on adult studies. The mean survival is 4.6 years ranging from 6 months to 24 years. Mortality is site dependent: 13% mortality rate for soft tissue tumors, 35% for liver tumors, and 65% for lung tumors. Overall survival (OS) is 73% at 5 years [52]. However, the OS following progressive disease is only 24% [52]. Long-term surveillance for local and distant recurrence is required for this aggressive lesion [38].

Angiosarcoma

The term "angiosarcoma" unofficially includes two entities: "hemangiosarcoma" (classic angiosarcoma) and "lymphangiosarcoma" (angiosarcoma arising from lymphatic endothelium in an area of chronic lymphedema, described first in 1948) [53]. Lymphangiosarcoma will be discussed separately and has not been acknowledged as a distinct diagnosis either by WHO or by the ICD-10 (US medical coding).

Angiosarcoma represents about 2% of soft tissue sarcomas [54], with 600 cases diagnosed in the United States per year, approximately 2 cases per million. It mostly affects elderly adults, and it has been described very rarely in children. Reports of its association to the vinyl chloride exposure [55] and previous radiation [56] have been published.

In adults, the most common location of presentation is the head and neck (sun-exposed areas) or the breast following irradiation for breast cancer, but it may arise in any location. In children, angiosarcomas may have a cutaneous localization or may develop in the deep tissue or viscera. For the cutaneous lesions, there appears to be a significant correlation with pre-existing conditions affecting the same area as the tumor [57], such as xeroderma pigmentosum [58–61] or a previous history of local radiation for another primary tumor. Even though radiotherapy is standard of care for a multitude of primary malignancies, radiation-induced angiosarcoma after irradiation of the breasts for carcinoma dominates the medical literature [62] with only sparse reports in other locations. Furthermore, it was noted that c-myc amplification is a specific marker for radiation-induced angiosarcoma of the breast [63, 64] and can be used to differentiate from other atypical vascular lesions arising after radiation for breast cancer [65].

Clinically, angiosarcomas present as a rapidly enlarging purple plaque or nodule that eventually ulcerates and may ooze serosanguinous fluid. Frequently noted are multiple satellite papules or nodules with same characteristics [66].

Ninety-six percent of adult cutaneous angiosarcomas present in the head and neck region, while in children the lower extremities seem to be more commonly affected. In adults, males are the most commonly affected, while in pediatrics, females dominate the number of cases.

Deep angiosarcomas do not appear to have a predilection for a specific location and have been described in the pericardium, the heart, the liver, the spleen, inside of pelvis, etc. Hepatic angiosarcomas will be discussed separately due to their interesting features. Histologically, angiosarcomas manifest some heterogeneity and sometimes offer significant diagnostic challenges to the pathologist. In the classical case, they are composed of racemose and arborizing vessels, exhibiting cytologic atypia with an elevated mitotic index (up to 27 mitotic figures per 10 high power fields in some publications). They may manifest endothelial stratification and while most have an epithelioid morphology (in children), some contain spindle cells.

Immunohistochemically, angiosarcoma stains positive for CD31 and CD34 (endothelial markers) and for *Ulex europaeus* and von Willebrand factor. As approximately 20% of hepatic angiosarcoma is Glut-1 positive and some of the intermediate malignant forms are still labeled as infantile hemangiomas due to this Glut-1 positivity, more studies and consensus among vascular pathology specialists are needed to identify the correct classification and best set of immunostains required for full characterization of these tumors [67].

Necrosis and hemorrhage within the tumor are very common and may affect large portions of the mass. Occasionally, angiosarcoma cells are aneuploid (especially if arising in a cutaneous area post-radiation).

The preferred imaging method is MRI with contrast of the affected area. Full metastatic evaluation including at least pulmonary CT should be obtained at initial presentation and then at reassessment time points due to its high predilection for lung metastases.

In children with hepatic hemangiomas, US with Doppler may be monitored routinely, and if the lesions do not respect the typical clinical course (proliferation, stabilization, involution at the normal age – please see chapter on infantile hemangioma for full details), MRI with contrast should be obtained.

Due to the rapid progression of angiosarcoma with local and metastatic invasion, multiple therapeutic measures are attempted. Surgical complete resection is always considered but rarely possible due to the extent of disease at diagnosis. Amputation of an extremity or complete resection of localized tumor has been described and when combined with intense systemic chemotherapy, appears to have a better outcome.

For the most cases though, after partial resection, chemotherapy with ifosfamide/doxorubicin/vincristine or gemcitabine/docetaxel has been effectively employed (see details in the hepatic angiosarcoma section). Radiotherapy has been indicated, mostly in primary cutaneous angiosarcoma, with limited efficacy.

Molecular studies of angiosarcoma tissue samples proved to have activation of PI3K/mTOR and MAPK pathways. Through mouse models of angiosarcoma exhibiting these activating mutations, it was recently shown that combined treatment with mTOR inhibitors (like sirolimus) and MEK inhibitors (like trametinib) was able to induce significant tumor regression and prevent metastases. Hopefully, in the future, similar treatment schemas may improve prognosis in patients [68].

The prognosis currently is very poor with a progression-free survival of 3–7 months, median overall survival of 14–18 months, and 5-year OS of 20–35% [54]. The numbers vary among publications, but all indicate that angiosarcoma is highly metastatic and very aggressive, with a high mortality rate. Most metastases involve the lungs and liver. Interestingly, when primary and secondary angiosarcomas were compared, the outcome was very similar despite few variations. One would think that secondary angiosarcoma (arising in an area that was previously radiated or in a patient that has received chemotherapy already for another primary malignant process) would be more aggressive, but differences were not statistically significant, making primary angiosarcoma as morbid as secondary [56].

Hepatic Angiosarcoma

Recent case reports of hepatic angiosarcoma diagnosed in early childhood and their interesting features deserve special attention [67].

Patients present most commonly between 1 and 5 years of age (with a median of 3 years). The clinical complaints include abdominal distension, abdominal pain, constipation, vomiting, fever, jaundice, or difficulty of breathing due to large abdominal volume. Frequently a history of cutaneous infantile hemangiomas during infancy with normal involution is obtained [69]. Sometimes, history includes an infantile hepatic hemangioma (IHH) treated with steroids or propranolol for a period of time prior to the diagnosis of angiosarcoma.

Multiple articles describe typical cases of childhood hepatic angiosarcoma coexisting with IHH (previously called hemangioendothelioma type I) [70, 71], and others recapitulate malignant transformation of hemangioma toward angiosarcoma [72]. This observation differentiates the hepatic angiosarcoma presenting in childhood from adult hepatic angiosarcoma, where the coexistence of the two vascular entities (benign and malignant) was never described.

Interestingly, in patients with both cutaneous and hepatic infantile hemangiomas, only the hepatic lesions appear to progress to angiosarcoma, while the cutaneous ones respect the natural history of IH and undergo involution as expected. Also, from the considerably larger number of very aggressive, complicated IHs present in any other location than the liver, none was described to progress to angiosarcoma, suggesting the hepatic environment itself may play a role in the transformation.

Regarding the evaluation and diagnosis of a hepatic angiosarcoma, MRI with contrast by a dynamic protocol to assess filling pattern is the imaging of choice. For any new hepatic tumor, the differential diagnosis includes hepatoblastoma, mesenchymal hamartoma, hepatic hemangioma (either infantile or congenital), focal nodular hyperplasia, hepatic arteriovenous malformation, or secondary metastases. In angiosarcoma, the mass (unique or multifocal) demonstrates hyperintense T2 signal and hypointense T1 signal. It has intense diffusion restriction and heterogenous enhancement throughout suggesting intense vascularity (Fig. 7.1a, b). Intralesional hemorrhage and necrosis are common.

Patients may present with anemia and/or thrombocytopenia due to intralesional bleeding. Alpha-fetoprotein (AFP) is normal or only minimally elevated (differential diagnosis with hepatoblastoma). Liver function tests may be affected, but it is rare that the child presents in full liver failure.

Due to the critical importance of assigning the correct diagnosis, a biopsy will be almost always performed (Fig. 7.1c). This may be a complicated procedure, due to the high vascularity within the lesion and the potential risk of rupture causing intra-abdominal bleeding.

The natural history of a hepatic angiosarcoma is to metastasize quickly (especially to the lungs) Fig. 7.1d. Local invasion is also extremely common with new foci of tumor appearing in the unaffected hepatic lobe.

Whenever possible complete surgical resection of the tumor should be attempted and systemic chemotherapy initiated. Various treatment schemas have been utilized and most frequently reported including ifosfamide/doxorubicin/vincristine or gemcitabine/docetaxel [72]. The former is usually effective in soft tissue sarcomas. Six cycles of every 3-week treatments are recommended with frequent assessments.

Gemcitabine/docetaxel is also effective and it appears to be better tolerated as mostly outpatient therapy. Unfortunately, due to the very limited number of cases, there is no comparative study between the two protocols and the choice of first-line therapy is left to institutional preference.

Frequently, other anti-angiogenic agents are added to the regimen, and bevacizumab, sorafenib, sirolimus, and even propranolol have been tried with varying results. Hepatic angiosarcoma is not eligible for liver transplant in most institutions due to its highly metastatic potential even in patients with localized disease. Complete cure is rare, and chemotherapy and surgical interventions unfortunately only delay the inevitable.

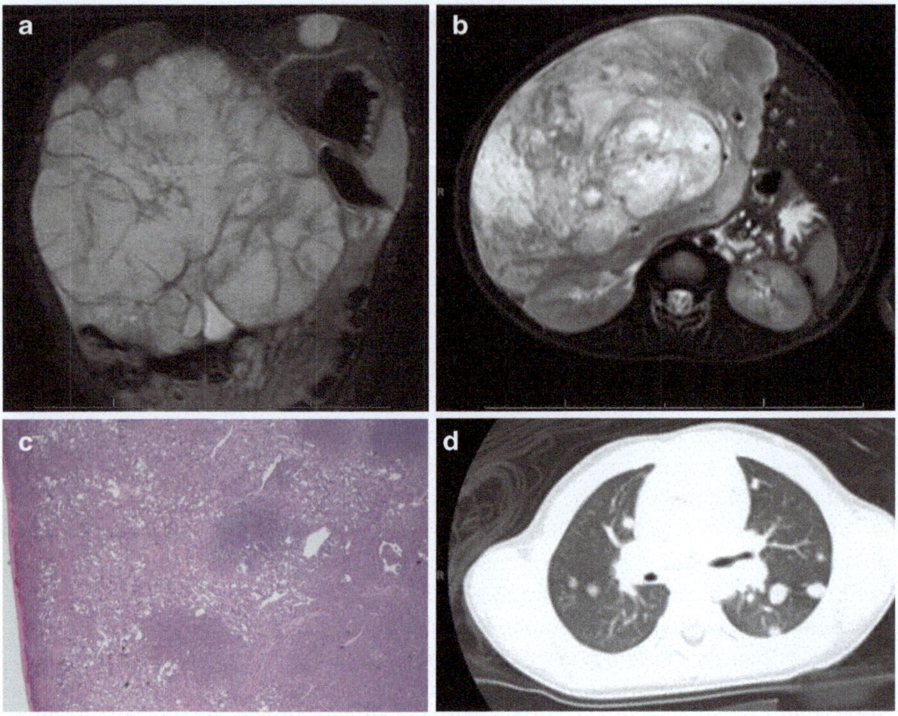

Fig. 7.1 Hepatic angiosarcoma. (**a**) 3 years old female with multifocal hepatic tumors proven to be angiosarcoma. (**b**) 3 years old male with unifocal large hepatic angiosarcoma. (**c**) H&E stain showing low-grade neoplasm alternating with solid, nodular areas highly proliferative. (**d**) Pulmonary metastases at diagnosis for patient b

Due to the above-described correlation between the IHH and the angiosarcoma, in the recently published hepatic hemangioma guidelines for diagnosis and monitoring [73], the consensus paper recommends monitoring a child with infantile liver hemangiomas until the hemangioma involution is complete.

Lymphangiosarcoma

Lymphangiosarcoma as a new entity was first described in patients with upper extremity chronic lymphedema due to breast cancer therapy [53]. The clear relationship with inadequate lymphatic drainage was confirmed by multiple case reports and small case series from the adult literature. Due to the significantly high incidence of breast cancer and resulting lymphedema, secondary lymphangiosarcoma dominates the medical literature with almost none describing primary lesions (without chronic lymphedema [74, 75] or lymphatic malformation present years prior to the malignant transformation). In the pediatric population, breast cancer is very rarely encountered, and the management of other forms of cancer almost never results in lymphedema leaving lymphatic malformations as the major predisposing factor for lymphangiosarcoma.

The clinical presentation of a cutaneous lymphangiosarcoma closely resembles angiosarcoma with one or more reddish-purple indurated areas or nodules that develop chronic ulceration and ooze serosanguinous fluid. Pain is present and sometimes difficult to manage. When the lymphangiosarcoma does not have a cutaneous component but develops in the context of chylothorax or chylous ascites, the diagnosis is even more difficult to make and requires a high index of suspicion [76].

Lymphangiosarcoma histology resembles angiosarcoma with a dissecting growth pattern of atypical vessels lined by epithelioid cells. High mitotic index, necrosis, and hemorrhage are highly prevalent within the tumor. The immunohistochemistry may differentiate the two entities: lymphangiosarcoma is strongly positive for lymphatic markers: Prox-1 and/or podoplanin (D2-40) and less intense or completely negative for CD31 and CD34 (endothelial markers). Mouse model experiments found that constitutive activation of mTORC1 in endothelial cells may lead to the development and progression of lymphangiosarcoma through VEGF signaling [77]. Also, lymphangiosarcoma appears to have the same c-myc amplification identified in post-radiation angiosarcoma of the breast. [64]

Lymphangiosarcoma shares many features with hemangiosarcoma, including imaging characteristics, sarcoma-type attempted treatment, and poor prognosis. As majority of cases affect the extremities, complete surgical resection with amputation is commonly described. Still, due to the high metastatic potential to the liver, lungs, and bones, many cases present with metastases at diagnosis and continue to progress regardless of therapy. Chemotherapy regimens include ifosfamide/doxorubicin, gemcitabine/docetaxel, and multiple targeted anti-angiogenic drugs such sorafenib, sunitinib, bevacizumab, and the mTOR inhibitor sirolimus.

Chronic lymphedema secondary to cancer management is rare in children, but the complex lymphatic malformations where lymphedema, chylothorax, and chylous ascites are part of the condition have started to be recognized earlier especially in the multidisciplinary vascular centers. At least theoretically, if generalized lymphatic anomaly (GLA) is managed carefully from diagnosis in the pediatric years, with medical therapy (like mTOR inhibitors) to reduce the amount of effusions present, compression, and complete decongestive therapy with lymphatic massage, it is hoped that the incidence of lymphangiosarcoma will be reduced [78].

References

1. Fletcher CDM, Bridge JA, Hogendoorn PCW, Mertens F. WHO classification of tumours of soft tissue and bone: IARC Press; 2013.
2. Dasgupta R, Fishman SJ. ISSVA classification. Semin Pediatr Surg. 2014;23(4):158–61.
3. Wells GC, Whimster IW. Subcutaneous angiolymphoid hyperplasia with eosinophilia. Br J Dermatol. 1969;81(1):1–14.
4. Kleck CJ, Seidel MJ. Epithelioid hemangioma of the distal humerus with pathologic fracture. Orthopedics. 2012;35(1):e116–9.
5. Ko JS, Billings SD. Diagnostically challenging epithelioid vascular tumors. Surg Pathol Clin. 2015;8(3):331–51.

6. Schenker K, Blumer S, Jaramillo D, Treece AL, Bhatia A. Epithelioid hemangioma of bone: radiologic and magnetic resonance imaging characteristics with histopathological correlation. Pediatr Radiol. 2017;47(12):1631–7.
7. Fetsch JF, Sesterhenn IA, Miettinen M, Davis CJ Jr. Epithelioid hemangioma of the penis: a clinicopathologic and immunohistochemical analysis of 19 cases, with special reference to exuberant examples often confused with epithelioid hemangioendothelioma and epithelioid angiosarcoma. Am J Surg Pathol. 2004;28(4):523–33.
8. Liu KX, Duggan EM, Al-Ibraheemi A, Shaikh R, Adams DM. Characterization of long-term outcomes for pediatric patients with epithelioid hemangioma. Pediatr Blood Cancer. 2019;66(1):e27451.
9. Huang SC, Zhang L, Sung YS, et al. Frequent FOS gene rearrangements in epithelioid hemangioma: a molecular study of 58 cases with morphologic reappraisal. Am J Surg Pathol. 2015;39(10):1313–21.
10. Pagliai KA, Cohen BA. Pyogenic granuloma in children. Pediatr Dermatol. 2004;21(1):10–3.
11. Baselga E, Wassef M, Lopez S, Hoffman W, Cordisco M, Frieden IJ. Agminated, eruptive pyogenic granuloma-like lesions developing over congenital vascular stains. Pediatr Dermatol. 2012;29(2):186–90.
12. Browning JC, Eldin KW, Kozakewich HP, Mulliken JB, Bree AF. Congenital disseminated pyogenic granuloma. Pediatr Dermatol. 2009;26(3):323–7.
13. Hoeger PH, Colmenero I. Vascular tumours in infants. Part I: benign vascular tumours other than infantile haemangioma. Br J Dermatol. 2014;171(3):466–73.
14. Sud AR, Tan ST. Pyogenic granuloma-treatment by shave-excision and/or pulsed-dye laser. J Plast Reconstr Aesthet Surg. 2010;63(8):1364–8.
15. Ghodsi SZ, Raziei M, Taheri A, Karami M, Mansoori P, Farnaghi F. Comparison of cryotherapy and curettage for the treatment of pyogenic granuloma: a randomized trial. Br J Dermatol. 2006;154(4):671–5.
16. Tritton SM, Smith S, Wong LC, Zagarella S, Fischer G. Pyogenic granuloma in ten children treated with topical imiquimod. Pediatr Dermatol. 2009;26(3):269–72.
17. Neri I, Baraldi C, Balestri R, Piraccini BM, Patrizi A. Topical 1% propranolol ointment with occlusion in treatment of pyogenic granulomas: an open-label study in 22 children. Pediatr Dermatol. 2018;35(1):117–20.
18. Lim YH, Douglas SR, KO CJ, et al. Somatic activating RAS mutations cause vascular tumors including pyogenic granuloma. J Invest Dermatol. 135(6):1698–1700.
19. Calonje E, Fletcher CD, Wilson-Jones E, Rosai J. Retiform hemangioendothelioma. A distinctive form of low-grade angiosarcoma delineated in a series of 15 cases. Am J Surg Pathol. 1994;18(2):115–25.
20. Duke D, Dvorak A, Harris TJ, Cohen LM. Multiple retiform hemangioendotheliomas. A low-grade angiosarcoma. Am J Dermatopathol. 1996;18(6):606–10.
21. Requena L, Kutzner H. Hemangioendothelioma. Semin Diagn Pathol. 2013;30(1):29–44.
22. Sanz-Trelles A, Rodrigo-Fernandez I, Ayala-Carbonero A, Contreras-Rubio F. Retiform hemangioendothelioma. A new case in a child with diffuse endovascular papillary endothelial proliferation. J Cutan Pathol. 1997;24(7):440–4.
23. Emberger M, Laimer M, Steiner H, Zelger B. Retiform hemangioendothelioma: presentation of a case expressing D2-40. J Cutan Pathol. 2009;36(9):987–90.
24. Parsons A, Sheehan DJ, Sangueza OP. Retiform hemangioendotheliomas usually do not express D2-40 and VEGFR-3. Am J Dermatopathol. 2008;30(1):31–3.
25. Requena L, Luis Diaz J, Manzarbeitia F, Carrillo R, Fernandez-Herrera J, Kutzner H. Cutaneous composite hemangioendothelioma with satellitosis and lymph node metastases. J Cutan Pathol. 2008;35(2):225–30.
26. Dabska M. Malignant endovascular papillary angioendothelioma of the skin in childhood. Clinicopathologic study of 6 cases. Cancer. 1969;24(3):503–10.
27. Quecedo E, Martinez-Escribano JA, Febrer I, Oliver V, Velasco M, Aliaga A. Dabska tumor developing within a preexisting vascular malformation. Am J Dermatopathol. 1996;18(3):302–7.

28. Morgan J, Robinson MJ, Rosen LB, Unger H, Niven J. Malignant endovascular papillary angioendothelioma (Dabska tumor). A case report and review of the literature. Am J Dermatopathol. 1989;11(1):64–8.
29. Fanburg-Smith JC, Michal M, Partanen TA, Alitalo K, Miettinen M. Papillary intralymphatic angioendothelioma (PILA): a report of twelve cases of a distinctive vascular tumor with phenotypic features of lymphatic vessels. Am J Surg Pathol. 1999;23(9):1004–10.
30. Neves RI, Stevenson J, Hancey MJ, et al. Endovascular papillary angioendothelioma (Dabska tumor): underrecognized malignant tumor in childhood. J Pediatr Surg. 2011;46(1):e25–8.
31. Nayler SJ, Rubin BP, Calonje E, Chan JK, Fletcher CD. Composite hemangioendothelioma: a complex, low-grade vascular lesion mimicking angiosarcoma. Am J Surg Pathol. 2000;24(3):352–61.
32. Leen SL, Clarke PM, Chapman J, Fisher C, Thway K. Composite Hemangioendothelioma of the submandibular region. Head Neck Pathol. 2015;9(4):519–24.
33. Rubin BP. Pathology and genetics of tumors of soft tissue and bone. In: Fletcher CDM, Mertens F, editors. World Health Organization classification of tumours. Lyon, France: IARC Press; 2002. p. 168–9.
34. Bridge J, Hogendoorn, P. WHO classification of soft tissue and bone. 2013.; http://ebookcentral.proquest.com.
35. McNab PM, Quigley BC, Glass LF, Jukic DM. Composite hemangioendothelioma and its classification as a low-grade malignancy. Am J Dermatopathol. 2013;35(4):517–22.
36. Weiss SW, Ishak KG, Dail DH, Sweet DE, Enzinger FM. Epithelioid hemangioendothelioma and related lesions. Semin Diagn Pathol. 1986;3(4):259–87.
37. Sardaro A, Bardoscia L, Petruzzelli MF, Nikolaou A, Detti B, Angelelli G. Pulmonary epithelioid hemangioendothelioma presenting with vertebral metastases: a case report. J Med Case Rep. 2014;8:201.
38. Sardaro A, Bardoscia L, Petruzzelli MF, Portaluri M. Epithelioid hemangioendothelioma: an overview and update on a rare vascular tumor. Oncol Rev. 2014;8(2):259.
39. Colmenero I, Hoeger PH. Vascular tumours in infants. Part II: vascular tumours of intermediate malignancy [corrected] and malignant tumours. Br J Dermatol. 2014;171(3):474–84.
40. Anderson T, Zhang L, Hameed M, Rusch V, Travis WD, Antonescu CR. Thoracic epithelioid malignant vascular tumors: a clinicopathologic study of 52 cases with emphasis on pathologic grading and molecular studies of WWTR1-CAMTA1 fusions. Am J Surg Pathol. 2015;39(1):132–9.
41. Rest CC, Botton E, Robinet G, Conan-Charlet V, Bizais Y, Visvikis D. FDG PET in epithelioid hemangioendothelioma. Clin Nucl Med. 2004;29(12):789–92.
42. Lee WW, So Y, Kang SY, et al. F-18 fluorodeoxyglucose positron emission tomography for differential diagnosis and prognosis prediction of vascular tumors. Oncol Lett. 2017;14(1):665–72.
43. Tanas MR, Sboner A, Oliveira AM, et al. Identification of a disease-defining gene fusion in epithelioid hemangioendothelioma. Sci Transl Med. 2011;3(98):98ra82.
44. Antonescu CR, Le Loarer F, Mosquera JM, et al. Novel YAP1-TFE3 fusion defines a distinct subset of epithelioid hemangioendothelioma. Genes Chromosomes Cancer. 2013;52(8):775–84.
45. Lee SJ, Yang WI, Chung WS, Kim SK. Epithelioid hemangioendotheliomas with TFE3 gene translocations are compossible with CAMTA1 gene rearrangements. Oncotarget. 2016;7(7):7480–8.
46. Tsarouha H, Kyriazoglou AI, Ribeiro FR, Teixeira MR, Agnantis N, Pandis N. Chromosome analysis and molecular cytogenetic investigations of an epithelioid hemangioendothelioma. Cancer Genet Cytogenet. 2006;169(2):164–8.
47. Saste A, Cabrera Fernandez DF, Gulati R, et al. A trimodality approach in the management of metastatic low-grade epithelioid hemangioendothelioma of the bone. Case Rep. 2015;2015:bcr2015210196.
48. Watanabe S, Yano F, Kita T, et al. 18F-FDG-PET/CT as an indicator for resection of pulmonary epithelioid hemangioendothelioma. Ann Nucl Med. 2008;22(6):521–4.
49. Aquilina K, Lim C, Kamel MH, Marks CJ, O'Sullivan MG, Keohane C. Epithelioid hemangioendothelioma of the spine. Report of two cases. J Neurosurg Spine. 2005;3(5):393–9.

50. Saada E, Saint Paul MC, Gugenheim J, Follana P, Francois E. Metastatic hepatic epithelioid hemangio-endothelioma: long-term response to sunitinib malate. Oncol Res Treat. 2014;37(3):124–6.
51. Cournoyer E, Al-Ibraheemi A, Engel E, et al. Clinical characterization and long-term outcomes in pediatric epithelioid hemangioendothelioma. Pediatr Blood Cancer. 2020;67(2):e28045.
52. Lau K, Massad M, Pollak C, et al. Clinical patterns and outcome in epithelioid hemangioendothelioma with or without pulmonary involvement: insights from an internet registry in the study of a rare cancer. Chest. 2011;140(5):1312–8.
53. Stewart FW, Treves N. Lymphangiosarcoma in postmastectomy lymphedema; a report of six cases in elephantiasis chirurgica. Cancer. 1948;1(1):64–81.
54. Cioffi A, Reichert S, Antonescu CR, Maki RG. Angiosarcomas and other sarcomas of endothelial origin. Hematol Oncol Clin North Am. 2013;27(5):975–88.
55. Elliott P, Kleinschmidt I. Angiosarcoma of the liver in Great Britain in proximity to vinyl chloride sites. Occup Environ Med. 1997;54(1):14–8.
56. Hillenbrand T, Menge F, Hohenberger P, Kasper B. Primary and secondary angiosarcomas: a comparative single-center analysis. Clin Sarcoma Res. 2015;5:14.
57. Oskrochi Y, Razi K, Stebbing J, Crane J. Angiosarcoma and dialysis-related arteriovenous fistulae: a comprehensive review. Eur J Vasc Endovasc Surg. 2016;51(1):127–33.
58. De Silva BD, Nawroz I, Doherty VR. Angiosarcoma of the head and neck associated with xeroderma pigmentosum variant. Br J Dermatol. 1999;141(1):166–7.
59. Leake J, Sheehan MP, Rampling D, Ramani P, Atherton DJ. Angiosarcoma complicating xeroderma pigmentosum. Histopathology. 1992;21(2):179–81.
60. Ludolph-Hauser D, Thoma-Greber E, Sander C, Sommerhoff CP, Rocken M. Mast cells in an angiosarcoma complicating xeroderma pigmentosum in a 13-year-old girl. J Am Acad Dermatol. 2000;43(5 Pt 2):900–2.
61. Marcon I, Collini P, Casanova M, Meazza C, Ferrari A. Cutaneous angiosarcoma in a patient with xeroderma pigmentosum. Pediatr Hematol Oncol. 2004;21(1):23–6.
62. Salminen SH, Sampo MM, Bohling TO, Tuomikoski L, Tarkkanen M, Blomqvist CP. Radiation-associated sarcoma after breast cancer in a nationwide population: increasing risk of angiosarcoma. Cancer Med. 2018;7:4825.
63. Requena C, Rubio L, Lavernia J, et al. Immunohistochemical and fluorescence in situ hybridization analysis of MYC in a series of 17 cutaneous angiosarcomas: a single-center study. Am J Dermatopathol. 2018;40(5):349–54.
64. Udager AM, Ishikawa MK, Lucas DR, McHugh JB, Patel RM. MYC immunohistochemistry in angiosarcoma and atypical vascular lesions: practical considerations based on a single institutional experience. Pathology. 2016;48(7):697–704.
65. Fraga-Guedes C, Andre S, Mastropasqua MG, et al. Angiosarcoma and atypical vascular lesions of the breast: diagnostic and prognostic role of MYC gene amplification and protein expression. Breast Cancer Res Treat. 2015;151(1):131–40.
66. Deyrup AT, Miettinen M, North PE, et al. Pediatric cutaneous angiosarcomas: a clinicopathologic study of 10 cases. Am J Surg Pathol. 2011;35(1):70–5.
67. Grassia KL, Peterman CM, Iacobas I, et al. Clinical case series of pediatric hepatic angiosarcoma. Pediatr Blood Cancer. 2017;64(11) https://doi.org/10.1002/pbc.26627.
68. Chadwick ML, Lane A, Thomas D, et al. Combined mTOR and MEK inhibition is an effective therapy in a novel mouse model for angiosarcoma. Oncotarget. 2018;9(37):24750–65.
69. Selby DM, Stocker JT, Ishak KG. Angiosarcoma of the liver in childhood: a clinicopathologic and follow-up study of 10 cases. Pediatr Pathol. 1992;12(4):485–98.
70. Weinberg AG, Finegold MJ. Primary hepatic tumors of childhood. Hum Pathol. 1983;14(6):512–37.
71. Falk H, Herbert JT, Edmonds L, Heath CW Jr, Thomas LB, Popper H. Review of four cases of childhood hepatic angiosarcoma–elevated environmental arsenic exposure in one case. Cancer. 1981;47(2):382–91.

72. Jeng MR, Fuh B, Blatt J, et al. Malignant transformation of infantile hemangioma to angiosarcoma: response to chemotherapy with bevacizumab. Pediatr Blood Cancer. 2014;61(11):2115–7.
73. Iacobas I, Phung TL, Adams DM, et al. Guidance document for hepatic hemangioma (infantile and congenital) evaluation and monitoring. J Pediatr. 2018;203:294–300.. e292
74. Agale SV, Khan WA, Chawlani K. Chronic lymphedema of filarial origin: a very rare etiology of cutaneous lymphangiosarcoma. Indian J Dermatol. 2013;58(1):71–3.
75. Brittain JM, Nymark T, Hildebrandt MG, Hovgaard D, Andersen KF. Stewart-Treves syndrome on the lower extremity associated to idiopathic chronic lymphedema visualized on FDG PET/CT. Clin Nucl Med. 2017;42(12):e519–22.
76. Quarmyne MO, Gupta A, Adams DM. Lymphangiosarcoma of the thorax and thoracic vertebrae in a 16-year-old girl. J Clin Oncol. 2012;30(29):e294–8.
77. Sun S, Chen S, Liu F, et al. Constitutive activation of mTORC1 in endothelial cells leads to the development and progression of lymphangiosarcoma through VEGF autocrine signaling. Cancer Cell. 2015;28(6):758–72.
78. Felmerer G, Dowlatshahi AS, Stark GB, et al. Lymphangiosarcoma: is Stewart-Treves syndrome a preventable condition? Lymphat Res Biol. 2016;14(1):35–9.

Capillary Malformations and Associated Syndromes

8

Megha M. Tollefson and Adrienne M. Hammill

Abbreviations

AVM	Arteriovenous malformation
CLOVES	Congenital lipomatous overgrowth and vascular malformation with epidermal nevus and skeletal abnormalities
CM	Capillary malformation
CMTC	Cutis marmorata telangiectatica congenita
CNS	Central nervous system
CT	Computed tomography
CVM	Capillary venous malformation
DCMO	Diffuse capillary malformation with overgrowth
KTS	Klippel-Trenaunay syndrome
M-CM	Macrocephaly-capillary malformation syndrome
MRA	Magnetic resonance arteriography
MRI	Magnetic resonance imaging
MRV	Magnetic resonance venography
PDL	Pulsed-dye laser
PPV	Phakomatosis pigmentovascularis
PWB	Port-wine birthmark
PWS	Port-wine stain
SWS	Sturge-Weber syndrome

M. M. Tollefson
Division of Pediatric Dermatology, Mayo Clinic, Rochester, MN, USA
e-mail: Tollefson.Megha@mayo.edu

A. M. Hammill (✉)
Division of Hematology, Hemangioma and Vascular Malformation Center, University of Cincinnati College of Medicine, Cincinnati Children's Hospital Medical Center, Cincinnati, OH, USA
e-mail: adrienne.hammill@cchmc.org

C. C. Trenor III, D. M. Adams (eds.), *Vascular Anomalies*,
https://doi.org/10.1007/978-3-030-25624-1_8

Capillary Malformations

Port-Wine Birthmark

The terms capillary malformation (Table 8.1) and port-wine stain (PWS) or more recently port-wine birthmark (PWB) are often used interchangeably. PWB, also referred to as a *nevus flammeus*, is the most common type of capillary malformation. PWB occur in 0.3% of all newborns and are present at birth [1], although may initially be misdiagnosed as a bruise or other birth trauma. They are flat, well-demarcated, and usually located on one side of the body respecting the midline and

Table 8.1 Capillary malformations and associated syndromes

Lesion	Pattern	Associations	Prognosis	Treatment
Capillary malformation (CM)	Flat, well-demarcated, homogeneous	Facial/forehead involvement: Sturge-Weber syndrome	Do not fade; may darken and thicken over time	None or PDL
Nevus simplex	Faint, pink, characteristic locations	None	Forehead and eyelids commonly fade	None needed
Sturge-Weber syndrome (SWS)	Homogeneous facial capillary malformation	Glaucoma, seizures, developmental delay	Central nervous system and ophthal mologic complications	PDL for CM, appropriate subspecialty treatment of seizures and glaucoma
CMTC	Fixed reticulate coarse vascular pattern	Soft tissue atrophy, ulceration	Capillary malformation will often lighten with age	Rarely needed
DCMO	Diffuse (multiple discontinuous body regions), often reticular pattern, prominent superficial veins (1/3)	Overgrowth, possible leg length inequality	May lighten somewhat	Orthopedic referral for leg length issues as indicated
CVM	Capillary malformation borders less defined, venous dilation most commonly superficial veins, deep system intact	Overgrowth, possible limb length inequality	Significant coagulopathy not common	Orthopedic referral for leg length issues Supportive care: compression therapy Sclerotherapy, endovascular laser, or radiofrequency ablation
PPV	Variable clinical findings, all with capillary malformation	Variable	Variable	Laser treatment of cutaneous findings

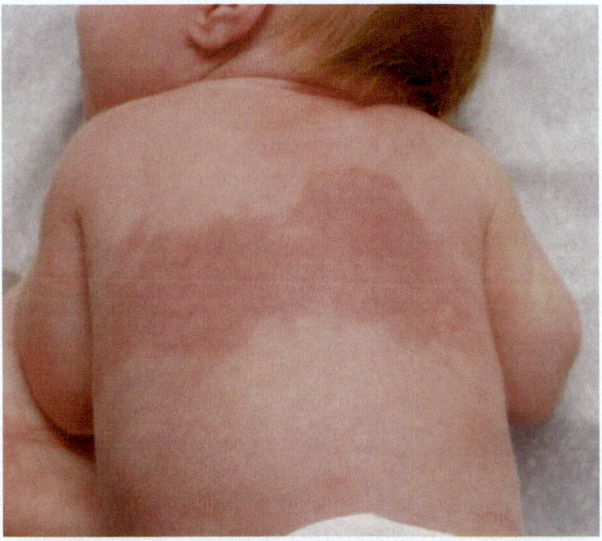

Fig. 8.1 Capillary malformation. Well-defined capillary malformation on the trunk of a child

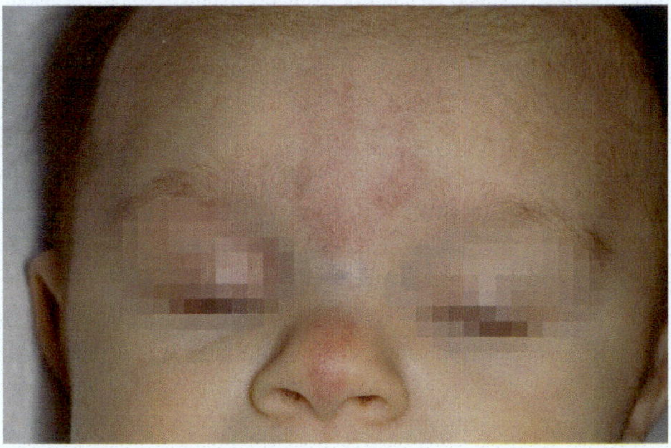

Fig. 8.2 Glabellar and eyelid nevus simplex

grow in proportion to the child but early on may be confused for infantile hemangiomas or nevus simplex (Fig. 8.1). A somatic activating mutation in GNAQ has been found to be responsible for the development of classic PWB in both Sturge-Weber syndrome and in non-syndromic PWB. These mutations are enriched within, but not limited to, blood vessel endothelial cells in skin [2, 3] and brain [4]. In addition, mutations in the closely related GNA11 gene have been identified in some GNAQ-negative capillary malformations [5].

Unlike PWB, infantile hemangiomas undergo a rapid growth phase in early infancy, followed by gradual spontaneous resolution. Nevus simplex, also known as "stork bites" or "angel kisses," are present in 30–40% of newborns at birth, commonly involve the glabella, nape of the neck, and eyelids, and generally fade within the first 2 years of life (Fig. 8.2) [6, 7]. Some, particularly those on the nape of the neck, may persist into adulthood. While not a true malformation, they are composed of ectatic capillaries and felt by most to be a form of persistent fetal circulation. Although faint, more salmon pink in color, and often midline, they may sometimes be mistaken for PWB, particularly when less common sites are involved. When additional sites such as the scalp, nose, lip, lumbosacral skin, and back are involved in addition to the more common sites, the term "nevus simplex complex" has been proposed [7].

A PWB may occur at any location of the body, most often on the face where they may extend to mucosal surfaces, may range in size from small to extremely large, and may be present as one patch or as multiple patches. PWB and other CMs may be associated with certain congenital syndromes, several of which will be discussed in this chapter. The appearance and location of PWB can be important when considering associations and underlying syndromes; those that have a more "geographic" appearance are more likely to be associated with underlying abnormalities particularly when involving a limb [8]. PWB present on the face may require evaluation for ocular and neurologic associations [9]. Those present in the lumbosacral area may be associated with underlying spinal dysraphism (especially when seen with another associated anomaly such as a lipoma or hair tuft), while those in the cervical area may be associated with an underlying mass or pit [10, 11]. They may be slightly warm but significant warmth on exam should suggest another diagnosis, including hemangioma or a combined malformation involving an arteriovenous malformation (AVM), as in CM-AVM.

The diagnosis of a PWB is usually a clinical one, but when biopsied or excised, histopathology shows an increased number of ectatic capillaries primarily located in the superficial dermis. There may also be impaired neural control of these blood vessels, which then leads to progressive dilation of the vessels and altered vascular flow [12]. While ultrasound evaluation is often not necessary in the diagnosis of a PWB, it can be helpful in ruling out an underlying or associated arteriovenous malformation (AVM) if one is suspected, as a PWB will show slow-flow and an AVM will have high-flow on Doppler interrogation.

PWB persist throughout life. Although benign, several complications may occur directly related to the CM. A common complication is the development of overlying dermatitis. This should be treated, especially in those undergoing treatment for the CM, and usually responds to skin-directed therapy with moisturizer and topical steroids. While initially flat and macular, PWB may darken, thicken, and become more nodular during adulthood. This can happen at any location of the body, but is more common with PWB involving the head and neck, where 2/3 develop soft tissue or bony hypertrophy or nodule formation [13, 14]. In one study of head and neck PWB, without treatment, soft tissue hypertrophy began at 9 years of age particularly when involving the mid-face. Fourteen percent of patients had associated bony hypertrophy starting at 15 years of age, and 44% developed nodules at an average of 22 years of age [14]. Treatment (discussed below) is often recommended in an effort to prevent these complications. Trunk and limb PWB may also develop thickening and hypertrophy, as well as vascular bleb formation often in association with an underlying lymphatic or venolymphatic malformation [8]. Pyogenic granulomas, benign but friable vascular tumors, may also develop within PWB and should be treated appropriately [15].

Sturge-Weber Syndrome

Sturge-Weber syndrome (SWS), also known as encephalotrigeminal angiomatosis, is a triad first described in 1879 consisting of a facial capillary malformation, ocular vascular malformations leading to glaucoma and buphthalmos, and leptomeningeal/central nervous system (CNS) vascular malformation predisposing to seizures and developmental delay. Historically it was hypothesized that SWS is caused by a somatic mosaic mutation, and indeed whole exome sequencing from three patients with SWS confirmed a causative somatic activating mutation in GNAQ [16]. These findings were confirmed in another study that found this same GNAQ mutation in 80% of patients with sporadic SWS [17].

Skin Manifestations

A child who has any facial PWB has up to a 6% chance of having SWS (Fig. 8.3) [18]. Historically, those with a PWB in the distribution of the trigeminal nerve, particularly V1, were felt to be at highest risk for the development of SWS, with approximately

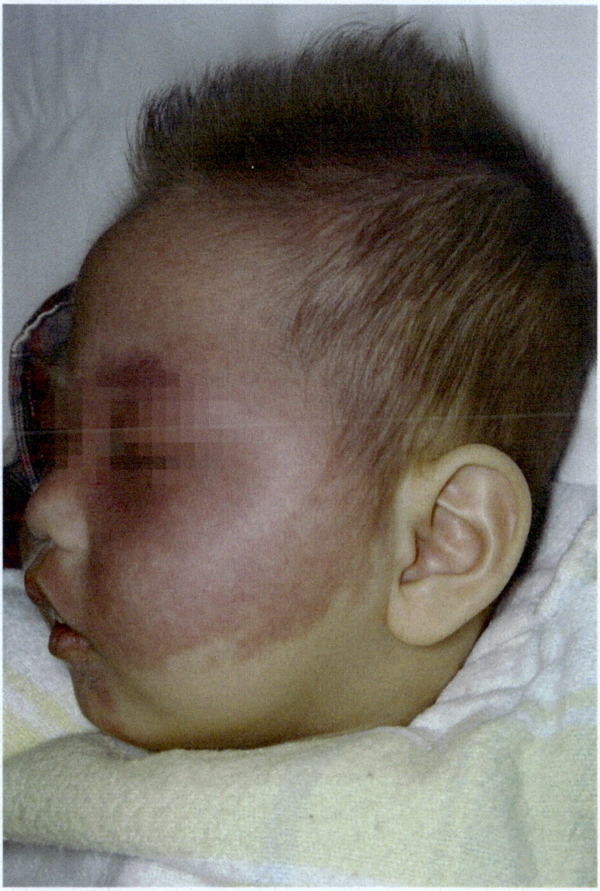

Fig. 8.3 Facial port-wine birthmark in a patient with Sturge-Weber syndrome

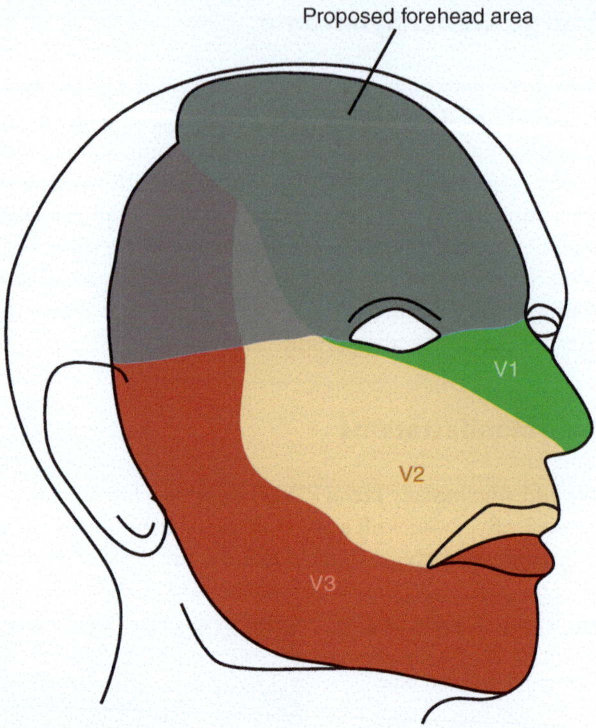

Fig. 8.4 Forehead area at high risk for Sturge-Weber syndrome. Distribution of the "forehead," defined as any part of the forehead from the midline to an imaginary line between the outer canthus of the eye and the top of the ear including the upper eyelids. (Reused with permission from Waelchli et al. [21]; http://onlinelibrary.wiley.com/doi/10.1111/bjd.13203/full#bjd13203-fig-0001)

8% having SWS [19]. Newer studies suggest that patterns of facial PWB distribution that correspond to vascular patterns of mosaicism, especially when involving the forehead, are associated with an increased risk of SWS (Fig. 8.4) [20, 21]. Out of 192 patients with a facial PWB, when the forehead was not involved, not a single patient had seizures, abnormal neurologic development, abnormalities on MRI, nor glaucoma; in all of those who had one or more of those abnormalities, the forehead was invariably involved, with the defined forehead area involving portions of all three branches of the trigeminal nerve [21].

The CM present in SWS may extend onto mucosal surfaces and may result in gingival hypertrophy; this may be more pronounced in those with SWS being treated with phenytoin for seizures. Maxillary bone hypertrophy may also be seen, especially in those patients with overlying PWB. Macrochelia, or lip overgrowth, has recently been related to the presence of GNAQ mutation in lip [22].

Ocular Manifestations

The most common ocular abnormality seen in SWS is glaucoma, with a prevalence of 50–60% [23]. Presence of the CM on the eyelid increases the risk for glaucoma. The precise mechanism for its development is unknown, but it is usually ipsilateral to the intraocular vascular malformation (may be bilateral especially in those with bilateral PWB) with mechanical pressure or increased venous pressure as possible reasons. Two-thirds of patients develop glaucoma at birth or in early infancy, but the risk of development is lifelong with a mean age of diagnosis of 2.9 years; thus patients must continue to be monitored for early detection and treatment [23]. In those that are at risk, recommendations are for first ophthalmological examination in the neonatal period and if normal, then re-evaluation frequently for the first 2 years, followed by at least annually thereafter. Corneal clouding at birth is an indication of acute angle glaucoma and should be treated emergently. Those with congenital or early-onset glaucoma may develop buphthalmos.

CNS Manifestations

Seizures are the most common neurologic manifestation of SWS, present in up to 90% of patients [24] and more common in those with bilateral PWB. Similar to glaucoma, seizures usually develop within the first year of life but may also develop later [25]. Later age of seizure onset correlates with lower prevalence of developmental delay and fewer special educational needs [26]. Developmental delay and intellectual impairment are common in patients with SWS; the underlying mechanisms appear to be multifactorial. Abnormal venous drainage can lead to venous stasis and microvascular thrombosis. Recurrent seizures, along with inappropriate autonomic response to those seizures, can lead to ischemic damage. Transient stroke-like or hemiplegia episodes have also been seen in up to 30% of patients with SWS and seem to be more common in toddlers who suffer minor head injuries [25]. Headaches are also a common complaint in patients with SWS, with 28% of patients reporting symptoms of migraine headache [27].

CNS imaging is often helpful in establishing the diagnosis and in delineating the extent of SWS, although routine imaging in infancy in the absence of neurologic symptoms has not been universally recommended as it may give false negative results before the age 1 year and the majority of infants with a facial port-wine birthmark do not have brain involvement. Contrast-enhanced MRI remains the gold standard for diagnosis of intracranial involvement because the characteristic "tram track" intracranial calcifications, visible by CT scan or plain x-ray films, often do not appear until 2 years of age or later. MRI should be performed with gadolinium contrast and should also interrogate the vascular anatomy of the brain with MRV. Susceptibility-weighted imaging and post-contrast flair provide increased sensitivity in demonstrating the extent of involvement with abnormal leptomeningeal and deep draining vessels. In addition, diffusion sequences should be performed, as well as spectroscopy if possible [28, 29]. Findings of leptomeningeal enhancement, choroid plexus enlargement, with or without venous anomalies, extensive deep draining vessels, or cortical atrophy would be consistent with a diagnosis of Sturge-Weber syndrome in an infant or young child.

Care of the patient with SWS must be multidisciplinary. Its treatment is primarily aimed at control of neurologic and ocular symptoms, though increasing attention is being paid to the role of thrombosis in the pathogenesis of SWS. Low-dose aspirin is increasingly used in these patients with some improvement in their symptoms, including seizure frequency [30, 31]. Patients should be counseled on the importance of good hydration and prompt fever control. Furthermore, because prolonged seizures worsen cerebral perfusion in SWS, aggressive seizure management is critical. Treatment options for the CM will be discussed below. Patients may also be directed to The Sturge-Weber Foundation (www.sturge-weber.com) for resources and support.

Cutis Marmorata Telangiectatica Congenita (CMTC)

CMTC is an uncommon but clinically distinctive cutaneous vascular malformation. It is present at birth and mimics the physiologic cutis marmorata (mottling) which is commonly seen in young infants, particularly when they are cold; however, there are some distinctive distinguishing features. It may also resemble a reticular PWB. CMTC has a fixed reticulate coarse vascular pattern (Fig. 8.5) that can also be accentuated by cold, accompanied by varying amounts of telangiectasia, soft tissue atrophy, and potentially, ulceration [32, 33]. Unlike with cutis marmorata, the erythema does not resolve with warming. There may also be varying amounts of subcutaneous atrophy, particularly over joints, with resulting skin breakdown.

CMTC may be generalized but more commonly involves only one extremity (the leg in 75% of cases) and respects the midline [34]. It is most often an isolated finding but in some cases, congenital anomalies have been reported. Congenital anomalies may be associated in up to 50% of patients although that is likely an overestimation due to referral and reporting bias [34]. The most commonly

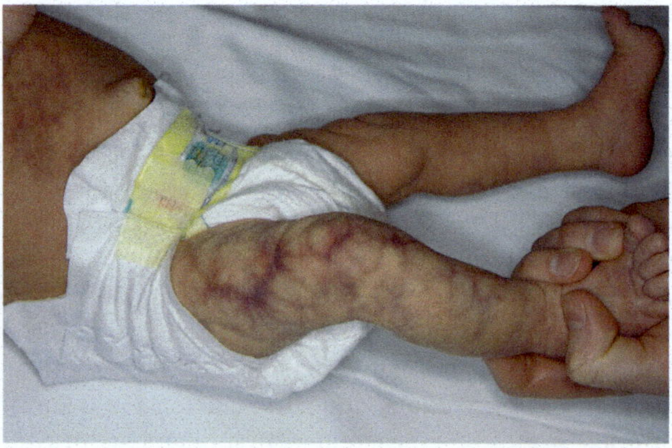

Fig. 8.5 Cutis marmorata telangiectatica congenita. Note distinct coarse reticular pattern of the trunk and leg

associated abnormality is limb atrophy (usually the one that is affected), but other associations may include hyperplasia (overgrowth) of the limb, aplasia cutis congenita, asymmetry of the skull, macrocephaly, syndactyly, scoliosis, hypothyroidism, developmental delay, and anogenital anomalies, among others, although many of these may due to the presence of alternative diagnoses such as macrocephaly-capillary malformation (M-CM, discussed further in the Overgrowth Syndromes chapter) [35]. CMTC is seen in Adams-Oliver syndrome, which consists of limb defects and aplasia cutis congenita.

Histopathology findings in CMTC are variable but often consist of an increased number of dilated capillaries in the dermis and subcutaneous tissues. However, the diagnosis is primarily a clinical one. An etiology for the development of CMTC is unknown, although genetic mosaicism has been proposed. No active treatment is indicated in the majority of cases. CMTC usually lightens with age in the majority of patients, usually by age 2, although some residual reticulate erythema usually persists [36]. In cases of ulceration, the ulcer should be treated with supportive care.

Diffuse Capillary Malformation with Overgrowth (DCMO)

DCMO has recently been suggested as a distinct clinical entity, in order to differentiate it from other capillary malformation overgrowth syndromes which have higher likelihoods of complications and significant morbidity [37]. Specifically, DCMO has been defined as diffuse capillary malformation, involving multiple body regions in discontinuum, and often having a reticular pattern (Fig. 8.6). It tends to lighten some with age but rarely as significantly as true CMTC. Prominent superficial veins are noted to be involved in approximately one-third of patients.

Overgrowth does not necessarily correlate with areas of CM, and growth remains proportionate throughout life. With overgrowth of one of the lower extremities, patients should be monitored for limb length inequality through puberty; 55% of patients in the initial series were found to have limb length discrepancies. Thirty percent of patients have abnormalities of the digits, including soft tissue syndactyly, "sandal gap" deformity, and macrodactyly. Of note, such abnormalities are also described in CLOVES syndrome (see Overgrowth Syndromes chapter). In addition, some patients have unilateral facial overgrowth and are frequently noted to have accelerated dental eruption on the hypertrophic side, even in the absence of any capillary malformation in the area.

No patient in the initial series of 73 had any developmental delays. There were no abdominal malignancies detected, even with 11% (7 of 73) having total hemihypertrophy. At least one patient was noted to have a Chiari I, and those patients with capillary staining crossing midline should be considered for workup of spinal anomalies.

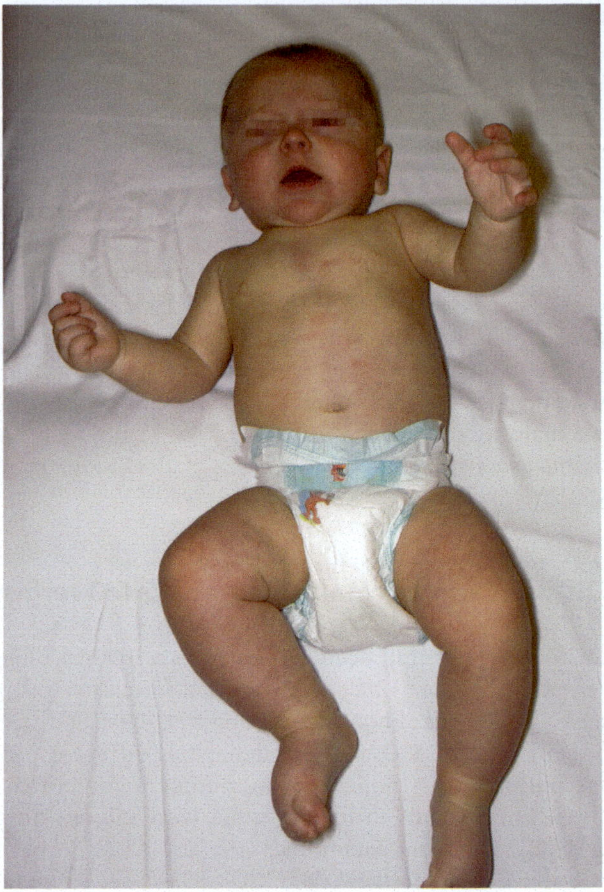

Fig. 8.6 Diffuse capillary malformation with overgrowth

Capillary Venous Malformation (CVM)

Capillary malformations may also be associated with venous distention. This may occur even in otherwise "simple" PWB, with increased visibility of draining veins, but is most clear in large regional capillary malformations. Venous distention becomes more visible with time and with height gain (due to an increased effect of gravity), so may not be recognized in early childhood. Many of these patients will go on to have distended and/or ectatic veins visible below the capillary malformation and sometimes even peripheral to the CM (Fig. 8.7).

These are likely distinct from malformations seen in Klippel-Trenaunay syndrome (KTS), as they do not contain any lymphatic component, and the capillary lesions tend to have less defined borders [38]. Dilation of veins occurs most commonly in superficial veins, but may also be seen in deep veins and

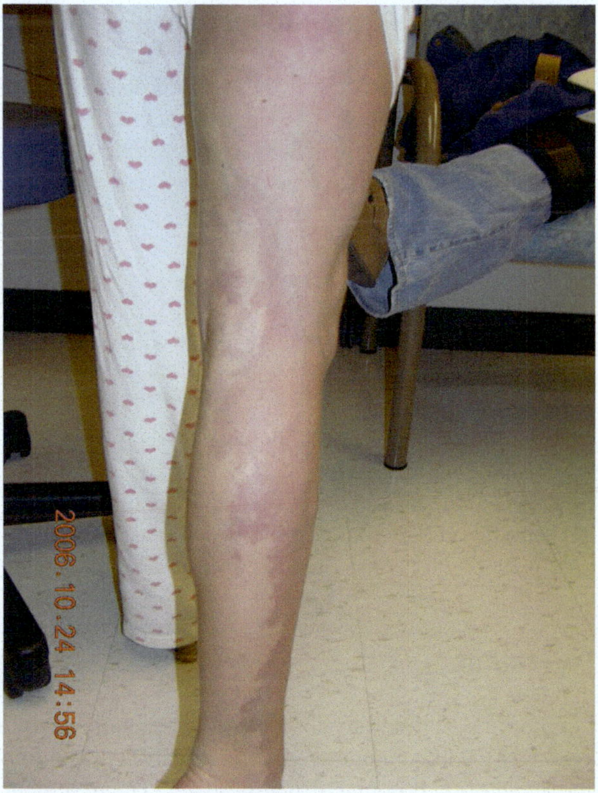

Fig. 8.7 Capillary venous malformation

intramuscular vessels. The most frequent areas for distention are the popliteal fossa and the dorsal foot.

Venous distention becomes symptomatic in some, but not all, patients over time. This generally presents as pain within the distended veins, but has alternately been described as pressure or burning, and may be accompanied by swelling. The symptomatic distention can be treated with supportive care, including compression therapy, or with sclerotherapy. In time, endovascular laser or radiofrequency ablation may have an increasing role in these patients, as those with CVM generally have an intact deep venous system, in contrast to those with KTS (discussed further in Overgrowth Syndromes). Leg length inequality is also noted in a majority of patients, including both overgrowth and undergrowth of the involved bones. Depending on the degree of discrepancy, this can be treated with noninvasive intervention such as use of a shoe lift for the shorter leg or more invasive procedures such as epiphysiodesis of the longer limb.

Of note, this group of patients does not seem to have increased prevalence of coagulopathy, thrombophlebitis, or bleeding and thus may portend a significantly less symptomatic prognosis than for KTS.

Phakomatosis Pigmentovascularis (PPV)

PPV is a term used to describe a group of disorders consisting of an extensive CM, along with a melanocytic or epidermal nevus. There are five types described in the classification depending on the particular findings. Extracutaneous findings, including neurologic and ocular abnormalities, may also be present [39].

- Type I: CM + epidermal nevus
- Type II: CM + dermal melanocytosis, with or without nevus anemicus (most common, accounts for 70–80% of PPV)
- Type III: CM + nevus spilus, with or without nevus anemicus
- Type IV: CM + dermal melanocytosis + nevus spilus, with or without nevus anemicus
- Type V: CMTC + dermal melanocytosis [40]

This is a rare group of disorders that are thought to be sporadic, although slightly more common in females [41]. Treatment is generally supportive, although laser treatment may be considered for the cutaneous findings.

Treatment

Capillary malformations do not resolve spontaneously, and their persistence can be associated with a number of complications, including medical ones described above, and psychosocial difficulties [42]. The treatment of choice is the pulsed dye laser (PDL). Treatment of the CM before it begins to thicken and hypertrophy may prevent or delay thickening and nodularity later in life, and for that reason, many advocate for treatment early in childhood [43]. However, whether or not early treatment results in a better cosmetic outcome as compared to later treatment is still controversial with authors on both sides of the argument. The timing of treatment, however, must be weighed with the possible risks of general anesthesia early in life. In very young infants, treatment can sometimes be accomplished with swaddling and topical anesthetic agents alone if the CM is localized. Older children are often able to tolerate PDL with only topical anesthesia if the CM is not extensive and does not involve the eyelid.

The PDL targets intravascular hemoglobin and as a result ablates target vasculature with minimal collateral damage. Multiple treatments spaced 6–8 weeks apart are necessary. While complete clearance is generally unattainable, most treated lesions demonstrate 50 to 90% lightening, with some variation largely based on location of the lesion; the centrofacial area and limb lesions are generally less responsive to treatment possibly due to relatively increased blood vessel density and diameter [44, 45]. Maintenance treatment throughout life may be required, with repeat laser procedures as indicated.

There is a subset of CMs that are "PDL-resistant." In these patients novel, laser and light therapies are being utilized and studied, including intense pulsed light and the long-pulsed tunable dye, alexandrite, and Nd:YAG lasers [46]. In addition, several studies now suggest that topical sirolimus may be a helpful adjunctive treatment option in patients undergoing laser treatment for their CMs, to prevent revascularization in the immediate posttreatment period [47, 48].

In patients with visible CMs, specialty cosmetic cover-up can be used to camouflage the affected area; this has been shown to improve quality of life in affected patients [49].

References

1. Jacobs AH, Walton RG. The incidence of birthmarks in the neonate. Pediatrics. 1976;58:218–22.
2. Couto JA, et al. Endothelial cells from capillary malformations are enriched for somatic GNAQ mutations. Plast Reconstr Surg. 2016;137:77e–82e. https://doi.org/10.1097/PRS.0000000000001868.
3. Tan W, et al. The somatic GNAQ mutation (R183Q) is primarily located within the blood vessels of port wine stains. J Am Acad Dermatol. 2016;74:380–3. https://doi.org/10.1016/j.jaad.2015.09.063.
4. Huang L, et al. Somatic GNAQ mutation is enriched in brain endothelial cells in Sturge-Weber syndrome. Pediatr Neurol. 2017;67:59–63. https://doi.org/10.1016/j.pediatrneurol.2016.10.010.
5. Couto JA, et al. A somatic GNA11 mutation is associated with extremity capillary malformation and overgrowth. Angiogenesis. 2017;20:303–6. https://doi.org/10.1007/s10456-016-9538-1.
6. Alper JC, Holmes LB. The incidence and significance of birthmarks in a cohort of 4,641 newborns. Pediatr Dermatol. 1983;1:58–68.
7. Juern AM, Glick ZR, Drolet BA, Frieden IJ. Nevus simplex: a reconsideration of nomenclature, sites of involvement, and disease associations. J Am Acad Dermatol. 2010;63:805–14. https://doi.org/10.1016/j.jaad.2009.08.066.
8. Maari C, Frieden IJ. Klippel-Trenaunay syndrome: the importance of "geographic stains" in identifying lymphatic disease and risk of complications. J Am Acad Dermatol. 2004;51:391–8. https://doi.org/10.1016/j.jaad.2003.12.017.
9. Tallman B, et al. Location of port-wine stains and the likelihood of ophthalmic and/or central nervous system complications. Pediatrics. 1991;87:323–7.
10. Davis DA, Cohen PR, George RE. Cutaneous stigmata of occult spinal dysraphism. J Am Acad Dermatol. 1994;31:892–6.
11. Enjolras O, Boukobza M, Jdid R. Cervical occult spinal dysraphism: MRI findings and the value of a vascular birthmark. Pediatr Dermatol. 1995;12:256–9.
12. Smoller BR, Rosen S. Port-wine stains. A disease of altered neural modulation of blood vessels? Arch Dermatol. 1986;122:177–9.
13. Cordoro KM, Speetzen LS, Koerper MA, Frieden IJ. Physiologic changes in vascular birthmarks during early infancy: mechanisms and clinical implications. J Am Acad Dermatol. 2009;60:669–75. https://doi.org/10.1016/j.jaad.2008.11.020.
14. Lee JW, Chung HY, Cerrati EW, O TM, Waner M. The natural history of soft tissue hypertrophy, bony hypertrophy, and nodule formation in patients with untreated head and neck capillary malformations. Dermatol Surg. 2015;41:1241–5. https://doi.org/10.1097/DSS.0000000000000525.
15. Garzon MC, Enjolras O, Frieden IJ. Vascular tumors and vascular malformations: evidence for an association. J Am Acad Dermatol. 2000;42:275–9. https://doi.org/10.1016/S0190-9622(00)90138-5.
16. Shirley MD, et al. Sturge-Weber syndrome and port-wine stains caused by somatic mutation in GNAQ. N Engl J Med. 2013;368:1971–9. https://doi.org/10.1056/NEJMoa1213507.

17. Nakashima M, et al. The somatic GNAQ mutation c.548G>A (p.R183Q) is consistently found in Sturge-Weber syndrome. J Hum Genet. 2014;59:691–3. https://doi.org/10.1038/jhg.2014.95.
18. Piram M, et al. Sturge-Weber syndrome in patients with facial port-wine stain. Pediatr Dermatol. 2012;29:32–7. https://doi.org/10.1111/j.1525-1470.2011.01485.x.
19. Enjolras O, Riche MC, Merland JJ. Facial port-wine stains and Sturge-Weber syndrome. Pediatrics. 1985;76:48–51.
20. Dutkiewicz AS, et al. A prospective study of risk for Sturge-Weber syndrome in children with upper facial port-wine stain. J Am Acad Dermatol. 2015;72:473–80. https://doi.org/10.1016/j.jaad.2014.11.009.
21. Waelchli R, et al. New vascular classification of port-wine stains: improving prediction of Sturge-Weber risk. Br J Dermatol. 2014;171:861–7. https://doi.org/10.1111/bjd.13203.
22. Ma G, Liu F, Cai R, Liu Y, Lin X. Somatic GNAQ mutation in different structures of Port-wine Macrocheilia. J Invest Dermatol. 2018;138:S218.
23. Sharan S, et al. Port-wine vascular malformations and glaucoma risk in Sturge-Weber syndrome. J AAPOS. 2009;13:374–8. https://doi.org/10.1016/j.jaapos.2009.04.007.
24. Paller AS. The Sturge-Weber syndrome. Pediatr Dermatol. 1987;4:300–4.
25. Lo W, et al. Updates and future horizons on the understanding, diagnosis, and treatment of Sturge-Weber syndrome brain involvement. Dev Med Child Neurol. 2012;54:214–23. https://doi.org/10.1111/j.1469-8749.2011.04169.x.
26. Comi A, Roach ES, Bodensteiner JB. In: Bodensteiner JB, Roach ES, editors.. Ch. 4, p. 69–93 Sturge-Weber Syndrome: The Sturge-Weber Foundation; 2010.
27. Cambon H, et al. Focal chronic ischemia and concomitant migraine: an atypical form of Sturge-Weber angiomatosis? Rev Neurol. 1987;143:588–94.
28. Lin DD, Barker PB, Hatfield LA, Comi AM. Dynamic MR perfusion and proton MR spectroscopic imaging in Sturge-Weber syndrome: correlation with neurological symptoms. J Magn Reson Imaging. 2006;24:274–81. https://doi.org/10.1002/jmri.20627.
29. Lin DD, Barker PB, Kraut MA, Comi A. Early characteristics of Sturge-Weber syndrome shown by perfusion MR imaging and proton MR spectroscopic imaging. AJNR Am J Neuroradiol. 2003;24:1912–5.
30. Bay MJ, Kossoff EH, Lehmann CU, Zabel TA, Comi AM. Survey of aspirin use in Sturge-Weber syndrome. J Child Neurol. 2011;26:692–702. https://doi.org/10.1177/0883073810388646.
31. Lance EI, Sreenivasan AK, Zabel TA, Kossoff EH, Comi AM. Aspirin use in Sturge-Weber syndrome: side effects and clinical outcomes. J Child Neurol. 2013;28:213–8. https://doi.org/10.1177/0883073812463607.
32. Picascia DD, Esterly NB. Cutis marmorata telangiectatica congenita: report of 22 cases. J Am Acad Dermatol. 1989;20:1098–104.
33. South DA, Jacobs AH. Cutis marmorata telangiectatica congenita (congenital generalized phlebectasia). J Pediatr. 1978;93:944–9.
34. Kienast AK, Hoeger PH. Cutis marmorata telangiectatica congenita: a prospective study of 27 cases and review of the literature with proposal of diagnostic criteria. Clin Exp Dermatol. 2009;34:319–23. https://doi.org/10.1111/j.1365-2230.2008.03074.x.
35. Garzon MC, Huang JT, Enjolras O, Frieden IJ. Vascular malformations. Part II: associated syndromes. J Am Acad Dermatol. 2007;56:541–64. https://doi.org/10.1016/j.jaad.2006.05.066.
36. Enjolras O. Cutis marmorata telangiectatica congenitaAnnales de dermatologie et de venereologie. 2001;128:161–6.
37. Lee MS, Liang MG, Mulliken JB. Diffuse capillary malformation with overgrowth: a clinical subtype of vascular anomalies with hypertrophy. J Am Acad Dermatol. 2013;69:589–94. https://doi.org/10.1016/j.jaad.2013.05.030.
38. Uihlein LC, Liang MG, Fishman SJ, Alomari AI, Mulliken JB. Capillary-venous malformation in the lower limb. Pediatr Dermatol. 2013;30:541–8. https://doi.org/10.1111/pde.12186.
39. Ruiz-Maldonado R, Tamayo L, Laterza AM, Brawn G, Lopez A. Phacomatosis pigmentovascularis: a new syndrome? Report of four cases. Pediatr Dermatol. 1987;4:189–96.

40. Fernandez-Guarino M, et al. Phakomatosis pigmentovascularis: clinical findings in 15 patients and review of the literature. J Am Acad Dermatol. 2008;58:88–93. https://doi.org/10.1016/j.jaad.2007.08.012.
41. Happle R. Phacomatosis pigmentovascularis revisited and reclassified. Arch Dermatol. 2005;141:385–8. https://doi.org/10.1001/archderm.141.3.385.
42. Strauss RP, Resnick SD. Pulsed dye laser therapy for port-wine stains in children: psychosocial and ethical issues. J Pediatr. 1993;122:505–10.
43. van der Horst CM, Koster PH, de Borgie CA, Bossuyt PM, van Gemert MJ. Effect of the timing of treatment of port-wine stains with the flash-lamp-pumped pulsed-dye laser. N Engl J Med. 1998;338:1028–33. https://doi.org/10.1056/NEJM199804093381504.
44. Renfro L, Geronemus RG. Anatomical differences of port-wine stains in response to treatment with the pulsed dye laser. Arch Dermatol. 1993;129:182–8.
45. Selim MM, et al. Confocal microscopy study of nerves and blood vessels in untreated and treated port wine stains: preliminary observations. Dermatol Surg. 2004;30:892–7. https://doi.org/10.1111/j.1524-4725.2004.30259.x.
46. Savas JA, Ledon JA, Franca K, Chacon A, Nouri K. Pulsed dye laser-resistant port-wine stains: mechanisms of resistance and implications for treatment. Br J Dermatol. 2013;168:941–53. https://doi.org/10.1111/bjd.12204.
47. Marques L, et al. Topical rapamycin combined with pulsed dye laser in the treatment of capillary vascular malformations in Sturge-Weber syndrome: phase II, randomized, double-blind, intraindividual placebo-controlled clinical trial. J Am Acad Dermatol. 2015;72:151–158.e151. https://doi.org/10.1016/j.jaad.2014.10.011.
48. Nelson JS, Jia W, Phung TL, Mihm MC Jr. Observations on enhanced port wine stain blanching induced by combined pulsed dye laser and rapamycin administration. Lasers Surg Med. 2011;43:939–42. https://doi.org/10.1002/lsm.21141.
49. Ramien ML, et al. Quality of life in pediatric patients before and after cosmetic camouflage of visible skin conditions. J Am Acad Dermatol. 2014;71:935–40. https://doi.org/10.1016/j.jaad.2014.07.029.

Venous Malformations and Associated Syndromes: Diagnosis and Management

9

Ann M. Kulungowski, Manish N. Patel, and Steven J. Fishman

Introduction

Venous malformations arise due to errors in vascular development during the first trimester of pregnancy. Venous malformations are present at birth though may not be readily apparent. Commonly, incorrectly labeled "cavernous hemangioma," venous malformations are not vascular tumors as the suffix *–oma* implies tumor. This terminology is confusing and should be avoided. The abnormal collections of veins may be localized or diffuse and can occur anywhere in the body, including the viscera such as brain and liver. Venous malformations frequently involve the skin and subcutaneous tissue with variable extension into the skeletal muscle and even bone. They can be associated with other vascular anomaly syndromes.

The presentation of venous malformations is variable, presenting as simple varicosities and ectasias, discrete masses, or a complex collection of channels infiltrating tissue or an organ system (Fig. 9.1). Venous malformations commonly present as a soft, compressible bluish mass with characteristic enlargement when placed in a dependent position. They are classified as focal, multifocal, or diffuse. Venous

A. M. Kulungowski (✉)
Division of Pediatric Surgery, Vascular Anomalies Center, University of Colorado School of Medicine, Children's Hospital Colorado, Aurora, CO, USA
e-mail: ann.kulungowski@childrenscolorado.org

M. N. Patel
Department of Radiology and Medical Imaging, Hemangioma and Vascular Malformation Center, University of Cincinnati School of Medicine, Cincinnati Children's Hospital Medical Center, Cincinnati, OH, USA
e-mail: manish.patel@cchmc.org

S. J. Fishman
Department of Surgery, Vascular Anomalies Center, Harvard Medical School, Children's Hospital Boston, Boston, MA, USA
e-mail: steven.fishman@childrens.harvard.edu

C. C. Trenor III, D. M. Adams (eds.), *Vascular Anomalies*,
https://doi.org/10.1007/978-3-030-25624-1_9

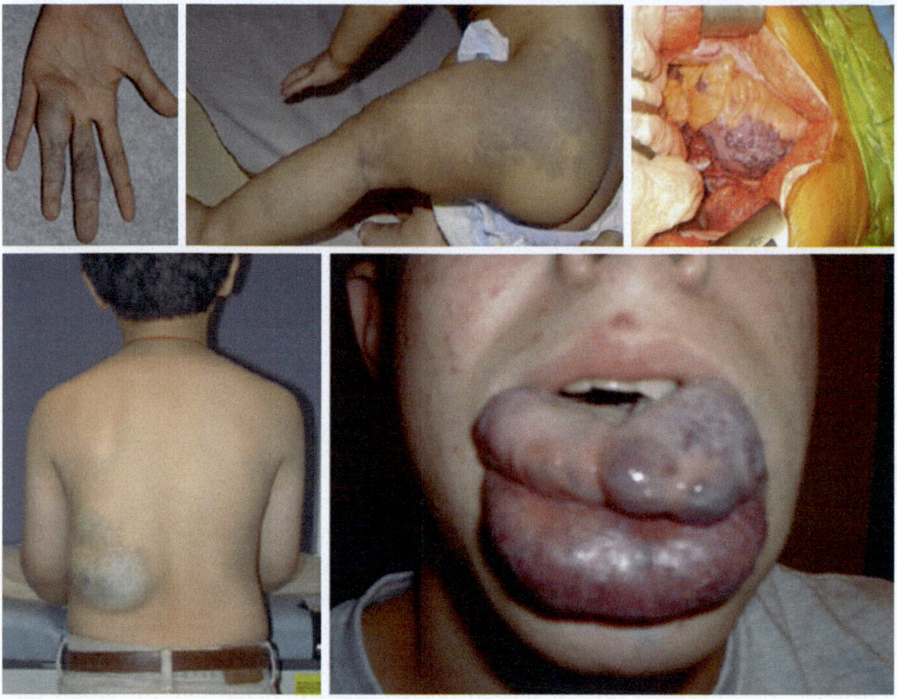

Fig. 9.1 Variable appearance of venous malformations involving the hand (*top, left*), left buttock and extremity (*top, middle*), colorectum (*top, right*), left flank (*bottom, left*), and tongue and lower lip (*bottom, right*)

malformations, as with other vascular malformations, grow proportionately with the child. Slow expansion and progression of venous malformations is observed with time, particularly during adolescence [1].

Histopathology

Sporadic venous malformations are composed of irregular channels, lined by a flat, inactive endothelium. The mural architecture is distorted with focally absent or scant smooth muscle. The diminished smooth muscle likely contributes to the observed expansion of venous malformations with time. Luminal diameter ranges from small to large. Venous channels present in a variety of shapes from round to clusters. The lumens are often filled with blood but are sometimes empty or contain protein.

Luminal thrombi in various stages of organization are often present. Phleboliths can be observed. Sometimes the venous malformation appears to have recanalized itself and demonstrates intravascular papillary, endothelial hyperplasia. This phenomenon also is known as a Masson's tumor or vegetant intravascular hemangioendothelioma [2]. The endothelium undergoes hyperplasia in response to thrombosis [3].

The histologic appearance of venous malformations associated with unique locations or with other syndromes may exhibit additional characteristics. Glomuvenous malformation is characterized by variably sized dysplastic venous-like channels. At least one of the layers of a glomuvenous malformation (GVM) is composed of uniform, cuboidal eosinophilic glomus cells. Smooth muscle of variable thickness is present in some channels. Organizing thrombus and phleboliths also are observed.

Cutaneomucosal venous malformations histopathologically are very thin walled with organizing thrombi. The channels are small to medium in size and are devoid of a smooth muscle layer except very focally [3].

The superficial cutaneous venous malformations in blue rubber bleb nevus syndrome (BRBNS) appear as large venous-like channels that lack smooth muscle. Deeper anomalous channels tend to have smooth muscle. The venous-like channels are separated by fibrous tissue. Thrombi and calcifications are frequently present. The intestinal lesions of blue rubber bleb nevus syndrome have a similar histologic appearance. The venous malformations tend to involve the submucosa mostly, though some are full thickness and can extend into the mesentery [3].

Histopathologic features of fibroadipose vascular anomaly (FAVA) include dense fibrous tissue, fat, and lymphoplasmacytic aggregates within atrophied muscle [4]. Large and sometimes smaller, irregular, and occasionally abnormally muscularized venous channels are present. Organizing thrombi, lymphatic components, and atrophied skeletal muscle can be observed. Dense fibrous tissue encircles the nerves. There is no evidence of arteriovenous shunting in the vasculature of fibroadipose vascular anomaly. Nerves, thick coiled arteries, and metaplastic bone are observed in some specimens [3].

Genetics

Most venous malformations are sporadic (99%), solitary, and localized [5]. Somatic mutations in the gene for the endothelial tyrosine kinase receptor TIE2 have been identified in approximately 60% of sporadic venous malformations [6–9]. TIE2 mutations cause chronic activation of the MAPK pathway which causes alterations in the normal endothelial cell layer due to fibronectin deficiency in the extracellular matrix. Plasminogen/plasmin pathway is also upregulated [8]. PIK3CA mutations are identified in 20% of sporadic venous malformations involving the subcutis [9]. Most patients with Klippel-Trenaunay (capillary/lymphaticovenous malformation with overgrowth) and congenital lipomatous overgrowth, vascular malformations, epidermal nevi, and skeletal anomalies (CLOVES) syndromes as well as FAVA have somatic mosaic PIK3CA mutations.

Cutaneomucosal venous malformations are caused by a gain-of-function mutation that inappropriately activates the TIE2 receptor [10]. *TIE2* causes defective veins likely by affecting endothelial cell behaviors such as proliferation, migration, tube formation, and other activities [10, 11]. TIE2 signaling is involved in signaling between endothelial and smooth muscle cells [12]. Penetrance is high (94%) and occurs equally between the genders [13].

BRBNS is caused by postzygotic activating TIE2 mutations [7]. There is no gender bias.

GVM is caused by mutations in the glomulin (GLMN) gene [14–16]. Not much is known about the function of glomulin. Glomuvenous malformations are mostly inherited in an autosomal dominant fashion [5]. One half of the inherited GVM go undiagnosed at birth and appear later in life. Sporadic GVM are present at birth [17]. Penetrance is high, approximately 90%, for heritable glomuvenous malformations [14]. There is no gender predilection. Inherited GVM tend to be smaller, multiple, and located all over the body.

Types and Unique Locations

Sporadic Venous Malformation

Venous malformations can arise in any tissue, including the muscle, bone, and hollow and solid viscera. They are most commonly found in the skin and soft tissues. Venous malformations usually are present at birth. They may not become apparent until later in life depending upon location. Their presentation is heterogeneous ranging from blue, soft, compressible masses to a diffuse network of venous channels that permeate an organ or tissue. Venous malformations grow proportionately with the child. The lesions tend to expand with time likely due to altered hemodynamics and disorganized muscular walls. Phlebothrombosis is common and can cause pain. Phleboliths may be palpable within the venous malformation. Clinical manifestations of venous malformations vary by anatomic location.

Head and Neck

Venous malformations of the head and neck are usually unilateral. They can be disfiguring and cause distortion of facial features. Dental malocclusion is common. Cervical venous malformations may cause obstruction of the pharynx, especially in the recumbent position. Airway compression can occur. Oropharyngeal lesions present significant risk of hemorrhage during procedures such as tooth extraction or tonsillectomy.

Extremities

Venous malformations of the extremities can be superficial, involving skin and subcutaneous tissue, or deep, involving the muscle and even bone. A limb length discrepancy may be present. The limb with the venous malformation may be longer or shorter. Intramuscular venous malformations can be debilitating due to pain. FAVA can present with contractures [4]. Venous malformations of the extremity may extend into the joints. Intra-articular lesions cause pain, swelling, contractures, weakness, and hemarthrosis [18, 19]. The joint is affected because the venous malformation forms a mass or results in arthritis. Synovium involved with venous malformation is prone to bleeding and swelling. The arthritis is likely due to generalized synovial inflammation and/or rapid cartilage degeneration. Arthropathy is a serious complication of repeated bloody effusions in joints with venous malformation. The synovial lining becomes fibrotic, and hyaline cartilage disintegrates causing pain, deformity, and functional impairment [20].

Diffuse phlebectasia of Bockenheimer is a particularly severe form of venous malformation affecting an extremity. Features include phlebectasia of all veins, superficial and deep, of the limb, muscular wasting, and near complete replacement of the muscle with venous malformation. The bones are often involved by venous malformation and are thin and prone to fracture.

Gastrointestinal

Venous malformations can occur in the solid and hollow viscera. Venous malformations of the hollow viscera can occur anywhere from mouth to anus. They can be solitary or multifocal and range in size from minute to massive. A faint blue stain in the perineum may indicate an underlying pelvic venous malformation. Gastrointestinal venous malformations most commonly occur as transmural lesions of the left colon and rectum with variable local extension into pelvic structures (Fig. 9.1) [21–23]. Mesenteric and portal venous anomalies may be associated. A rectal venous malformation associated with ectasia of mesenteric veins is a risk factor for portomesenteric venous thrombosis [24].

Gastrointestinal bleeding is the most common presenting symptom of hollow visceral venous malformations. Hematemesis is rare. The bleeding is usually per rectum in the form of hematochezia or melena. Chronic bleeding can go unrecognized. Anemia of unknown etiology can be the initial manifestation. The bleeding is usually slow and does not cause hemodynamic compromise. Colorectal lesions can cause spasmodic abdominal pain. Intestinal obstruction by a venous malformation is rare. Intussusception can occur with intestinal venous malformations.

Hepatic

Hepatic venous malformations are commonly, improperly referred to as "hemangiomas" or "hemangioendotheliomas." Due to confusion regarding nomenclature, patients have received erroneous therapies such as corticosteroid or embolization. Hepatic hemangiomas are true tumors of infancy. Hepatic venous malformations are typically identified during adulthood. They likely arise due to slow, gradual expansion from smaller lesions. Autopsy series report a prevalence of 0.4–7.5% [25]. Some hepatic venous malformations can be massive. They may cause pain. Rupture is exceedingly rare. Concern arises during pregnancy with large lesions due to increases, especially during labor, of intra-abdominal pressure. Planning for a cesarean section can be considered for a symptomatic patient; there is little objective data regarding management [26]. Observation with serial ultrasonography can be performed to follow the venous malformations. Asymptomatic lesions can be followed at less frequent intervals.

Genitourinary

Venous malformations can occur in any of the structures of the genitourinary tract. The renal pyramids and pelvis, ureters, and bladder can be involved [27]. Bladder venous malformations occur in isolation or as a component of a more extensive

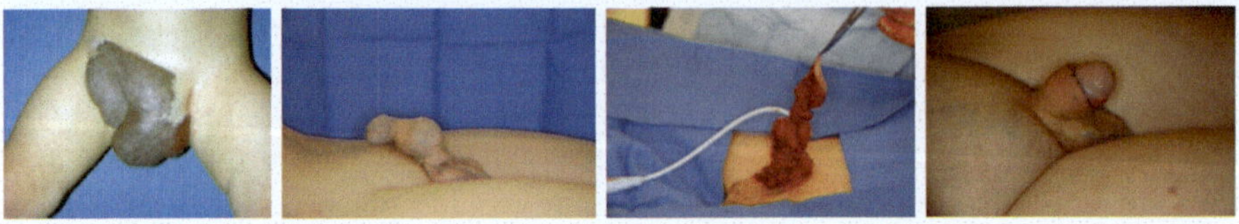

Fig. 9.2 Genital venous malformations. Venous malformations of the labia majora and perineum causing expansion and distortion of the labia (*left*). Penile shaft and scrotal venous malformation (*left, middle*) undergoing debulking surgery (*right, middle*). Final appearance of the penis after resection (*right*)

vascular malformation of the pelvis and/or lower extremities. Genitourinary venous malformations can be asymptomatic or cause hematuria. Renal colic can arise if larger clots are passed.

Venous malformations of the genitalia do occur (Fig. 9.2). In girls and women, the uterus and vagina can be involved. Excessive bleeding with menstruation or intercourse is the exception. Involvement of the external genitalia can cause psychological distress for the patient and family. Pain is a common complaint due to near constant dependency. Venous malformations in women may block the introitus, making urination and intercourse difficult. The penis and scrotum can be affected (Fig. 9.2). Impotence in men is uncommon, as the corpora cavernosum are generally intact. Hematuria and hematospermia can occur if there is urethral involvement.

Bone

Intraosseous venous malformations can be present as solitary lesions or be associated with extremity venous malformations. Bony venous malformations mostly occur in the cranium, vertebrae, scapulae, ribs, pelvis, and long bones. Diagnosis without a biopsy is challenging as the venous malformations cannot always be distinguished from other benign tumors, cysts, and granulomas. The continued application of the term "hemangioma" to describe intraosseous venous malformation adds to the diagnostic conundrum [28].

Glomuvenous Malformations (GVM)

Glomuvenous malformations almost always are superficial, occurring in the skin and subcutaneous fat. The trunk and extremities are typical locations. The face can be affected [29]. Glomuvenous malformations are variable in their presentation with regard to size and color. Some present as nodular and scattered or plaque-like and regional, covering an extremity [30]. The inherited glomuvenous malformations tend to be smaller lesions scattered throughout the body. The color can be pink, purple, or dark blue. Pain is a common symptom. Compression does not decompress a glomuvenous malformation and tends to exacerbate discomfort.

Cutaneomucosal Venous Malformation

Cutaneoumucosal venous malformations tend to be small, less than 5 cm in diameter, and multiple. A solitary lesion is identified in approximately 25% of patients. About half of the venous malformations occur in cervicofacial area; 37% occur on the extremities [5]. The lesions are usually superficial and rarely extend into the muscle. Joints are not involved. Cutaneomucosal venous malformations have been found in gastrointestinal tract, brain, and lungs [31].

Blue Rubber Bleb Nevus Syndrome (BRBNS)

The venous malformations in blue rubber bleb nevus syndrome consist of multifocal lesions that affect the skin and gastrointestinal tract (Fig. 9.3) [32, 33]. The cutaneous venous malformations in blue rubber bleb nevus syndrome are true venous malformations and not nevi. There is commonly a dominant, large cutaneous lesion associated with multiple smaller venous malformations in the palmoplantar surfaces. The venous malformations are typically 1–2 cm in size and range in color from blue to purple.

The gastrointestinal lesions are more clinically relevant than the venous malformations of the skin and soft tissue [34]. The venous malformations in the gastrointestinal tract are similar in their appearance to the cutaneous lesions. There is a direct correlation between the number of cutaneous and visceral lesions [34]. The gastrointestinal venous malformations can cause gastrointestinal bleeding at a young age. The bleeding can continue throughout the patient's life. Massive sudden hemorrhage is rare. Rather, the patients are chronically anemic, requiring lifelong iron replacement and repeated blood transfusions if not treated [34]. The gastrointestinal lesions can serve as a lead point for small bowel intussusception. This complication can be self-limited, causing intermittent crampy abdominal pain, or result in intestinal obstruction, necessitating operative intervention [35, 36].

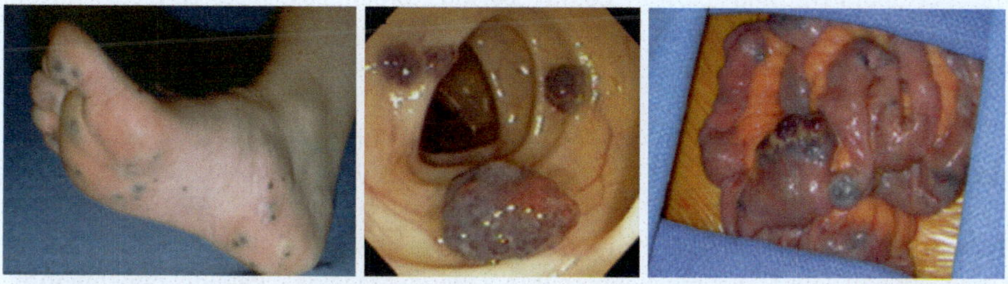

Fig. 9.3 Blue rubber bleb nevus syndrome. The characteristic appearances of multifocal venous malformation involving the sole of the foot (*left*), colon during endoscopy (*middle*), and small intestine at time of laparotomy (*right*)

Fibroadipose Vascular Anomaly (FAVA)

Fibroadipose vascular anomaly most commonly presents with a painful intramuscular mass of an extremity [4]. The calf is most commonly involved; the upper extremity can be affected. There is fibrofatty overgrowth and phlebectasia. The muscle features fibrotic replacement. Presentation ranges from birth to adulthood. Contracture of the affected extremity is common.

Venous Ectasia

Focal venous ectasia of the internal and/or external jugular veins is a form of venous malformation. The patient usually presents with a compressible, painless neck mass that increases in size with a Valsalva maneuver. The neck mass can be of considerable size [37].

Venous ectasias are also observed in patients with some combined, complex, and syndromic vascular anomalies such as in Klippel-Trenaunay and CLOVES (congenital lipomatous overgrowth, vascular malformations, epidermal nevi, and skeletal anomalies) syndromes. Persistent embryonic veins are found in the lower extremities of patients with Klippel-Trenaunay syndrome (Fig. 9.4). The marginal venous system is a network of embryologic veins originating in the dorsum of the foot and ascending the lateral aspect of the calf and thigh. The system terminates in the femoral or iliac veins or the inferior vena cava. Phlebectasias in CLOVES syndrome are located in the limbs, centrally, and thorax. The involved veins can be orthotopic or persistent embryonic veins. Potentially involved orthotopic veins include the jugular, axillary, subclavian, innominate, intercostal, azygous, and short saphenous veins. The vena cava, superior and inferior, portions can also be involved. These large orthotopic or embryonic veins can dilate with time. Due to capaciousness and direct connection to larger veins, embryologic and phlebectatic veins predispose patients to the risk of deep venous thrombosis and pulmonary embolism [38]. Risk of deep venous thrombosis and pulmonary embolism is increased during the perioperative and periprocedural period, pregnancy, bed rest, or travel. Periprocedural thromboembolism for patients with Klippel-Trenaunay and CLOVES syndromes is approximately 10% [39].

Assessment

Pain is the most common symptom associated with venous malformations. Congestive discomfort is most apparent in dependent lesions. Patients may mention a sense of heaviness, especially more so with dependency, in the area of a venous malformation. Venous malformations are problematic as they can cause disfigurement or apply pressure on neighboring structures. Life-threatening hemorrhage from a venous malformation after minor trauma is uncommon.

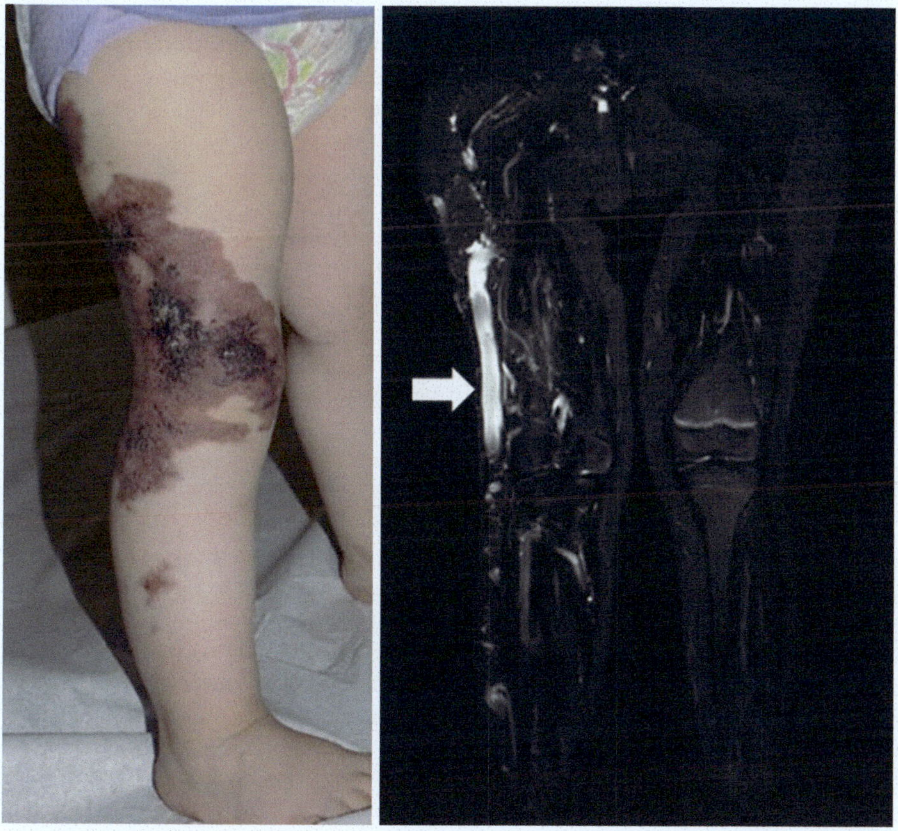

Fig. 9.4 Toddler with Klippel-Trenaunay syndrome of the right lower extremity with laterally placed capillary and lymphatic malformations (*left*). Coronal STIR MRI sequence of the right leg shows a lateral marginal vein (*right, arrow*)

A localized intravascular coagulopathy can be associated with large, extensive venous malformations ($\geq$10 cm^2) and multifocal lesions [40]. Constant activation of coagulation due do stagnation of blood within the venous malformation leads to consumption of coagulation factors. Thrombin is produced and converts fibrinogen into fibrin. Fibrinolysis elevates fibrin degradation products. Fibrinogen, factor V, factor VIII, factor XIII, and antithrombin III also are low. The chronic consumptive coagulopathy causes episodes of thrombosis, leading to the formation of phleboliths, or bleeding. The coagulopathy can be exacerbated by discontinuation of compression, intervention (sclerotherapy or surgical procedure), menses, or pregnancy.

Coagulation studies (prothrombin time, activated partial thromboplastin time, and D-dimer and fibrinogen levels) should be assessed in patients with diffuse and multifocal venous malformations, especially prior to invasive procedures. Patients at higher risk of bleeding and clotting have higher D-dimers and lower fibrinogen. Low von Willebrand factor (vWF) also occurs in patients with large venous malformations especially of the limbs and trunk [41]. Platelet counts can also be slightly decreased in the 100,000 to 150,000/mm^3 range. Localized intravascular coagulopathy should not be confused with Kasabach-Merritt phenomenon that is observed with kaposiform hemangioendothelioma. (See Coagulation chapter.)

Imaging

Most vascular malformations can be accurately diagnosed by history and physical examination. Imaging is an invaluable adjunct as it provides diagnostic confirmation, documents the size and the extent of the lesion, and assists with therapeutic planning.

Conventional plain film radiographs of venous malformations are not required. They can be used to document leg length discrepancy. Bony destruction and distortion can be seen. Phleboliths are identified by plain films when present.

Gray-scale and color Doppler ultrasound with spectral analysis provide a rapid, minimally invasive method for evaluating vascular anomalies. Focal venous malformations are compressible with ultrasound and generally appear as hypoechoic channels or masses with multiple septations (Fig. 9.5). Little to no flow is present within a venous malformation unless the lesion is compressed or augmented. The malformation refills when the pressure is released. Phleboliths appear as focal areas of increased echogenicity with acoustic shadowing. No arteriovenous shunting should be present within a venous malformation. Ultrasound does not define the depth or the extent of a large, deep venous malformation but can adequately image superficial lesions.

Magnetic resonance imaging (MRI) is the preferred imaging modality for the evaluation of vascular malformations. Venous malformations typically are bright on T2-weighted sequences (Figs. 9.5 and 9.6). MRI accurately defines the location and extent of the lesion and provides information regarding adjacent structures including nerves, joint space involvement, and venous inflow and outflow (Figs. 9.5 and 9.6). Gradient echo sequences help distinguish slow flow versus fast flow lesions. Contrast-enhanced sequences are useful to distinguish venous from lymphatic malformations. Venous malformations tend to have more diffuse enhancement compared to septal enhancement of macrocystic lymphatic malformations. Microcystic lymphatic malformations can be at times difficult to distinguish from VM. Fibroadipose vascular anomaly (FAVA) MRI characteristics include heterogeneous high T1-weighted signal (due to the fatty component) with increased intensity on T2-weighted sequences (Fig. 9.7) [4]. Contrast-enhanced MRI of fibroadipose vascular anomaly shows moderate to strong enhancement of the affected muscle. A fatty component can be seen within the intrafascial/intramuscular compartment and within the subcutis [4].

Magnetic resonance angiography and venography can provide supplemental information regarding flow and mapping of venous channels. Limitations of MRI include the potential need for a general anesthetic dependent upon patient age and/

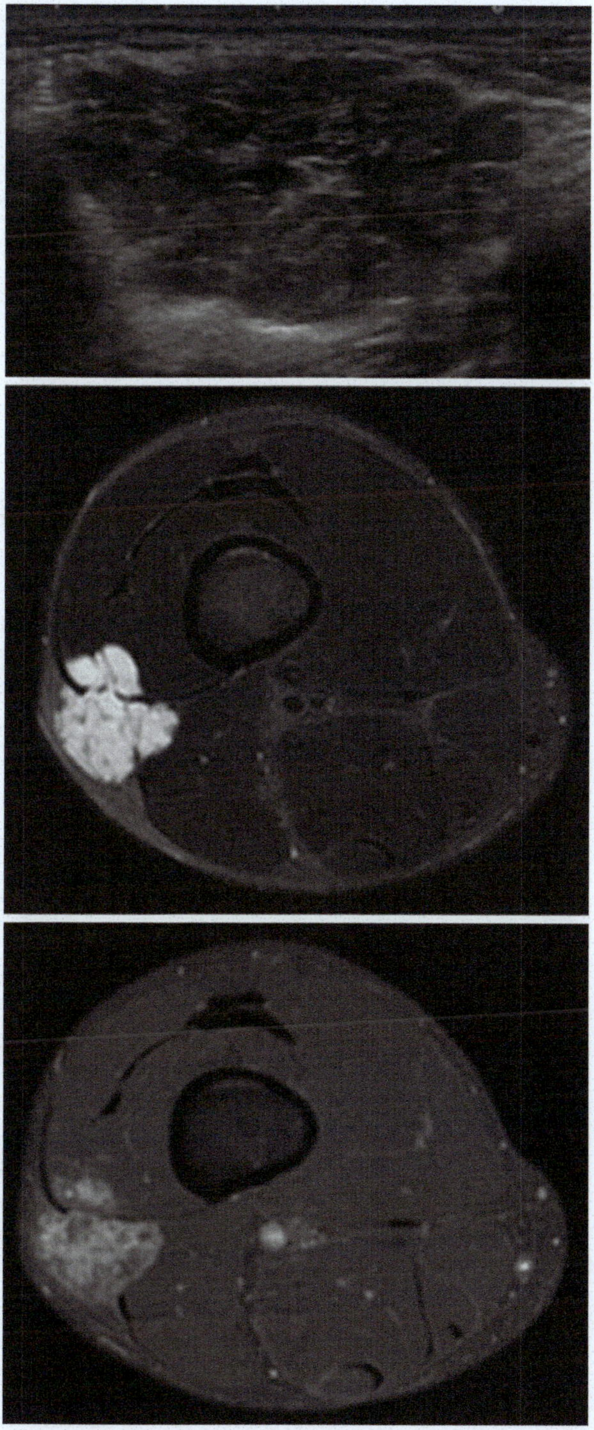

Fig. 9.5 Venous malformation of the thigh within the subcutaneous fat with extension into the vastus lateralis muscle. The venous malformation is predominately hypoechoic on ultrasound (*top*) with multiple internal septations. The venous malformation is bright on T2-weighted MRI (*middle*) with generalized enhancement on contrast-enhanced MRI (*bottom*). Internal septations within the lesion are also noted on MRI

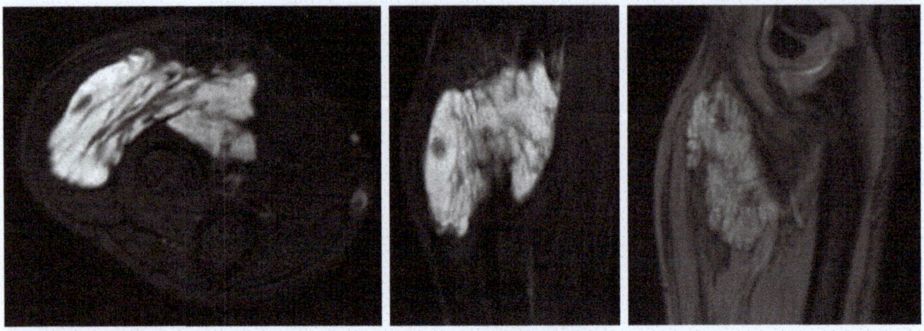

Fig. 9.6 Intramuscular venous malformation of the forearm. Axial (*left*) and coronal (*middle*) T2-weighted MRI (*right*) demonstrate a venous malformation of increased T2 signal. The venous malformation has multiple septations with phleboliths. Diffuse enhancement (*right*) is noted on contrast-enhanced sequences

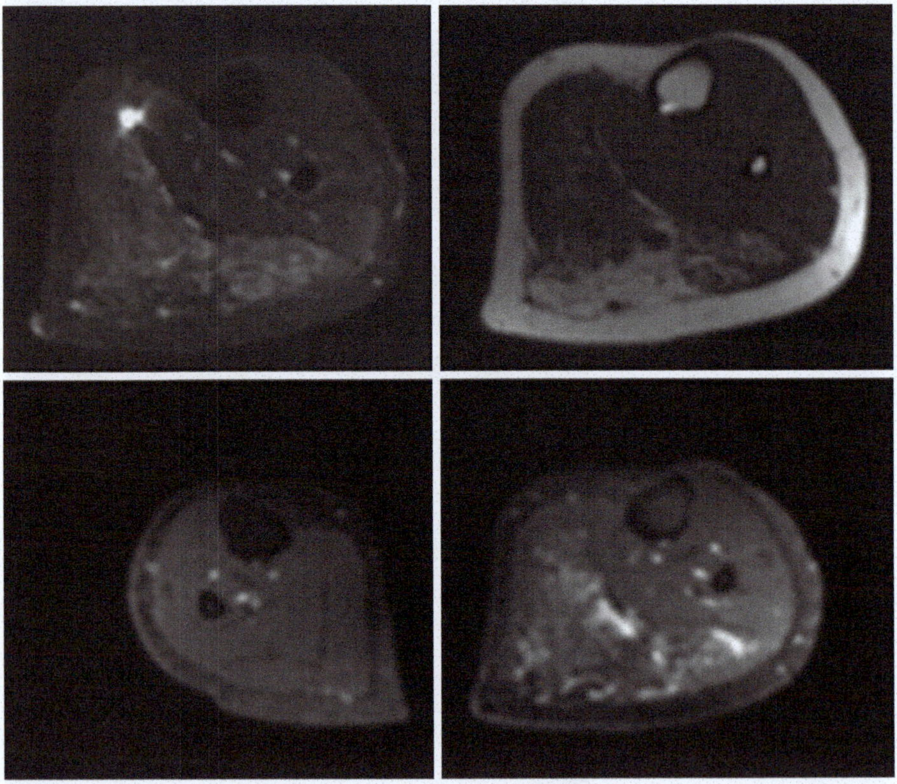

Fig. 9.7 Fibroadipose vascular anomaly (FAVA) of the left calf. Patient presented with chronic pain and swelling of left calf. Axial T2- (*top, left*), T1- (*top, right*), and post-contrast T2-weighted (*bottom*) MR images showing fat containing intramuscular lesion of the posterior musculature of the calf with heterogeneous T2 signal (*top, left*) and enhancement of post-contrast images (*bottom*) consistent with FAVA. (Images courtesy of Dr. Gulraiz Chaudry)

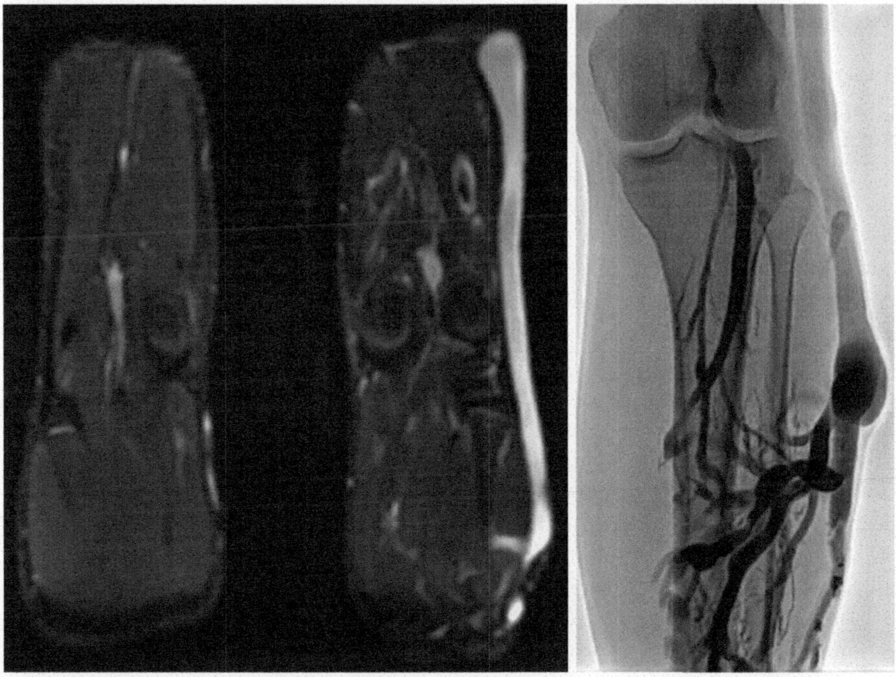

Fig. 9.8 Teenager with an extensive capillary venolymphatic malformation involving his left lower extremity. T2-weighted coronal MRI (*left*) and conventional venogram (*right*) demonstrate a prominent marginal vein along the lateral aspect of the leg. Numerous ectatic venous channels are seen on the conventional venogram draining into the marginal vein. Additionally, a deep venous system was present and patient had eventual thermal ablation of this marginal vein

or length of study, intravenous access particularly when contrast is administered, and exposure to gadolinium-based contrast agents. Nephrogenic systemic fibrosis is a rare reaction to gadolinium contrast-based agents. Patients especially susceptible are those with moderate to end-stage renal failure.

Computed tomography is rarely indicated. In general, computed tomography is inferior to magnetic resonance imaging. The density of venous malformation is similar to that of muscle and shows slow, heterogeneous enhancement. The presence of phleboliths may confirm the diagnosis.

Conventional venography by direct puncture followed by contrast injection demonstrates the morphology, interconnections, and draining veins of the venous malformation (Fig. 9.8). The channels are variable in their appearance. Diffuse intramuscular venous malformations can have the appearance of channels or "lakes." Embryonic or phlebectatic veins can present as fusiform channels.

Management

Coagulopathy and Thrombosis (I Have Not Seen the Coagulation Chapter but if Management Is Included in that Chapter the Chapter Should Be Referred to and All of this Taken Out)

A chronic consumptive coagulopathy can contribute to thrombosis or bleeding. Phleboliths form as a result of thrombosis. Bleeding risk is increased due to a concomitant reduction in von Willebrand factor and platelets. All patients with an extensive, either diffuse or multifocal, venous malformation should have evaluation with laboratories prior to any surgical or interventional procedure or pregnancy. Laboratory tests include a complete blood count, prothrombin time, activated partial thromboplastin time, D-dimer, and fibrinogen levels. A prothrombotic assessment should be included to identify patients at increased risk of thrombotic events if needed. These laboratories include proteins C and S, prothrombin gene mutation, thrombin-antithrombin, factor V Leiden, PAI-1 polymorphism, factor VIII, homocysteine level, lupus anticoagulant, anticardiolipin antibody, and antithrombin III [42]. A hematologic consultation is recommended for patients with abnormal laboratories, especially prior to any procedures or pregnancy.

Consideration should be given to treatment with low-molecular-weight heparin to improve the coagulation profile for patients with elevated D-dimer levels during the perioperative period, pregnancy, bed rest, or travel. Low-molecular-weight heparin is initiated 2 weeks prior to an operation or intervention and for 2 weeks thereafter [42]. Dosing during pregnancy should be managed by a hematologist and maternal-fetal specialist.

Pulmonary Arterial Hypertension (Need to See if this Is in the Coagulation Chapter)

Extensive venous malformations can lead to pulmonary arterial hypertension. Chronic thromboembolic pulmonary hypertension is due to recurrent or unresolved pulmonary embolism caused by localized intravascular coagulopathy and a hypercoagulable state. Elevated D-dimer correlates to an increase risk of pulmonary arterial hypertension in patients with extensive venous malformations [43]. Echocardiography is critical for evaluation of these patients.

Treatment

Treatment can broadly be divided into medical, interventional, surgical, and combined approaches. Pain, bleeding, disfigurement, and intra-articular involvement are reasons to consider treatment.

Medical Management

Compression Garments

Compression is the mainstay of therapy for venous malformations, especially for a lesion of the extremity. Graded elastic compression garments can be worn while upright during the day and removed during the night. The garments should be customized for the patient. For growing children and adolescents, garments should be resized to account for growth at approximately 6-month intervals. At least two garments should be available to increase compliance.

Anti-inflammatory Medication

There is no known systemic pharmacologic agent known to treat reduce the size of venous malformations. Current medical management is used to target side effects. Anti-inflammatory medications and aspirin can be used for pain and swelling. Narcotics should be limited [44].

Anticoagulants

Low-molecular-weight heparin is used to treat localized intravascular coagulopathy associated with venous malformations. It also is used to manage chronic pain caused by inflammation, thrombosis, and formation of phleboliths in large venous malformations. Patients receiving long-term low-molecular-weight heparin should have their heparin levels (anti-factor Xa) followed. A dexa scan is recommended during chronic low-molecular-weight heparin use to evaluate for osteopenia.

Sirolimus

The phosphatidylinositol 3-kinase (PI3K)/AKT signaling pathway which is essential for cell growth and survival directs vascular development and angiogenesis. Sirolimus, a mammalian target of rapamycin (mTOR), combines signals from the PI3K/AKT pathway to ensure proper cell growth and proliferation. Upregulation of mTOR signaling increases expression of vascular endothelial growth factor, essential for angiogenesis and lymphangiogenesis [45]. Disorders with inappropriate activation of the PI3K/AKT/mTOR pathway result in overgrowth in association with vascular anomalies. Sirolimus has shown promise for patient with complicated vascular anomalies such as Klippel-Trenaunay and CLOVES syndromes with regard to symptom control. Similarly, fibroadipose vascular anomaly responds to sirolimus with improvement in pain and quality of life [46]. Sirolimus has been shown to ameliorate pain and transfusion requirements in patients with blue rubber bleb nevus syndrome [47]. Sirolimus has been shown to be effective in diffuse venous malformations such as TIE2 lesions and diffuse lesions by improving coagulations parameters and decreasing pain [48].

Iron

Patients who exhibit chronic blood loss anemia related to gastrointestinal bleeding may require lifelong iron replacement and repeat blood transfusions.

Interventional Management

Interventional treatment for venous malformations includes sclerotherapy, venous embolization, and endovenous ablation [49]. A pretreatment magnetic resonance image may be helpful prior to intervention as it illustrates the extent of the venous malformation. In general, focal, well-localized venous malformations without peripheral drainage are more easily treated, whereas diffuse venous malformations are more challenging to treat and often communicate with the main conducting veins which are often abnormal.

Sclerotherapy is the injection of a sclerosant directly into abnormal venous channels through a needle or short cannula (Figs. 9.9 and 9.10). Sclerosants are irritants that cause endothelial injury resulting in luminal obliteration due to thrombosis and fibrosis. Infants and children often require general anesthesia as injection of the sclerosant is painful. The venous malformation is accessed typically under ultrasonographic guidance. Contrast medium is injected under fluoroscopy (Figs. 9.9 and 9.10) to verify the lesion and document the venous outflow. The amount of sclerosant injected is usually less than the amount of contrast medium required to opacify the venous malformation [49] thought variable. Application of pressure and/or tourniquets can limit venous drainage and minimize systemic delivery of sclerosant during the procedure. Progressive induration of the soft tissues, indicative of thrombosis, may be palpable for more superficial venous malformations.

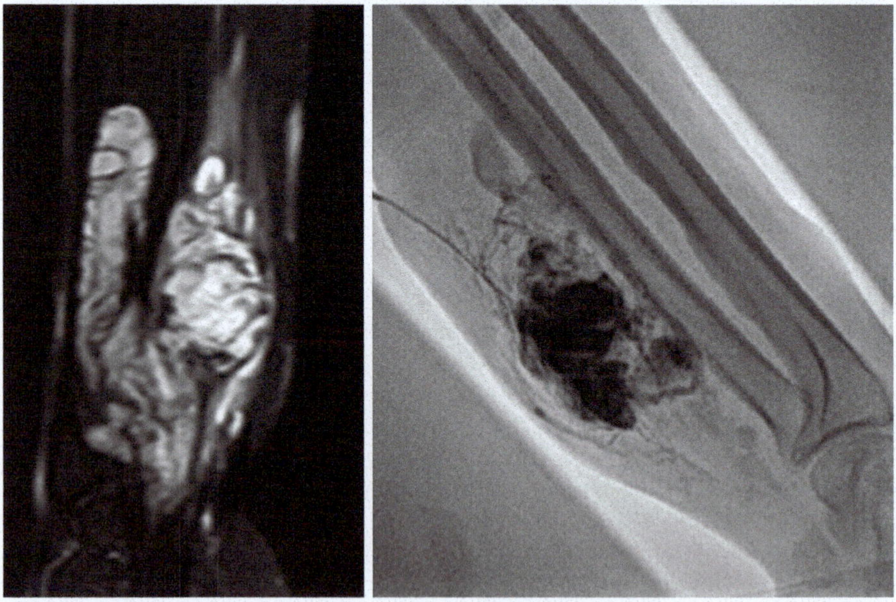

Fig. 9.9 Intramuscular venous malformation of the forearm. Lesion is hyperintense on T2-weighted imaging (*left*) with multiple septations and phleboliths. Selected image from sclerotherapy (*right*) demonstrates contrast opacification of the venous malformation with little wash out into the intramuscular or deep venous system

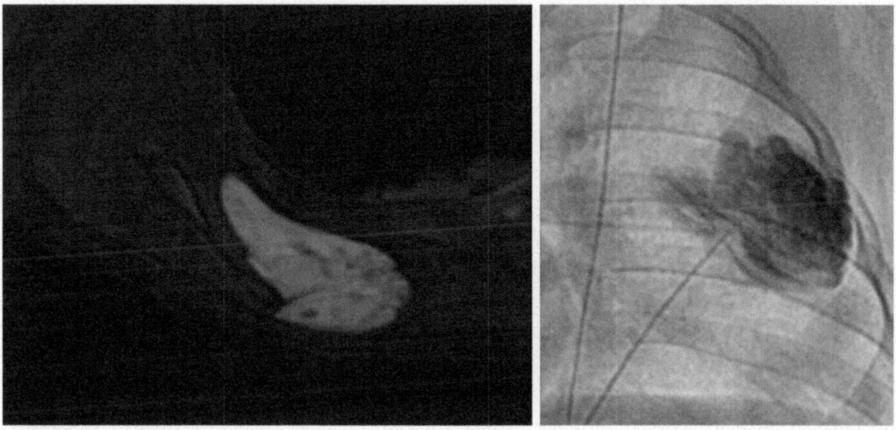

Fig. 9.10 Venous malformation of the chest wall located between the ribs and scapula. The lesion is bright on T2-weighted images (*left*). Multiple phleboliths are present within the multi-septated venous malformation. Selected image from a sclerotherapy procedure (*right*) shows contrast installation and opacification of the venous malformation

Venous embolization involves placement of a liquid embolic agent, coils, or occlusive devices into venous outflow channels through a catheter. This allows an effective way to keep the sclerosant within the venous malformation [50]. Sclerosant can then be injected so that the substance is sequestered within the malformation.

Common sclerosants include ethanol, sodium tetradecyl sulfate, and bleomycin. Foam sclerosant is made by mixing air or air and oily contrast medium (Lipiodol or Ethidol) with a surfactant sclerosant like sodium tetradecyl sulfate. Foam sclerosant mixtures are more efficacious in treating venous malformations as they increase the treatment surface area [51]. Foam sclerosant mixtures result in less risk of swelling, cardiovascular collapse, and nerve injury when compared to ethanol [51]. Bleomycin sclerotherapy results in less swelling of surrounding tissues than other sclerosants. It is ideal for locations where swelling is less well tolerated such as the airway, orbit, or perineum. Sclerotherapy should be administered by experienced practitioners with appropriate monitoring of the patient due to the risk of side effects.

Complications of sclerotherapy of venous malformations are infrequent but include skin breakdown and ulceration, deep venous thrombosis and pulmonary embolism, nerve injury, and compartment syndrome. These complications are more prevalent when ethanol is used as the sclerosant. The more common side effects include swelling, edema, and pain regardless of the sclerosant. Additional side effects of ethanol include pulmonary hypertension, cardiovascular collapse, and central nervous system depression requiring more care with its usage [49, 52]. Foam sclerosant mixtures result in less side effects but are not risk-free [49]. Bleomycin is associated with pulmonary fibrosis and require long-term dosage monitoring. In patients with underlying baseline coagulopathy and history of deep venous thrombosis, placement of IVC filters may be considered.

Advantages of sclerotherapy include no incisional scars, decreased risk of neurovascular injury compared to surgical excision, and opportunity for outpatient procedures. Disadvantages include the possible need for multiple procedures and radiation exposure. Sclerotherapy procedures are most effective when performed as a series of procedures, spaced 2–3 months apart [49].

Endovenous thermal ablation is a procedure that ablates prominent venous ectasias and persistent embryonic veins seen in Klippel-Trenaunay and CLOVES syndromes. Endovenous thermal ablation is typically performed with endovenous laser or radio frequency probes. Combining this technique with sclerotherapy and occlusion of the venous malformation's drainage enhances efficacy. Additionally, image-guided percutaneous cryoablation is a safe and effective treatment option for fibroadipose vascular anomalies [53].

After sclerotherapy and interventional procedures, compressive dressings are applied if possible. The treated site can be elevated and iced to help minimize swelling. Systemic corticosteroid can be administered for swelling in the head and neck. Patients at risk for airway obstruction, compartment syndrome, or those with baseline coagulopathy are admitted to the hospital for observation. If swelling around the airway is of concern, the patient may be left intubated [49]. Pain is managed with oral and/or systemic analgesic medications. Intravenous fluid is administered at twice maintenance during and after sclerotherapy to avoid hemoglobinuria. Hemoglobinuria occurs due to hemolysis, especially after injecting a large volume of sclerosant [54].

Preoperative embolization of venous malformations with n-butyl cyanoacrylate prior to surgical debulking has been shown to be safe and effective in children with the potential for minimizing blood loss and maximizing tissue and functional preservation [55, 56].

Surgical Management

Resection of venous malformations is indicated to reduce bulk, improve function, alter contour, reconstruct tissues altered or damaged by sclerotherapy, and to relieve pain. Surgical resection of venous malformations is ideal for focal lesions (Fig. 9.2). Preoperative sclerotherapy and glue embolization may allow resection of larger lesions and mitigate blood loss. Staged subtotal resections are often necessary for larger malformations. Operations near vital structures can be long and tedious. Preoperative planning is critical. Prior to the procedure, the surgeon should determine the extent of resection and abide by it. Dissection in the defined area of resection should be thorough to prevent reentry into scarred areas. Repeat excision of the same area is technically challenging and increases morbidity [21]. Partial dissection of large muscle groups in a piecemeal fashion increases the risk of contracture [57]. Major neurovascular structures should be preserved. Blood loss should be minimized with the use of compression and/or tourniquets when possible. A plan for blood and blood product replacement should be in place prior to commencement of the resection. Closed suction drainage of the resection cavity is usually necessary.

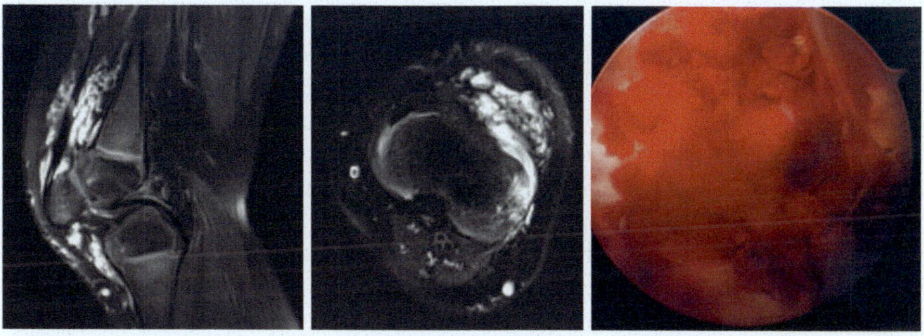

Fig. 9.11 Intra-articular venous malformation of the knee. T2-weighted sagittal (*left*) and axial (*right*) images of the knee demonstrate high signal within the intramuscular aspect of the knee with direct extension into the suprapatellar bursa and Hoffa's fat pad. Intra-articular appearance of venous malformation of the knee during arthroscopic resection (*right*)

Extremity venous malformation resection is generally reserved for those that are reasonably well localized in the subcutaneous tissues or a single muscle group, lesions with thrombosis, and those causing neurologic impairment or compressive problems [57]. For venous malformations with joint involvement, resection of the intra-articular component can treat pain and prevent joint destruction (Fig. 9.11). Eliminating recurrent hemarthroses helps prevent destruction of the articular cartilage. Joint synovectomy can be performed arthroscopically or with open resection. Bleeding may obscure visualization during an arthroscopic procedure. Open procedures are sometimes preferred to improve visualization and to maximize opportunity for a complete resection. Total joint arthroplasty is a salvage, end-stage procedure [20].

Gastrointestinal venous malformations that are asymptomatic can be managed expectantly. Gastrointestinal venous malformations that present with bleeding requiring transfusion, pain, intussusception, obstruction, and/or infection due to disruption of the mucosal barrier should be considered for surgical resection when technically feasible. Focal venous malformations limited to a specific region of a hollow viscus reliably can be resected [58]. Small, focal or multifocal, intraluminal venous malformations may be amenable to endoscopic or intraoperative sclerotherapy [22].

Patients with multifocal venous malformations of blue rubber bleb nevus syndrome resulting in anemia should be evaluated for surgical resection. These patients should have complete intraoperative gastrointestinal endoscopy, from mouth to anus, in order to identify all venous malformations. Upper endoscopy identifies lesions in the stomach, duodenum, and proximal jejunum. Small intestinal venous malformations can be identified during laparotomy by evaluating the luminal surface with a laparoscope. The laparoscope is placed through enterotomies made to remove full-thickness lesions, allowing visualization of a few feet of small intestine at a time. Colorectal lesions are detected with on-table, open-abdominal transanal colonoscopy. The venous malformations can be removed by wedge excision and polypectomy by intussusception of successive lengths of intestine. Bowel resection should be avoided to preserve intestinal length. This tedious approach is durable and can ameliorate transfusion dependence and anemia [34].

Diffuse colorectal venous malformations can be treated with colectomy, anorectal mucosectomy, and coloanal pull-through [59]. Fatal hemorrhage from the extrarectal venous malformation can occur if an attempt is made to resect the full-thickness of the rectum. Bleeding during the mucosectomy makes the dissection tedious. The mucosectomy is commenced approximately 1 to 2 centimeters above the dentate line to preserve endoanal sensation and maintain continence. Two teams can work simultaneously from the pelvis and transanal approaches to minimize the duration of the dissection.

Associated ectatic inferior mesenteric veins that accompany pelvic and colorectal venous malformations must be identified preoperatively. If bleeding is brisk enough from the associated colorectal venous malformation to necessitate surgical resection, the ectatic inferior mesenteric vein should be treated with prophylactic anticoagulation until the operation. The inferior mesenteric vein should be ligated proximally, simultaneous with the pull-through. If a pull-through is not warranted, proximal ligation of the inferior mesenteric vein should be performed to prevent portomesenteric thrombosis and portal hypertension [26].

Surgical intervention for hepatic and genitourinary venous malformations is sometimes necessary. Enucleation is favored over anatomic hepatic resection for symptomatic or rapidly expanding hepatic venous malformations. There is no definable size at which a hepatic venous malformation necessitates surgical treatment. Venous malformations of the urinary tract infrequently require surgery. Nephrectomy or partial nephrectomy is rarely necessary. Bleeding bladder venous malformations can be treated with cystoscopy and laser photocoagulation if superficial. More bulky symptomatic bladder lesions may require partial cystectomy. Visible genital venous malformations can be amenable to surgical debulking and contour resection. These procedures can improve pain and bring tremendous psychological benefit. If there are no functional limitations due to the presence of a genital venous malformation in infancy, it is prudent to delay treatment until structures are larger and closer to anatomical maturity [60].

Outcomes

Outcomes for patients with venous malformations are expressed in terms of symptom control [49]. "Cure" after interventional and surgical procedures is the exception. Venous malformations tend to recanalize and recur after treatment [61, 62]. Continued compression therapy should be utilized after treatment. Multimodality therapy combing interventional and surgical procedures can lead to improved results.

Conclusions

Venous malformations are heterogeneous in presentation. They can occur in isolation or in association with more complex syndromes. A multidisciplinary approach that allows for an individualized treatment plan improves patient satisfaction, outcomes, and potentially minimizes morbidity.

References

1. Hassanein AH, Mulliken JB, Fishman SJ, Alomari AI, Zurakowski D, Greene AK. Venous malformation: risk of progression during childhood and adolescence. Ann Plast Surg. 2012;68(2):198–201.
2. Masson P. Hemangioendotheliome vegetant intravasculaire. Anat Paris. 1923;93:517.
3. Kozakewich HPMJ. Histopathology of vascular malformations. In: Mulliken JB, Burrows P, Fishman SJ, editors. Mulliken and Young's vascular anomalies: hemangiomas and malformations. 2nd ed. New York: Oxford University Press; 2013. p. 480–507.
4. Alomari AI, Spencer SA, Arnold RW, et al. Fibro-adipose vascular anomaly: clinical-radiologic-pathologic features of a newly delineated disorder of the extremity. J Pediatr Orthop. 2014;34(1):109–17.
5. Boon LM, Mulliken JB, Enjolras O, Vikkula M. Glomuvenous malformation (glomangioma) and venous malformation: distinct clinicopathologic and genetic entities. Arch Dermatol. 2004;140(8):971–6.
6. Limaye N, Wouters V, Uebelhoer M, et al. Somatic mutations in angiopoietin receptor gene TEK cause solitary and multiple sporadic venous malformations. Nat Genet. 2009;41(1):118–24.
7. Soblet J, Limaye N, Uebelhoer M, Boon LM, Vikkula M. Variable somatic TIE2 mutations in half of sporadic venous malformations. Mol Syndromol. 2013;4(4):179–83.
8. Natynki M, Kangas J, Miinalainen I, et al. Common and specific effects of TIE2 mutations causing venous malformations. Hum Mol Genet. 2015;24(22):6374–89.
9. Greene AK, Goss JA. Vascular anomalies: from a clinicohistologic to a genetic framework. Plast Reconstr Surg. 2018;141(5):709e–17e.
10. Vikkula M, Boon LM, Carraway KL 3rd, et al. Vascular dysmorphogenesis caused by an activating mutation in the receptor tyrosine kinase TIE2. Cell. 1996;87(7):1181–90.
11. Vikkula M, Boon LM, Mulliken JB, Olsen BR. Molecular basis of vascular anomalies. Trends Cardiovasc Med. 1998;8(7):281–92.
12. Suri C, Jones PF, Patan S, et al. Requisite role of angiopoietin-1, a ligand for the TIE2 receptor, during embryonic angiogenesis. Cell. 1996;87(7):1171–80.
13. Wouters V, Limaye N, Uebelhoer M, et al. Hereditary cutaneomucosal venous malformations are caused by TIE2 mutations with widely variable hyper-phosphorylating effects. Eur J Hum Genet. 2010;18(4):414–20.
14. Brouillard P, Boon LM, Revencu N, et al. Genotypes and phenotypes of 162 families with a glomulin mutation. Mol Syndromol. 2013;4(4):157–64.
15. Boon LM, Brouillard P, Irrthum A, et al. A gene for inherited cutaneous venous anomalies ("glomangiomas") localizes to chromosome 1p21-22. Am J Hum Genet. 1999;65(1):125–33.
16. Brouillard P, Boon LM, Mulliken JB, et al. Mutations in a novel factor, glomulin, are responsible for glomuvenous malformations ("glomangiomas"). Am J Hum Genet. 2002;70(4):866–74.
17. Boon L, Vikkula M. Molecular genetics of vascular malformations. In: Mulliken J, Burrows P, Fishman S, editors. Mulliken and Youngs' vascular anomalies: hemangiomas and malformations. 2nd ed. New York: Oxford University Press; 2013. p. 327–75.
18. Cotten A, Flipo RM, Herbaux B, Gougeon F, Lecomte-Houcke M, Chastanet P. Synovial haemangioma of the knee: a frequently misdiagnosed lesion. Skelet Radiol. 1995;24(4):257–61.
19. Devaney K, Vinh TN, Sweet DE. Synovial hemangioma: a report of 20 cases with differential diagnostic considerations. Hum Pathol. 1993;24(7):737–45.
20. Spencer SA, Sorger J. Orthopedic issues in vascular anomalies. Semin Pediatr Surg. 2014;23(4):227–32.
21. Mulliken JB, Fishman SJ, Burrows PE. Vascular anomalies. Curr Probl Surg. 2000;37(8):517–84.
22. Fishman SJ, Fox VL. Visceral vascular anomalies. Gastrointest Endosc Clin N Am. 2001;11(4):813–34.. viii
23. Fishman SJ, Burrows PE, Leichtner AM, Mulliken JB. Gastrointestinal manifestations of vascular anomalies in childhood: varied etiologies require multiple therapeutic modalities. J Pediatr Surg. 1998;33(7):1163–7.

24. Kulungowski AM, Fox VL, Burrows PE, Alomari AI, Fishman SJ. Portomesenteric Venous Thrombosis Associated with Rectal Venous Malformation. J Pediatr Surg. 2010.(in press;45:1221.
25. MacSween RM, Anthony PP, Scheuer PJ. Pathology of the liver. New York: Churchill Livingstone; 1987.
26. Fishman S. Truncal, visceral, and genital vascular malformations. In: Mulliken J, Burrows P, Fishman S, editors. *Mulliken and Young's Vascular Anomalies: Hemangiomas and Malformations*. 2nd ed. New York: Oxford University Press; 2013. p. 966–1016.
27. Jahn H, Nissen HM. Haemangioma of the urinary tract: review of the literature. Br J Urol. 1991;68(2):113–7.
28. Greene AK, Rogers GF, Mulliken JB. Intraosseous "hemangiomas" are malformations and not tumors. Plast Reconstr Surg. 2007;119(6):1949–50; author reply 1950.
29. Mounayer C, Wassef M, Enjolras O, Boukobza M, Mulliken JB. Facial "glomangiomas": large facial venous malformations with glomus cells. J Am Acad Dermatol. 2001;45(2):239–45.
30. Mallory SB, Enjolras O, Boon LM, et al. Congenital plaque-type glomuvenous malformations presenting in childhood. Arch Dermatol. 2006;142(7):892–6.
31. Ardillon L, Lambert C, Eeckhoudt S, Boon LM, Hermans C. Dabigatran etexilate versus low-molecular weight heparin to control consumptive coagulopathy secondary to diffuse venous vascular malformations. Blood Coagul Fibrinolysis. 2015;27(2):216–9.
32. Bean W. Blue rubber-bleb nevi of the skin and gastrointestinal tract. In: Vascular spiders and related lesions of the skin, vol. 1958. Springfield: Charles C Thomas. p. 17–185.
33. Gascoyen M. Case of naevus involving the parotid gland and causing suffocation. Trans Pathol Soc (Lond). 1860;11:267.
34. Fishman SJ, Smithers CJ, Folkman J, et al. Blue rubber bleb nevus syndrome: surgical eradication of gastrointestinal bleeding. Ann Surg. 2005;241(3):523–8.
35. Beluffi G, Romano P, Matteotti C, Minniti S, Ceffa F, Morbini P. Jejunal intussusception in a 10-year-old boy with blue rubber bleb nevus syndrome. Pediatr Radiol. 2004;34(9):742–5.
36. Lee C, Debnath D, Whitburn T, Farrugia M, Gonzalez F. Synchronous multiple small bowel intussusceptions in an adult with blue rubber bleb naevus syndrome: report of a case and review of literature. World J Emerg Surg. 2008;3:3.
37. Fishman G, DeRowe A, Singhal V. Congenital internal and external jugular venous aneurysms in a child. Br J Plast Surg. 2004;57(2):165–7.
38. Kulungowski AM, Fishman SJ. Management of combined vascular malformations. Clin Plast Surg. 2011;38(1):107–20.
39. Reis J, Alomari AI, Trenor CC, et al. Pulmonary thromboembolic events in patients with congenital lipomatous overgrowth, vascular malformations, epidermal nevi, and spinal/skeletal abnormalities and Klippel-Trénaunay syndrome. J Vasc Surg Venous Lymphat Disord. 2018;6(4):511–6.
40. Enjolras O, Ciabrini D, Mazoyer E, Laurian C, Herbreteau D. Extensive pure venous malformations in the upper or lower limb: a review of 27 cases. J Am Acad Dermatol. 1997;36(2. Pt 1):219–25.
41. Mazoyer E, Enjolras O, Bisdorff A, Perdu J, Wassef M, Drouet L. Coagulation disorders in patients with venous malformation of the limbs and trunk: a case series of 118 patients. Arch Dermatol. 2008;144(7):861–7.
42. Adams D, Neufeld E. Coagulopathy and vascular malformations. In: Mulliken J, Burrows P, Fishman S, editors. Mulliken and Young's vascular anomalies: hemangiomas and malformations. 2nd ed. New York: Oxford University Press; 2013. p. 637–44.
43. Rodríguez-Mañero M, Aguado L, Redondo P. Pulmonary arterial hypertension in patients with slow-flow vascular malformations. Arch Dermatol. 2010;146(12):1347–52.
44. Nguyen JT, Koerper MA, Hess CP, et al. Aspirin therapy in venous malformation: a retrospective cohort study of benefits, side effects, and patient experiences. Pediatr Dermatol. 2014;31(5):556–60.
45. Lee DF, Hung MC. All roads lead to mTOR: integrating inflammation and tumor angiogenesis. Cell Cycle. 2007;6(24):3011–4.

46. Erickson J, McAuliffe W, Blennerhassett L, Halbert A. Fibroadipose vascular anomaly treated with sirolimus: Successful outcome in two patients. Pediatr Dermatol. 2017;34(6):e317–20.
47. Salloum R, Fox CE, Alvarez-Allende CR, et al. Response of blue rubber bleb nevus syndrome to Sirolimus treatment. Pediatr Blood Cancer. 2016;63(11):1911–4.
48. Hammer J, Seront E, Duez S, et al. Sirolimus is efficacious in treatment for extensive and/or complex slow-flow vascular malformations: a monocentric prospective phase II study. Orphanet J Rare Dis. 2018;13(1):191.
49. Burrows P. Percutaneous treatment of slow-flow vascular malformations. In: Mulliken J, Burrows P, Fishman S, editors. Mulliken and Young's vascular anomalies: hemangiomas and malformations. 2nd ed. New York: Oxford University Press; 2013. p. 661–709.
50. Burrows PE, Mason KP. Percutaneous treatment of low flow vascular malformations. J Vasc Interv Radiol. 2004;15(5):431–45.
51. Cabrera J, Cabrera J Jr, Garcia-Olmedo MA, Redondo P. Treatment of venous malformations with sclerosant in microfoam form. Arch Dermatol. 2003;139(11):1409–16.
52. Berenguer B, Burrows PE, Zurakowski D, Mulliken JB. Sclerotherapy of craniofacial venous malformations: complications and results. Plast Reconstr Surg. 1999;104(1):1–11; discussion 12–15.
53. Shaikh R, Alomari AI, Kerr CL, Miller P, Spencer SA. Cryoablation in fibro-adipose vascular anomaly (FAVA): a minimally invasive treatment option. Pediatr Radiol. 2016;46(8):1179–86.
54. Barranco-Pons R, Burrows PE, Landrigan-Ossar M, Trenor CC, Alomari AI. Gross hemoglobinuria and oliguria are common transient complications of sclerotherapy for venous malformations: review of 475 procedures. AJR Am J Roentgenol. 2012;199(3):691–4.
55. Uller W, El-Sobky S, Alomari AI, et al. Preoperative embolization of venous malformations using n-Butyl Cyanoacrylate. Vasc Endovasc Surg. 2018;52(4):269–74.
56. Tieu DD, Ghodke BV, Vo NJ, Perkins JA. Single-stage excision of localized head and neck venous malformations using preoperative glue embolization. Otolaryngol Head Neck Surg. 2013;148(4):678–84.
57. Upton IIIJ. Vascular malformations of the extremities. In: Mulliken J, Burrows P, Fishman S, editors. Mulliken and Young's vascular anomalies: hemangiomas and malformations. 2nd ed. New York: Oxford University Press; 2013. p. 903–65.
58. Borsellino A, Poggiani C, Alberti D, et al. Lower gastrointestinal bleeding in a newborn caused by isolated intestinal vascular malformation. Pediatr Radiol. 2003;33(1):41–3.
59. Fishman SJ, Shamberger RC, Fox VL, Burrows PE. Endorectal pull-through abates gastrointestinal hemorrhage from colorectal venous malformations. J Pediatr Surg. 2000;35(6):982–4.
60. Kulungowski AM, Schook CC, Alomari AI, Vogel AM, Mulliken JB, Fishman SJ. Vascular anomalies of the male genitalia. J Pediatr Surg. 2011;46(6):1214–21.
61. Smithers CJ, Vogel AM, Kozakewich HP, et al. An injectable tissue-engineered embolus prevents luminal recanalization after vascular sclerotherapy. J Pediatr Surg. 2005;40(6):920–5.
62. Kulungowski AM, Hassanein AH, Foster CC, Greene AK, Fishman SJ. Bevacizumab and interferon reduce venous recanalization following sclerotherapy. J Pediatr Surg. 2016;51(10):1670–3.

Lymphatic Anomalies

10

Gulraiz Chaudry, Cameron C. Trenor III, and Belinda Dickie

Lymphatic anomalies include varied disorders of lymphatic dysfunction, fluid collection, and involvement of bone and visceral tissues. Presentation of these disorders is dependent on anatomic location of involvement. As the lymphatic system is important to host immunity, lymphatic disorders often have risk of infections, and, when lymphatic fluid is lost, lymphopenia and hypogammaglobulinemia can occur. The nomenclature for lymphatic anomalies is evolving and often confused in the literature. In 2014, a consensus statement was published on the classification of lymphatic anomalies by the International Society for the Study of Vascular Anomalies. Within the new classification, lymphatic malformations were subsequently divided into several subsets. The overal ISSVA classification was then updated in 2018.

Further evolution of lymphatic disorder classification will likely occur as lymphangiography techniques have recently improved our understanding and visualization of these disorders.

G. Chaudry
Department of Radiology, Boston Children's Hospital, Harvard Medical School, Boston, MA, USA

C. C. Trenor III (✉)
Dana-Farber Cancer Institute, Boston Children's Hospital, Boston, MA, USA

Division of Hematology/Oncology, Vascular Anomalies Center, Harvard Medical School, Boston Children's Hospital, Boston, MA, USA
e-mail: Cameron.trenor@childrens.harvard.edu

B. Dickie
Department of Surgery, Boston Children's Hospital, Boston, MA, USA
Vascular Anomalies Center, Harvard Medical School, Boston, MA, USA

C. C. Trenor III, D. M. Adams (eds.), *Vascular Anomalies*,
https://doi.org/10.1007/978-3-030-25624-1_10

Lymphatic Tumors

Vascular tumors with immunostaining for lymphatic endothelial cells include kaposiform hemangioendothelioma, lymphangiosarcoma, and kaposiform lymphangiomatosis (KLA). The first two are covered in Chaps. 6 and 7, respectively.

KLA is a newly described, aggressive subtype of lymphatic anomaly [1]. KLA has imaging features overlapping with generalized lymphatic anomaly (see below), and mediastinal and/or pulmonary involvement occurs in most but not all cases [2]. The most common imaging features are enhancing infiltrating soft tissue disease in the mediastinum or retroperitoneum (Fig. 10.1). KLA has histologic overlap with spindle-shaped, D2-40-positive lymphatic endothelial cells classically seen in kaposiform hemangioendothelioma. It is unclear if KLA is a primary disorder or a worsening of GLA; the 2018 ISSVA classification [www.issva.org] considers KLA as a subset of GLA. KLA is associated with thrombocytopenia, hypofibrinogenemia, high D-dimer, and coagulopathy. These abnormalities are associated with bleeding, especially into areas of fluid collection. In patients with lymphatic disorders who have significant thrombocytopenia, coagulopathy, hemoptysis, or hemorrhage into fluid collections, KLA should be suspected. Diagnosis can be inferred clinically if biopsy is unsafe, but the diagnosis is confirmed by histology of soft tissue masses associated with KLA. Skin involvement can occur and is distinctively hyperpigmented and lacks the lymphatic vesicles and lymphedematous features of other lymphatic disorders. The 5-year survival rate for KLA is reported to be 51% [1]; of note this refers to patients with pulmonary and mediastinal involvement and predates the use of sirolimus. One case report describes improvement of a 9-year-old with KLA during sirolimus treatment [3], while others report variable response to sirolimus with two partial responses and two non-responders [4, 5]. The natural history of pulmonary KLA is progressive decline with episodes of exacerbation followed by incomplete recovery. Currently, patients are often maintained on sirolimus and often achieve disease stability (authors' experience). Some patients require the addition of vincristine, and/or pulses of steroids if sirolimus is insufficient. Other agents such as low-dose cyclophosphamide

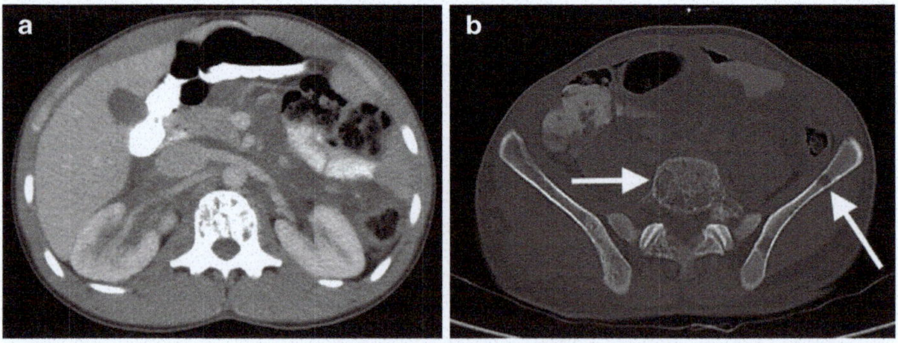

Fig. 10.1 Kaposiform lymphangiomatosis. A 20-year-old male with weight loss and intermittent bleeding from scrotum. (**a**) Contrast-enhanced CT scan of the abdomen. Low attenuation soft tissue is seen in the mesentery and retroperitoneum. (**b**) Multiple lytic lesions are noted in the vertebral body and ilium (arrows)

have also been used. A somatic activating mutation (Q61R) in NRAS has been described in 10/11 samples from KLA patients [6]. Studying primary cells from three patients with KLA, PI3K, and mTOR inhibitors were most effective at inhibiting cell proliferation [6]. To date, no reports of MEK, PI3K, or other targeted pathway inhibitors in KLA patients have been published.

Common Cystic Lymphatic Malformation (LM)

The most common manifestation of lymphatic malformations are congenital cystic lesions which can be identified on prenatal ultrasound. Macrocystic cervicofacial LM used to be called "cystic hygroma," but this term is now outdated. Cystic LMs can manifest as macrocysts, microcysts, or mixed type LMs. Frequent anatomic locations include the cervicofacial region, axilla, and mediastinum. LM is rare within skeletal muscle, although tongue involvement is relatively common.

On imaging, LM can appear vascular due to vessels within the septae between cysts, while flow of lymphatic fluid in the cysts is generally slow. Fluid-weighted (T2) sequences are bright, and enhancement is generally peripheral and delayed. In contrast, venous malformations enhance fully and rapidly and occur in other anatomic locations, including within muscle.

The typical natural history of LM is growth with the child. However, flares of growth can occur with intralesional hemorrhage, inflammation, or infection. Hemorrhage is common with trauma, but can occur unprovoked. Hemorrhage is suddenly painful and is diagnosed by ecchymosis, discoloration, or hyperechoic fluid on ultrasound. This is often treated supportively with compression and pain medication (e.g., ibuprofen, ketorolac, opiate). If erythema and fever accompany swelling and pain, inflammation or infection is more likely. Many clinicians and patients feel that many episodes are not infectious, but simply transient inflammation within LM cysts. However, this is clinically indistinguishable from bacterial cellulitis with risk of sepsis, so most episodes with suspicion of infection are treated with antibiotics. Empiric antibiotics generally target either skin (e.g., cephalexin or clindamycin if MRSA history or high risk) or oral flora (e.g., amoxicillin-clavulanate) depending on the location of the LM. Recurrence of symptoms may occur after 10–14 days of antibiotics, so clinicians often treat for a minimum of 21 days due to poor exposure of antibiotics within the LM. Recurrent hemorrhage or infection/inflammation is an indication for other treatment – sclerotherapy, resection, or sirolimus.

Cervicofacial LM has other complications related to this anatomic distribution, including airway compromise, visual impairment, challenges with oral hygiene, speech impediment, changes in face and jaw appearance, and other issues. Mandibular overgrowth, including increased mandible angle and bone thickening, is expected when adjacent LM is present. This appears unique to the mandible and is not related to direct bone invasion by LM. No data suggest that early treatment minimizes or prevents this complication, which may require orthodontia and reconstructive mandible surgery. Excellent dental care is critical to management of cervicofacial LM to prevent abscesses or caries as a source of chronic inflammation adjacent to the LM. Infection or inflammation near LM can cause expansion temporarily. This is particularly true of upper respiratory infections in cervicofacial LM.

In addition to supportive care described above, treatment directed at LM is optimized through discussion of surgical, sclerotherapy, and medical options. The treatment prescribed for LM is dependent on the anatomical type and location. The goals of management of these patients are to treat or prevent symptoms and complications and to preserve functionality. Treatment modalities are usually a combination of medical, surgical, and interventional radiology depending on the lesion. Guided by the location, size, and infiltrative nature of the lesion, a collaborative assessment and approach will lead to better outcomes for the patient. Patients and families should be counseled that LM can expand or incur further bleeding or infection complications following any intervention, and thus additional treatments may be required in the future.

Due to the success of other therapies and the infiltrative nature of LM, surgery is not usually the first-line treatment for lymphatic malformations, but is part of a multidisciplinary approach. Surgical options include excision, debulking, and laser therapy. When considering surgery, risks include blood loss, iatrogenic injury to neighboring structures, deformity, and scarring. There is also a chance of recurrence or expansion of remaining LM if incompletely excised. Thus, resection is usually reserved for symptomatic microcystic LM, for example, LM complicated by bleeding, infection, significant impairment of function, or deformity. Surgery is also favored for combined micro- and macrocystic LM with only residual microcystic component after sclerotherapy or for small, localized LM that can be completely excised.

Prior to consideration of debulking, a collaborative approach to timing of surgery and other treatment alternatives should be undertaken. For diffuse malformations, medical management (sirolimus) and sclerotherapy should be in the treatment algorithm together with surgery. For diffuse malformations, staged resection of defined anatomic areas is recommended. Subtotal resections of problematic areas should be performed in order to limit any residual deformity from surgery and to optimize function and cosmetic appearance. Periprocedural anticoagulation to control coagulopathy is rarely indicated in lymphatic malformations, as opposed to venous malformations where this practice may be indicated. Periprocedural sirolimus is increasingly used for partial debulking of LM. The intention of periprocedural sirolimus is to soften and potentially shrink LM prior to surgery, reduce intraoperative lymphatic leak, and create a "dry" operative field and to reduce the need or duration of percutaneous drains and wound complications from lymphatic fluid accumulation beneath the surgical wound.

Bleeding or leaking cutaneous vesicles may be managed by resection if they are localized and the wound can be closed primarily. However, vesicles often recur through the scar. Larger areas of vesicles that are symptomatic with leakage or bleeding are best managed with sclerotherapy of the underlying cysts and/or laser treatment (carbon dioxide, KTP) to the vesicles directly. If wide resection is done, closure may require skin grafting for coverage. Sirolimus, either systemic or topical, can also improve cutaneous lymphatic vesicles.

LM can be classified as macrocystic (Fig. 10.2), microcystic, or combined, and the subtype is relevant to sclerotherapy efficacy and sclerosant selection. The definition of microcysts is variable in the literature, but the term is best reserved for lesions with cysts that are too small to be accessed or aspirated individually (Fig. 10.3).

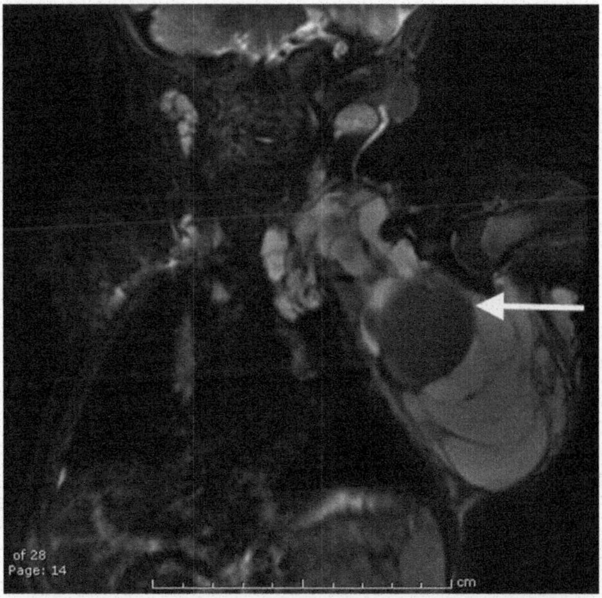

Fig. 10.2 Macrocystic LM. A 6-month-old girl with left axillary mass. T2-weighted coronal MRI demonstrates macrocystic lymphatic malformation, with evidence of intralesional hemorrhage (arrow)

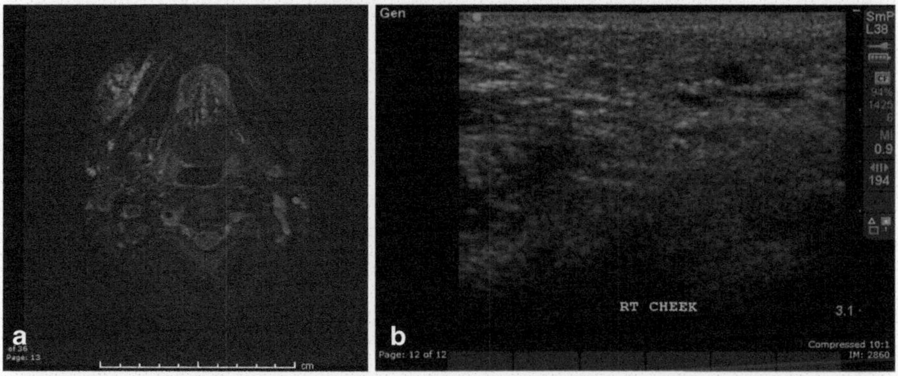

Fig. 10.3 Microcystic LM. A 17-year-old girl with right cheek swelling. (**a**) Axial T2-weighted MRI demonstrates infiltrative high signal disease within the right cheek and tongue. (**b**). Sonography of the right cheek confirms echogenic microcystic disease with no discrete macrocysts

Macrocystic LM generally responds well to intralesional sclerotherapy with doxycycline or sodium tetradecyl sulfate (STS). Microcystic LM has traditionally been treated by surgical debulking or resection, but sclerotherapy with bleomycin is increasingly utilized with over 100 reports in the literature. Bleomycin was first used as a sclerosant in pleural effusion and expanded to treat vascular malformations.

The expanded use of bleomycin has raised concerns for systemic complications, such as pulmonary fibrosis or acute pulmonary distress or skin hyperpigmentation. With judicious use of localized bleomycin therapy, the risk of systemic toxicity should be low although this was first reported in 1990 [7]. A review of 31 cases of microcystic or mixed LM treated with bleomycin did not identify any of these toxicities [8]. Systemic levels of bleomycin have been detected after localized use, and cases of toxicity, including hyperpigmentation [9, 10] and acute pulmonary toxicity [11], have been reported. Anecdotes of pulmonary fibrosis have been discussed at conferences, but none are yet reported. Further research is needed to understand the risk/benefit assessment and which patients are higher risk for bleomycin treatment of LM. Publication bias may influence the reporting of bleomycin efficacy, while patient-reported outcomes demonstrate a mixed response [12].

Isolated lymphatic endothelial cells have been utilized to identify somatic mosaic activating mutations in PIK3CA [13, 14]. Using RNASeq on blood samples from LM patients and controls, evidence of downstream activation of the PI3K/AKT pathway has been shown in circulation [15]. Now rationalized by recent genetic and biologic experiments, sirolimus has been increasingly used in LM, initially based on unmet need in refractory cases. Sirolimus medical therapy can reduce the size, firmness, T2 signal intensity, and frequency of hemorrhagic or infectious complications [16]. Mucosal response (oral, lingual, airway) to sirolimus has been excellent. Younger patients having received fewer prior procedures appear to be more responsive to sirolimus than older patients or those with a history of multiple sclerotherapy or surgical procedures [17]. In the future, therapies targeted somatic mutations may be used to treat LM, such as PI3K inhibitors for lesions with PIK3CA mutations.

Gorham-Stout Disease

Gorham-Stout disease (GSD) was first described in 1838 [18] as "disappearing bone syndrome" prior to the invention of the roentograph. GSD is eponymously named for the authors that associated osteolysis with vascular malformation, called hemangiomatosis at the time [19]. GSD does not refer to every lymphatic disorder of bone. Generalized lymphatic anomaly (GLA), kaposiform lymphangiomatosis (KLA), and central conducting lymphatic anomaly (CCLA) also have pathologic lymphatic bone involvement as discussed below. Using the classic definition, GSD is a disorder of peri-osseous expansion of lymphatic channels leading to progressive loss of cortical bone. Presentation may occur with pathologic fracture or as an incidental finding. The association with pathologic fracture and debate about the presence or absence of lymphatics in normal bone have led to the theory that trauma may trigger GSD; this is unproven, and incidental atraumatic cases have occurred. Progression can be rapid, but the natural history also includes years of disease stability. Two features distinguish GSD from other lymphatic disorders: (1) progressive loss of cortical bone and (2) regional involvement. GSD typically involves one to several adjacent bones, skipping intervening joints and tissues. Imaging and anatomic distinctions between GSD and GLA are described, with GSD having a general predilection for the axial skeleton and involving flat and long bones [20]. Involvement of thoracic bones can be associated with complicating pleural effusion. Involvement of the base of the skull can be complicated by cerebrospinal fluid leak.

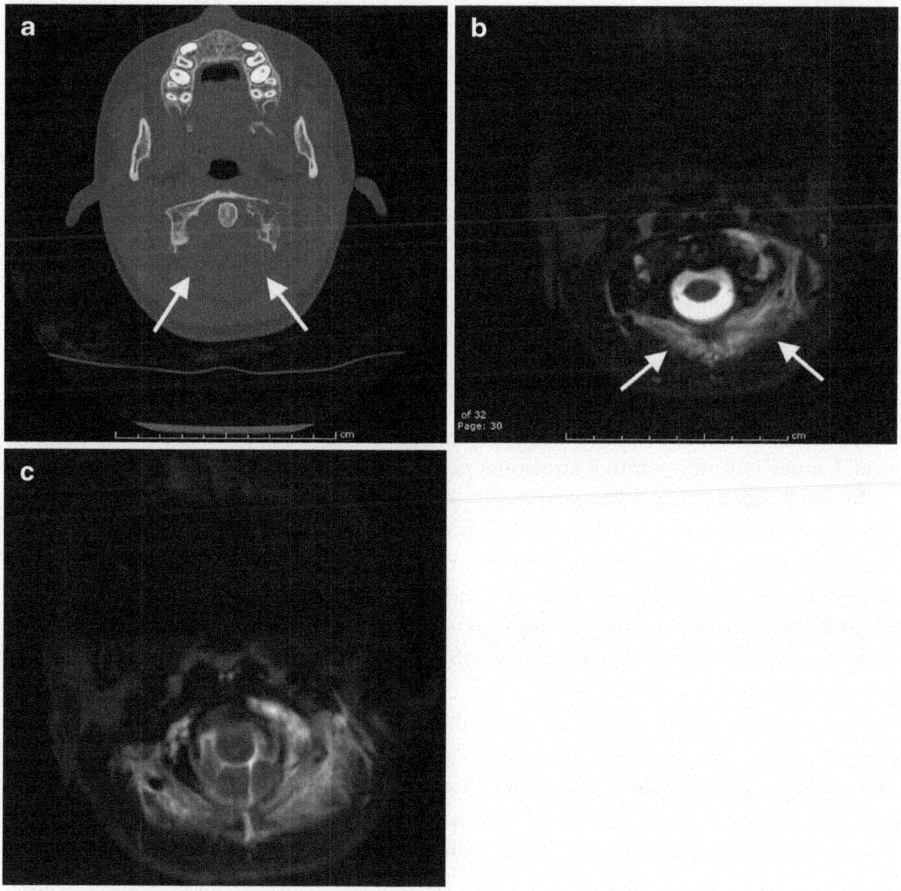

Fig. 10.4 Gorham-Stout disease. A 7-year-old-girl with headaches. (**a**) Axial CT scan demonstrates osteolysis of the posterior elements of C2 (arrows). (**b**) Axial T2-weighted MRI scan. Infiltrative high signal soft tissue mass is seen in the surrounding area (arrows). (**c**) Axial post-contrast T1 fat-saturated. Intense enhancement of the soft tissue mass is seen

The diagnosis of GSD is made by imaging, often serial. In addition to the bone findings above, peri-osseous infiltrative soft tissue is seen in the vast majority of patients [20]. On MRI, this soft tissue is bright on fluid-weighted sequences, with intense enhancement on administration of contrast (Fig. 10.4). Multiple reports of histologic features exist, but the location and timing of biopsy confound interpretation. Biopsy of areas of lost bone is often devoid of tissue, while biopsy of the edge of involved bone and surrounding soft tissues is confounded by timing. Early in disease or in incidental cases, osteoclast proliferation may be appreciated focally. Once symptomatic disease has progressed, lymphatic involvement within bone (i.e., positive D2-40 immunohistochemistry) may be seen, while osteoclast proliferation is more rare.

The genetic cause of GSD is currently unknown, but is presumed to be somatic as no familial cases are reported. Possible reasons that GSD genetics remain unknown are that genetic mutations are underrepresented in tissues submitted for sequencing (sampling error), mutation levels are below the limit of detection (sensitivity), or mutations are not in analyzed sequences (splicing mutation, epigenetic change). Many believe that periosteal lymphatics drive GSD progression. The existence of lymphatic channels in healthy bone remains controversial, supporting this theory. Better support comes from historical cases of attempts to surgically restore missing bone with autologous or cadaveric bone. This replaced bone is also resorbed if the primary lymphatic disease is not first controlled. Additionally, experience has taught us that hardware anchored in adjacent bone to support lost bone also fails when disease progression erodes bone around the anchoring screws. There are anecdotal cases of successful bone grafting or stabilization in GSD only when the disease is well controlled, including an illustrative case report of spine stabilization after 1 month of preoperative sirolimus [21].

Medical therapy has been used to control GSD. The most published regimen for therapy is interferon-alfa (2a or 2b), often in combination with bisphosphonates. Recent data also support the use of sirolimus in combination with bisphosphonates. In practice, dosing intensity, interval, and duration of bisphosphonates are highly variable, though zoledronate is the most common choice of bisphosphonate. The goal of therapy is to stabilize progressive disease and minimize complications; hence, medical therapy is generally reserved for cases with evidence of progressive disease or symptoms. The appropriate length of therapy, intensity of therapy, and long-term outcomes are currently unknown. Biomarkers of disease activity and response to therapy are urgently needed. As many case series of medical therapy reportedly for GSD also include GLA, it can be difficult to separate GSD response to therapy. These reports of medical therapies are summarized in the section on GLA below.

Generalized Lymphatic Anomaly (GLA)

GLA was adopted by the International Society for the Study of Vascular Anomalies (ISSVA) in 2014 as the new term for lymphangiomatosis. As the name implies, involvement is often widespread. Osteal involvement is common but distinct from GSD; GLA bone lesions are lytic in nature, without sclerotic (reactive) rim, but without loss of bone cortex characteristically seen with GSD (Fig. 10.5). In addition, the infiltrative peri-osseous soft tissue mass associated with GSD is not identified in GLA. Multifocal lytic bone lesions may also represent metastatic disease, so biopsy is often performed. The most common finding is the presence of lymphatic malformation (i.e., positive D2-40 immunohistochemistry) within bone. Biopsy of ribs is often considered, but should be avoided as rib biopsy in lymphatic disorders can lead to refractory iatrogenic pleural effusion. The ribs are the most common site of bony involvement in GLA followed by the spine. In contrast to GSD, lesions are also commonly seen in the appendicular skeleton. Pathologic fracture is uncommon given the preservation of cortical bone, but can occur with extensive bone

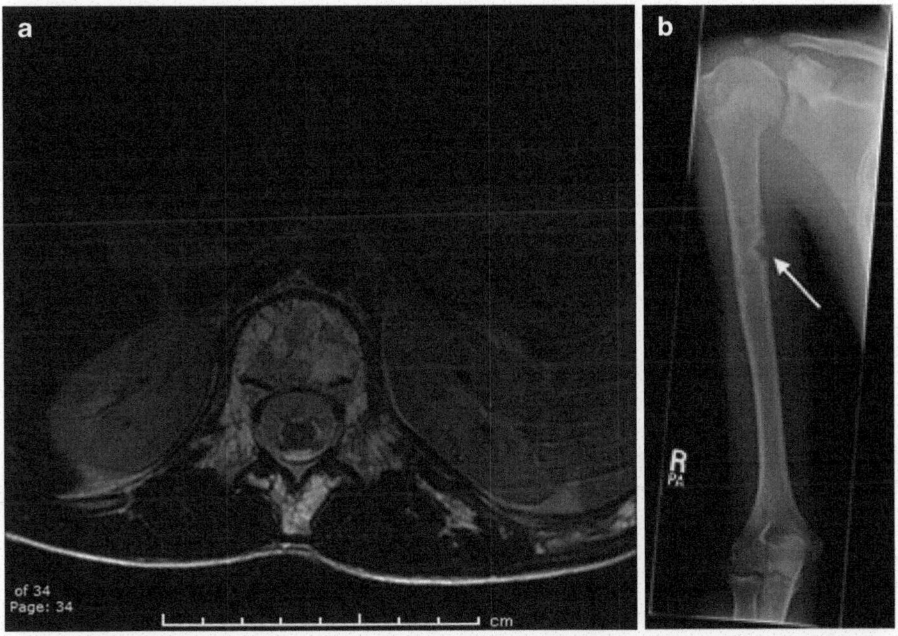

Fig. 10.5 Generalized lymphatic anomaly. A 7-year-old girl with bilateral pleural effusions. (**a**) Axial T2-weighted MRI. Diffuse infiltration of the vertebra and ribs. There is no surrounding soft tissue disease. (**b**) X-ray of the right humerus. Multiple discrete lytic lesions are seen in the right humerus (arrows) with preservation of the surrounding cortex

involvement (e.g., vertebral compression fracture) or trauma. GLA can also be accompanied by cystic LM, splenic lymphatic cysts, and lymphatic leak. Regional lymphatic channel dilation (i.e., lymphangiectasia) in pulmonary or intestinal viscera can occur without bone involvement. GLA has been an umbrella term for non-GSD complicated and disseminated lymphatic disease. The increasing utilization of lymphangiography has led recategorizing many GLA patients as having a primary disorder of faulty central lymphatic drainage leading to lymphatic reflux (see below as CCLA).

To date, there are two reports of genetics causes for GLA. Four hotspot mutations in PIK3CA have been reported in five of nine patients with GLA [22], consistent with GLA as a lymphatic disorder. One patient categorized as GLA was found to have a somatic NRAS mutation [23]. While there may be two genes related to GLA, the discovery of NRAS in 10 of 11 patients with KLA raises the possibility that KLA arises from patients with the phenotype of GLA, consistent with the ISSVA 2018 nomenclature.

The natural history of GLA is poorly understood, and long periods of stability on imaging are reported. Given the widespread involvement of GLA, focal procedures are generally limited to symptomatic complications, such as pleurocentesis or pleurodesis for pleural effusion. Medical therapy has been utilized in progressive or extensive disease, and treatment regimens are similar to those used in GSD. Most of the literature reports interferon with or without bisphosphonates, but sirolimus responses have also been recently reported. Due to relative potency and experience, zoledronate is the most common bisphosphonate utilized. The largest case series of GLA and GSD treated 18 patients (13 GLA and 5 GSD) with sirolimus, noting 15/18 had partial improvement more often in quality of life than in imaging and no patients had progressive disease on therapy [24]. The phase 2 study of sirolimus in complicated vascular anomalies included seven patients with GLA and three with GSD and reported 100% partial response at 6 months, though one GSD patient developed disease progression by 12 months on sirolimus monotherapy [16]. Low-dose sirolimus has also been reported in one patient with GLA [25]. Innovative regimens of imatinib in one GLA patient [26] and sunitinib and low-dose taxol in one GLA and one GSD patient [27] have also been reported.

Central Conducting Lymphatic Anomaly (CCLA)

In addition to the lymphatic malformations described above, there are other patients with a phenotype best described as resulting from lymphatic dysfunction. When the central lymphatics drain effectively but peripheral lymphatics do not, this results in lymphedema. When the central conducting lymphatics – thoracic duct, cisterna chyli, and other major channels – fail to drain the lymphatic system into the venous system, this results in CCLA. The lymphatic system is designed to return lymphatic fluid to the left subclavian vein through the valved thoracic duct outlet via an intricate system of vessels using peristalsis for antigravity flow. When channels are disrupted or peristalsis is impaired, lymphatic hypertension leads to distension of channels and leakage into other spaces. Lymphatic fluid collections are often chylous in CCLA, confirming the defect is cranial to the cisterna chylae. Chyle can be lost through intestinal villae, collect as ascites, pleural effusions or pericardial effusions, or reflux into bone or pulmonary parenchyma.

This diagnosis may be suspected on MRI with ectasia of lymphatics along the course of the central lymphatics, through the inguinal canal or along the tracheobronchial tree (Fig. 10.6). CCLA is confirmed by lymphangiography. Historically this was done by cutdown and microinjection into interphalangeal lymphatics of both feet. Most centers have now adopted intranodal injection in bilateral inguinal lymph nodes with imaging either by fluoroscopy in the interventional radiology suite or by MRI. As new imaging technologies emerge for study of lymphatic disorders, we hope to identify imaging biomarkers of disease severity, outcomes, and predictors or response to therapy. The term CCLA is being increasingly used as lymphangiography is applied to study other lymphatic disorders. The distinction between primary CCLA and abnormal lymphangiogram findings due to lymphatic dysfunction from other disorders is currently unclear. When lymphangiography demonstrates filling of the lymphatic system to the thoracic duct terminus, but lack of emptying into the left subclavian vein, this is interpreted as a failure of the terminal thoracic duct or valve. Microsurgical reimplantation of the terminal thoracic

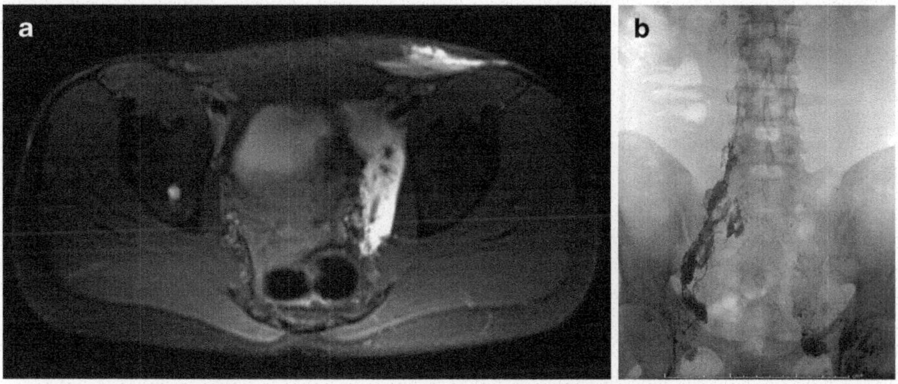

Fig. 10.6 Central conducting lymphatic anomaly. A 20-year-old male with left groin mass. (**a**) Axial MRI STIR. High signal perivascular lymphatic channels are seen, more prominent on the left, with infiltration into the subcutaneous fat. (**b**) Intranodal lymphangiogram. There is reflux of contrast in the left groin and pelvis, with minimal opacification of the central channels. Dilated lymphatic channels are also seen on the right

duct into another intrathoracic vein with valves has been reported to have corrected 5 patients completely and 3 partially, out of 14 attempts in patients with CCLA [28]. This technique requires further study to define predictors of responders and frequency of success, but offers hope to patients with few other options. Refluxing lymphatic channels can be targeted by embolization by interventional radiologists or surgical oversewing or ligation. For patients with global dysfunction of the central lymphatic channels, with failure to opacify the thoracic duct in some cases, the therapeutic options are much more limited.

A heterozygous splice site mutation in EPHB4 causing loss of function has been reported in one patient with CCLA [29]. Reports of medical therapy responses to sirolimus are mixed. Sirolimus has not been reported to be effective for 3 patients with CCLA [16] although one responder has been reported [30] and some cases of response after longer duration of therapy have occurred (personal cases of authors). Variable response may reflect length of therapy or poor understanding of variable mechanisms of disease grouped by abnormal lymphangiography.

Summary

As the lymphatic system is anatomically diffuse, and complications vary by location, extent, and impact on adjacent structures. Further, the lymphatic system is part of host immunity, and malformations are associated with an increased risk of infection. Treatment involves coordination of surgical, interventional radiology and medical options. The genetics of LM appear to group lymphatic malformations as PIK3CA-related and more aggressive conditions like KLA as NRAS-related. Lymphatic imaging has evolved significantly in recent years allowing visualization of abnormal lymphatic function and targeted therapies. Imaging and circulating biomarkers, robust outcome studies, and improved collaborative, multidisciplinary, prospective studies will further improve our understanding of these disorders and patient outcomes.

References

1. Croteau SE, Kozakewich HP, Perez-Atayde AR, et al. Kaposiform lymphangiomatosis: a distinct aggressive lymphatic anomaly. J Pediatr. 2014;164:383–8.
2. Goyal P, Alomari AI, Kozakewich HP, et al. Imaging features of kaposiform lymphangiomatosis. Pediatr Radiol. 2016;46:1282–90.
3. Wang Z, Li K, Yao W, Dong K, Xiao X, Zheng S. Successful treatment of kaposiform lymphangiomatosis with sirolimus. Pediatr Blood Cancer. 2015;62:1291–3.
4. Triana P, Dore M, Cerezo VN, et al. Sirolimus in the treatment of vascular anomalies. Eur J Pediatr Surg. 2017;27:86–90.
5. Ozeki M, Nozawa A, Yasue S, Endo S, Asada R, Hashimoto H, Fukao T. The impact of sirolimus on lesion size, clinical symptoms and quality of life of patients with lymphatic anomalies. Orphanet J Rare Dis. 2019;14:141.
6. Barclay SF, Inman KW, Luks VL, et al. A somatic activating NRAS variant associated with kaposiform lymphangiomatosis. Genet Med. 2019;21(7):1517–24.
7. Siegel RD, Schiffman FJ. Systemic toxicity following intracavitary administration of bleomycin. Chest. 1990;98:507.
8. Chaudry G, Guevara CJ, Rialon KL, et al. Safety and efficacy of bleomycin sclerotherapy for microcystic lymphatic malformation. Cardiovasc Intervent Radiol. 2014;37:1476–81.
9. Mack JM, Richter GT, Becton D, Salem O, Hill SEM, Crary SE. Short-term side effects and patient-reported outcomes of bleomycin sclerotherapy in vascular malformations. Pediatr Blood Cancer. 2018;65:e27008.
10. Milbar HC, Jeon H, Ward MA, Mitchell SE, Weiss CR, Cohen BA. Hyperpigmentation after foamed bleomycin sclerotherapy for vascular malformations. J Vasc Interv Radiol. 2019;30:1438–42.
11. Mendez-Echevarria A, Fernandez-Prieto A, de la Serna O, et al. Acute lung toxicity after Intralesional bleomycin sclerotherapy. Pediatrics. 2018;141:e20161787.
12. Horbach SER, van de Ven JS, Nieuwkerk PT, Spuls PI, van der Horst C, Reekers JA. Patient-reported outcomes of bleomycin sclerotherapy for low-flow vascular malformations and predictors of improvement. Cardiovasc Intervent Radiol. 2018;41:1494–504.
13. Glaser K, Dickie P, Neilson D, Osborn A, Dickie BH. Linkage of metabolic defects to activated PIK3CA alleles in endothelial cells derived from lymphatic malformation. Lymphat Res Biol. 2018;16:43–55.
14. Blesinger H, Kaulfuss S, Aung T, et al. PIK3CA mutations are specifically localized to lymphatic endothelial cells of lymphatic malformations. PLoS One. 2018;13:e0200343.
15. Kim T, Tafoya E, Chelliah MP, et al. Alterations of the MEK/ERK, BMP, and Wnt/beta-catenin pathways detected in the blood of individuals with lymphatic malformations. PLoS One. 2019;14:e0213872.
16. Adams DM, Trenor CC 3rd, Hammill AM, et al. Efficacy and safety of Sirolimus in the treatment of complicated vascular anomalies. Pediatrics. 2016;137:1–10.
17. Strychowsky JE, Rahbar R, O'Hare MJ, Irace AL, Padua H, Trenor CC 3rd. Sirolimus as treatment for 19 patients with refractory cervicofacial lymphatic malformation. Laryngoscope. 2018;128:269–76.
18. Jackson J. A boneless arm. Boston Med Surg J. 1838;18:368–9.
19. Gorham LW, Stout AP. Massive osteolysis (acute spontaneous absorption of bone, phantom bone, disappearing bone); its relation to hemangiomatosis. J Bone Joint Surg Am. 1955;37-A:985–1004.

20. Lala S, Mulliken JB, Alomari AI, Fishman SJ, Kozakewich HP, Chaudry G. Gorham-Stout disease and generalized lymphatic anomaly–clinical, radiologic, and histologic differentiation. Skelet Radiol. 2013;42:917–24.
21. Mo AZ, Trenor CC 3rd, Hedequist DJ. Sirolimus therapy as perioperative treatment of Gorham-Stout disease in the thoracic spine: a case report. JBJS Case Connect. 2018;8:e70.
22. Rodriguez-Laguna L, Agra N, Ibanez K, et al. Somatic activating mutations in PIK3CA cause generalized lymphatic anomaly. J Exp Med. 2019;216:407–18.
23. Manevitz-Mendelson E, Leichner GS, Barel O, et al. Somatic NRAS mutation in patient with generalized lymphatic anomaly. Angiogenesis. 2018;21:287–98.
24. Ricci KW, Hammill AM, Mobberley-Schuman P, et al. Efficacy of systemic sirolimus in the treatment of generalized lymphatic anomaly and Gorham-Stout disease. Pediatr Blood Cancer. 2019;66:e27614.
25. Dvorakova V, Rea D, O'Regan GM, Irvine AD. Generalized lymphatic anomaly successfully treated with long-term, low-dose sirolimus. Pediatr Dermatol. 2018;35:533–4.
26. Libby LJ, Narula N, Fernandes H, Gruden JF, Wolf DJ, Libby DM. Imatinib treatment of Lymphangiomatosis (generalized lymphatic anomaly). J Natl Compr Cancer Netw. 2016;14:383–6.
27. Rossler J, Saueressig U, Kayser G, von Winterfeld M, Klement GL. Personalized therapy for generalized lymphatic anomaly/Gorham-Stout disease with a combination of Sunitinib and Taxol. J Pediatr Hematol Oncol. 2015;37:e481–5.
28. Taghinia AH, Upton J, Trenor CC 3rd, et al. Lymphaticovenous bypass of the thoracic duct for the treatment of chylous leak in central conducting lymphatic anomalies. J Pediatr Surg. 2019;54:562–8.
29. Li D, Wenger TL, Seiler C, et al. Pathogenic variant in EPHB4 results in central conducting lymphatic anomaly. Hum Mol Genet. 2018;27:3233–45.
30. McCormick A, Rosenberg S, Tier K, Balest A. A case of a central conducting lymphatic anomaly responsive to Sirolimus. Pediatrics. 2016;137:e20152694.

11 Arteriovenous Malformation

Arin K. Greene and Patricia E. Burrows

Introduction

Arteriovenous malformation (AVM) is a fast-flow vascular malformation consisting of a network or nidus of abnormal blood vessels supplied by feeding arteries draining into veins. The lesional extent and angioarchitecture are extremely variable, as is the magnitude of the arteriovenous shunt. Unlike tumors, AVMs appear to replace the capillary bed of the affected tissue, causing an infiltrating lesion. AVM causes localized venous hypertension, reducing perfusion pressure to the involved and adjacent tissues, causing symptoms and signs of tissue ischemia. During childhood, AVM is usually associated with symmetrical overgrowth of the affected tissue, often with a capillary stain of the overlying skin (Fig. 11.1). Evolution occurs at a variable rate (Table 11.1, Schobinger staging system), although it is well-known that progression is stimulated by a number of events that stimulate somatic and angiogenic growth factors, such as trauma, puberty, and pregnancy [1, 2]. Over time, shunting increases, causing tissue ischemia with pain followed by tissue ulceration with bleeding (Schobinger stages III and IV) (Figs. 11.2 and 11.3). Extensive AVMs and those with large fistulas cause cardiac volume overload, potentially leading to high-output cardiac failure. AVMs outside of the central nervous system typically present with tissue overgrowth, pain, and ulcerative bleeding.

Most AVMs are somatic lesions and when located extracranially are usually the result of an *MAP2K1* mutation in endothelial cells [3]. AVMs are most frequently located intracranially often leading to neurological symptoms and/or hemorrhage; intracranial lesions are typically the result of a somatic *KRAS*

A. K. Greene
Department of Plastic and Oral Surgery, Boston Children's Hospital, Harvard Medical School, Boston, MA, USA

P. E. Burrows (✉)
Department of Radiology, Medical College of Wisconsin, St. Petersburg, FL, USA
e-mail: pburrows@mcw.edu

C. C. Trenor III, D. M. Adams (eds.), *Vascular Anomalies*,
https://doi.org/10.1007/978-3-030-25624-1_11

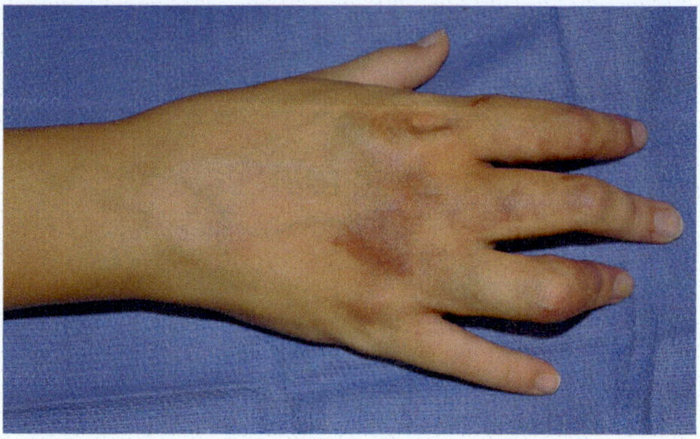

Fig. 11.1 Diffuse Schobinger stage III AVM of right hand of a 10-year-old girl who has undergone several embolizations. She has tissue overgrowth, swelling, patchy red stains, and dilated superficial veins. Flexion contractures of several fingers caused by ischemia. The diffuse AVM could not be embolized effectively

Table 11.1 Natural history of AVM

Stage 1	Warm, skin discoloration, fast-flow on Doppler
Stage 2	Growth, palpable pulsations, enlarged veins
Stage 3	Ulceration, bleeding, pain
Stage 4	Congestive heart failure

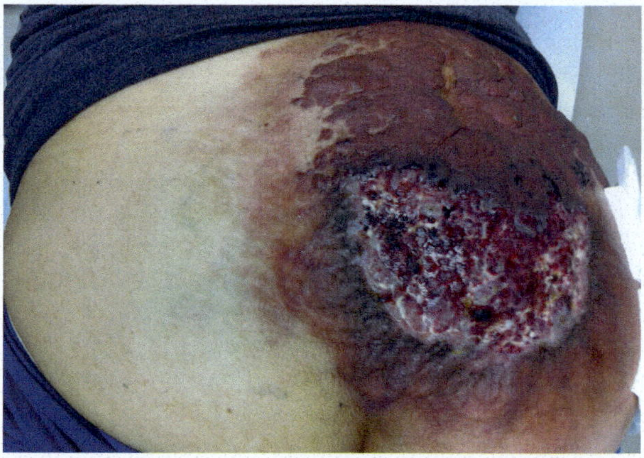

Fig. 11.2 Ulcerated, bleeding Schobinger stage III diffuse AVM of the right buttock in a 16-year-old girl, who was asymptomatic until 2 years earlier

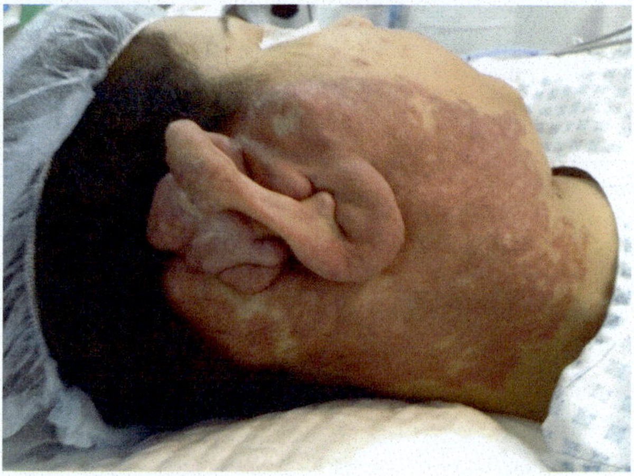

Fig. 11.3 Schobinger stage IV AVM of the pinna. A 20-year-old male with cardiac failure, ulceration, and bleeding. Note the huge varices behind the ear

mutation [4]. Congenital arteriovenous fistula [AVF] is a type of AVM, in which shunting occurs directly from artery to vein, without an intervening nidus. AVF can occur as an isolated defect or within a complex AVM. AVM and AVF are generally sporadic, although a small percentage of patients have hereditary forms. Hereditary forms are caused by germline mutations in *ACVRL*, *ENG*, *RASA1*, *EPHB4*, and *PTEN* [5]. AVM should be distinguished from vascular tumors that can contain arteriovenous shunts, such as infantile or congenital hemangiomas and certain malignancies. Usually, clinical and imaging features clearly differentiate AVM from tumor.

Diagnosis of AVM

Clinical findings in patients with AVM vary according to the extent and clinical stage. Generally, there is evidence of increased flow with prominent proximal pulsations, engorgement of draining veins, and increased skin temperature. With a large shunt, soft tissue pulsatility and/or venous thrill can be felt. The skin can be involved with a diffuse or patchy flat red stain. Over time, dark red keratotic macules called pseudo-kaposiform change may develop, especially in the lower extremities. The stain of AVM can easily be distinguished from isolated capillary malformation because of increased temperature. A portable Doppler probe can be used in the clinic to detect increased flow in the underlying tissues.

MRI with time-resolved contrast-enhanced MRA is the best diagnostic test to demonstrate extent and flow characteristics. Typically, standard MR images show some enlargement of the affected tissue with vascular flow voids representing dilated feeding arteries and draining veins (Fig. 11.4). With a few exceptions, the AVM does not have significant signal abnormality or mass effect. The lack of distinct soft tissue mass on fluid-sensitive sequences helps distinguish AVM from tumors. AVMs within a confined space, such as intramuscular AVMs, may demonstrate increased signal on T2-weighted sequences. Contrast enhancement may also be seen in AVMs composed of small channels. 2-D time-of-flight MRA is not reliable for diagnosing AVM, but may show enlargement of the feeding arteries. Time-resolved contrast-enhanced MRA, which obtains 3-D data sets every few seconds after intravenous contrast injection, is the best sequence to show arteriovenous shunting [6] (Fig. 11.5). In this study, veins draining an AVM will appear much sooner than normal veins. Unlike hemangioma, contrast washes out of the AVM quite quickly.

Ultrasonography with Doppler interrogation is a good method to confirm the presence of arteriovenous shunting. Involved tissue may appear normal or more echogenic than normal due to fibrofatty infiltration or edema. Feeding arteries will be dilated, with low-resistance waveform. Draining veins typically have turbulent, high velocity flow.

Catheter angiography is the best technique to delineate the specific angioarchitecture but, at least in children, is usually not performed unless intervention is planned during the same procedure. MRI often demonstrates tissue overgrowth and enlarged vascular flow voids, usually without a focal mass. MRA is helpful to show the anatomy of feeding and draining vessels. 2-D and 3-D time-of-flight MRA gives good resolution of the vascular anatomy, while dynamic time-resolved contrast-enhanced MRA confirms the present of a shunt, as well as better depiction of the venous anatomy. Knowledge of the angioarchitecture of an individual AVM is necessary to plan endovascular treatment and predict the likelihood of complete occlusion [7, 8]. A number of angiographic classifications have been proposed, based on an early paper describing dural AVMs [9]. There are three basic types of AVM angioarchitecture: direct arteriovenous fistula, arteriolovenous fistula, and arteriolovenular malformation. The direct arteriovenous fistula can be cured by placing an appropriate occluding device in the arteriovenous communication, either through a trans-arterial or transvenous approach. The arteriolovenous fistula is composed of

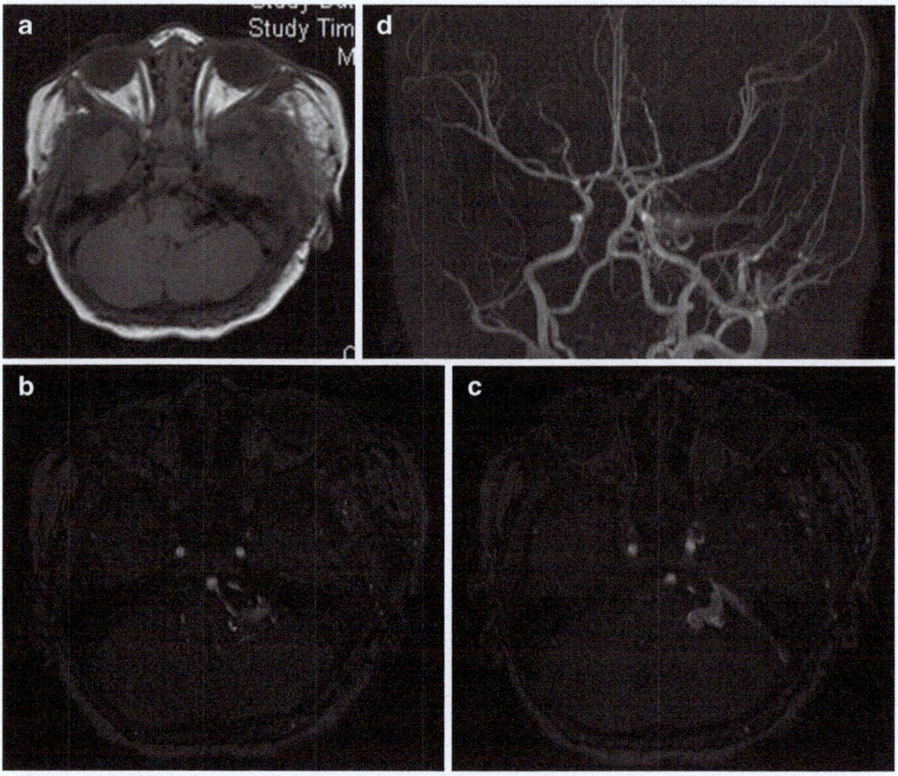

Fig. 11.4 Imaging of a patient with CM-AVM who had multiple CMs, Schobinger stage I small vessel AVM [arteriolovenular], and intracranial AVFs. (**a**) T1-weighted MR image through the face and posterior fossa shows dilated flow voids to the left of the brainstem representing AVF and increased thickness of temporalis muscle and subcutaneous fat in the left cheek. (**b**, **c**) Flow-senstive images through the posterior fossa show dilated vessels in the AVM and AVF. (**d**) 2-D time-of-flight MRA shows the dilation of the left external carotid branches, as well as visualization of an intracranial venous channel. (**e**) Right vertebral angiogram shows AVF in the left posterior fossa. (**f–h**) Serial angiographic images demonstrate the diffuse AVM of the left face

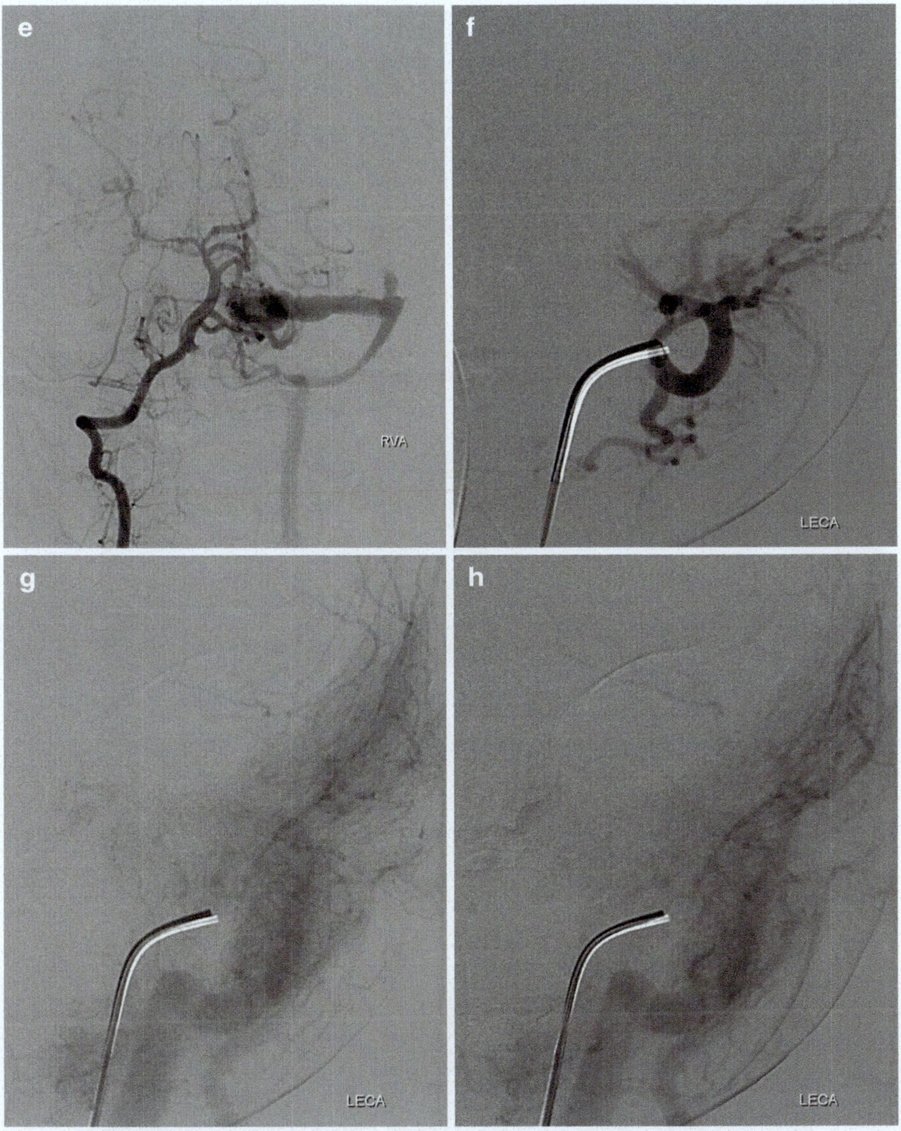

Fig. 4 (continued)

numerous arterial connections to a single outflow vein. It is best treated by packing or closing the immediate draining outflow vein, either by direct puncture or transvenous approach. This type of AVM also has a high rate of permanent occlusion. The arteriolovenular malformation, consisting of numerous arteries, nidus, and numerous draining veins, is usually managed transarterially or by direct puncture and has the lowest rate of complete occlusion by endovascular treatment.

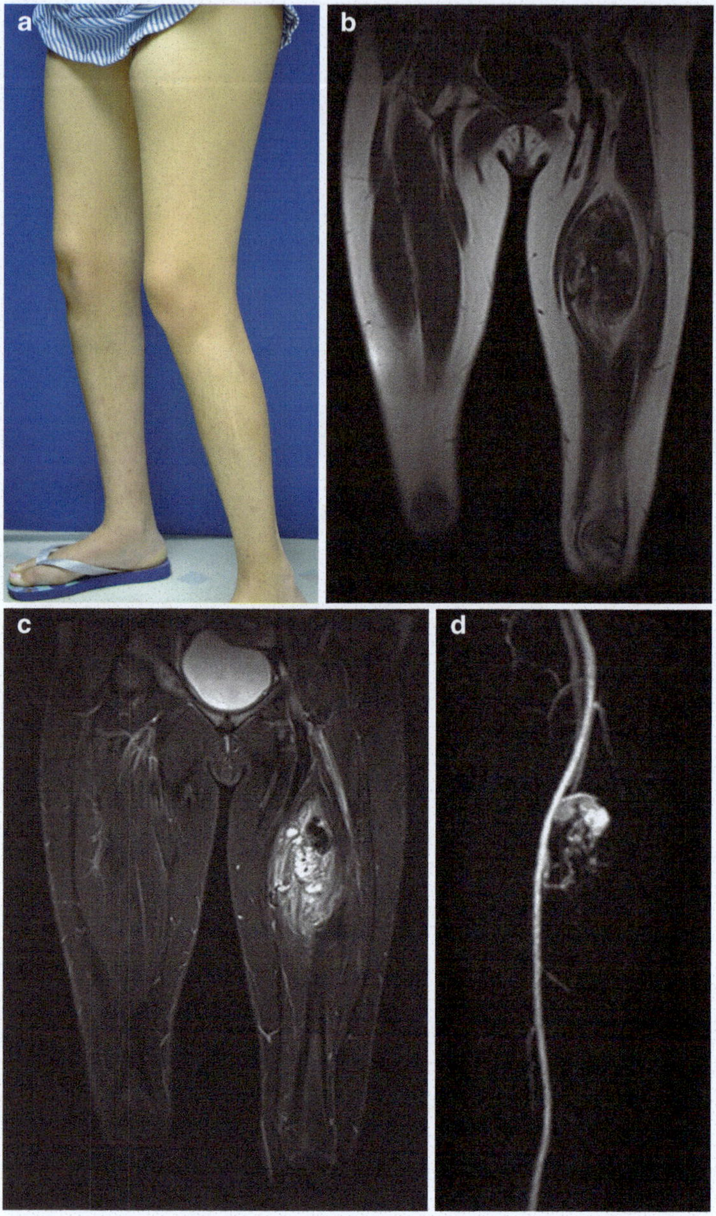

Fig. 11.5 PTEN tumor hamartoma syndrome in a 13-year-old girl with complex intramuscular AVM left thigh. (**a**) Photograph shows soft tissue mass of the anterior left thigh. (**b**) Coronal T1-weighted MR image of the thighs shows an intramuscular mass containing fat, soft tissue, and vascular flow voids. (**c**) Coronal T2-weighted image demonstrates increased signal within the mass and a large vascular flow void. Dilated left femoral vein confirms the presence of a shunt. (**d**, **e**) Early and late images from a contrast-enhanced time-resolved MRA show AVM with large varix draining to femoral vein. (**f**, **g**) Left femoral angiogram confirms AVM consisting of large AVF plus nidus. (**h**) Left femoral angiogram after embolization, using coils and NBCA in the venous components, and ethanol to close the remaining nidus, shows complete occlusion

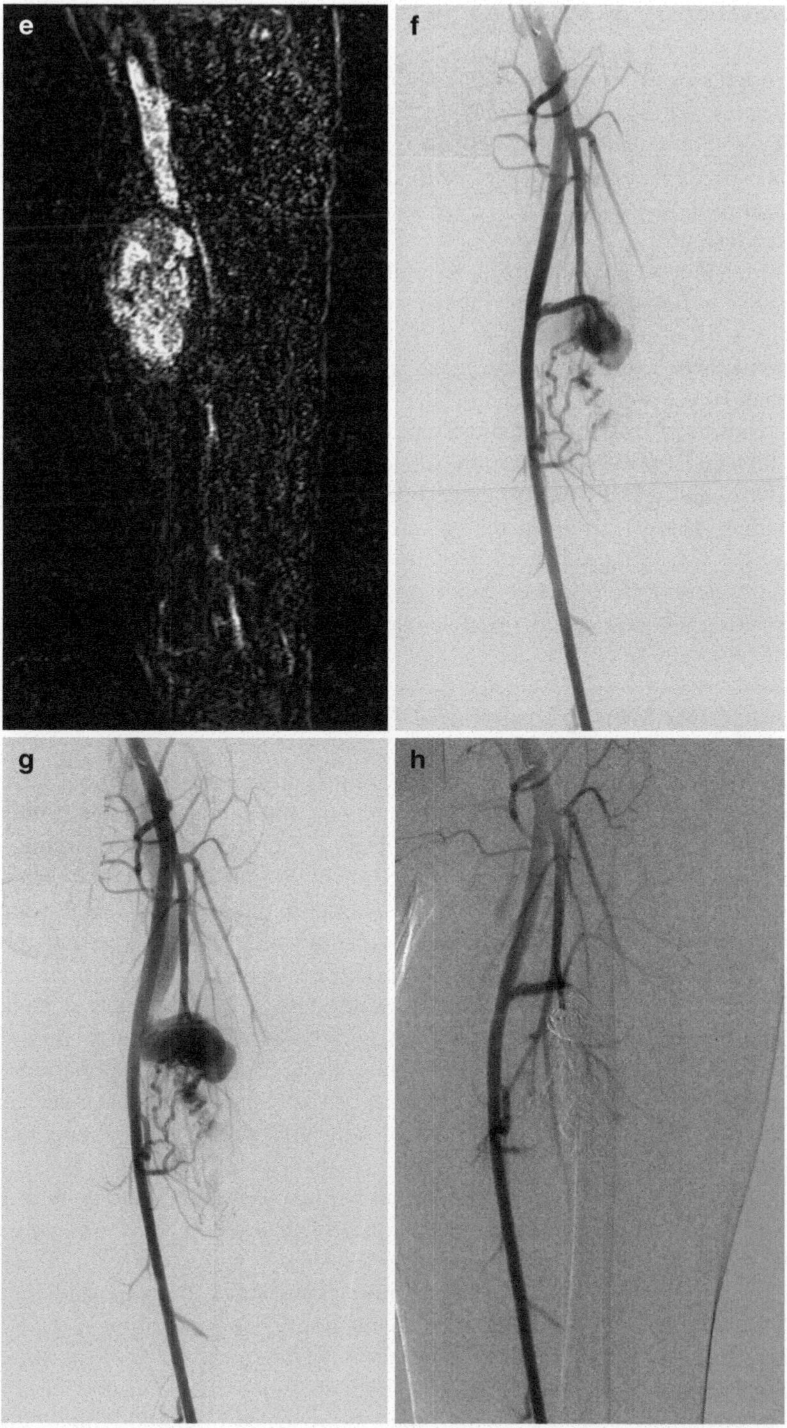

Fig. 5 (continued)

Natural History of AVM

AVM progresses over time and recurs after treatment. The evolution of AVM can be classified according to the Schobinger staging system (Table 11.1). Children with a stage 1 AVM have an approximately 50% risk of progression during childhood and an 82% risk during adolescence; 18% do not experience significant long-term growth until they are adults [10]. Diffuse AVMs are more likely to progress than localized lesions.

Despite subtotal and presumed "complete" extirpation, most AVMs re-enlarge after excision. Recurrence following resection typically occurs during the first year, and 86% will re-expand within 5 years. Patients not exhibiting regrowth 5 years later are likely to have long-term control. However, 5% will experience re-expansion more than 10 years postoperatively [10].

The cause of AVM enlargement is unknown. It may grow because of increased blood flow causing collateralization, dilatation of vessels, and thickening of adjacent arteries and veins. Arteriovenous shunts may open, stimulating hypertrophy of surrounding vessels from increased pressure. Alternatively, aneurysms might increase the size of these lesions. Because both males and females have a twofold risk of progression to a higher Schobinger stage in adolescence, circulating hormones during this period may promote expansion.

Endovascular Management of AVM

A variety of embolization materials and techniques are used for AVM treatment. It is inappropriate to compare results of embolization without consideration of the technique used. Transcatheter embolization of feeding arteries is the oldest technique, in which selective or supraselective catheterization of the arteries supplying the AVM is carried out. Embolization material, such as particles, microspheres, gelatin sponge, or NBCA glue, is injected with the goal of occluding the feeding arteries and decreasing flow. This technique is used preoperatively, 1 or 2 days before resection, to minimize blood loss. Because this method does not destroy or completely occlude the nidus and immediate draining veins, it has no long-term benefit and should not be used for palliative treatment without resection. Embolization of feeding arteries can lead to some ischemia of the surrounding tissue. Another technique that avoids proximal arterial occlusion is percutaneous embolization of the AVM nidus. Preoperatively, this is usually carried out with NBCA.

To achieve the best chance of long-term palliation or cure, endovascular treatment must selectively target the nidus and immediate draining veins. Absolute ethanol is the most effective agent for arteriolovenular malformations, because it penetrates the nidus and the immediate draining vein and destroys the endothelium. Ethanol can only be safely administered to the nidus. Any penetration of the normal capillary bed causes severe tissue destruction, leading to necrosis of the skin, soft tissue, and peripheral nerves. These procedures are time-consuming and, because of limits in ethanol volume per session, must be repeated numerous times. Ideally, embolization is repeated every month or every second month until the lesion is completely closed. With proper technique, normal vascularity to the affected tissues is retained. Complication rates are high, however, including tissue damage, peripheral nerve injury, pulmonary thromboembolism, and cardiovascular collapse.

AVF can be closed through an arterial or venous approach, as long as the exact communication between artery and vein is occluded [11]. Numerous mechanical occlusion devices, such as plugs, coils, or micro-coils, are available. Detachable coils and micro-coils can be positioned precisely before deployment. NBCA and Onyx are also effective in certain AVFs. Double-lumen balloon occlusion microcatheters are available for use with Onyx. Once a simple AVF is completely closed, recurrence is rare.

In arteriolovenous malformations, the single outflow vein is often occluded with a large number of coils, with or without additional ethanol or NBCA. This technique has excellent results, when applied to the appropriate lesion [12]. Permanent complete occlusion has been documented with 5-year and 10-year follow-up angiograms. Published series of patients undergoing primary embolization for peripheral AVM come mainly from the group at Samsung Medical Center in Seoul, Korea. This group reported an overall cure rate of 39%, with 10% major and 35% minor complications [8]. Extent of AVM and angiographic classification were the main predictors of outcome.

Small vessel AVMs [arteriolovenular] are the most difficult to treat. Localized small vessel AVMs can be treated with ethanol embolization. Staged bleomycin infiltration is also sometimes effective. However, diffuse small vessel AVMs do not respond well to embolization and often worsen.

Surgical Management of AVM

Operative Indications

Intervention for an AVM is not mandatory and should not leave a worse deformity than the appearance of the lesion [13]. Variables that determine whether an AVM should be resected are the stage, patient age, location of the lesion, and size of the AVM. If it is possible to completely resect a stage 1 or 2 AVM in an anatomically favorable area, then prophylactic excision and reconstruction should be considered before the lesion progresses [14]. However, if an AVM is located on the face and extirpation and reconstruction would leave a significant deformity, then it is generally best to wait until the lesion becomes very problematic before surgical intervention. Stage 3 and 4 AVMs require treatment for deformity, bleeding, pain, ulceration, and/or congestive heart failure.

Timing of Intervention

Stage 3–4 AVMs require immediate treatment, regardless of the age of the patient. Generally, an AVM should not be removed before 6 months of age. At this time the patient's risk of anesthesia is greater than for an adult. In addition, a young infant is less able to tolerate an operative procedure. If it is likely that a patient will require an operation, a common time to intervene is between 3 and 4 years of age. Because long-term memory and self-esteem begin to form at approximately 4 years of age, removing an AVM at this time will improve a deformity before the child's self-esteem begins to form, and the patient will likely not remember the procedure. Another period to extirpate an AVM is during late childhood/early adolescence when the child is able to communicate whether he/she would like to have a procedure.

Operative Approach

The operative strategy for an AVM is based on whether the lesion is localized, regional, or diffuse. A localized AVM involves 1–2 tissue planes (e.g., skin and subcutaneous tissue), is well-defined, and theoretically able to be entirely removed with linear closure. These lesions can sometimes be excised without preoperative embolization because bleeding is not significant. AVMs located in anatomically sensitive areas should have minimal or no margins taken. If a lesion is located in a nonsensitive area, then larger margins can be included as long as they don't significantly complicate the procedure.

Regional AVMs are large and/or involve >2 tissue planes. They usually cannot be reconstructed using local tissue; grafts or free-tissue transfer typically are required. Regional AVMs are managed by subtotal resection of a symptomatic area or complete extirpation and reconstruction with distant tissue. Lesions should have preoperative embolization to reduce intraoperative blood loss and facilitate the procedure. Skin grafts are best placed on a recipient site that is free of disease. If the underlying area contains AVM, then a graft has a high chance of failure and flap reconstruction is preferred.

Diffuse AVMs are unable to be entirely extirpated without causing significant morbidity. Patients are managed using embolization for palliation of bleeding, pain, and ulceration or undergo subtotal excisions of symptomatic areas. When resection is planned, patients have preoperative embolization. Operative intervention for a diffuse facial AVM should be focused on improving the patient's symptoms/appearance with localized staged procedures without causing a significant deformity. It is critical to avoid facial nerve injury. Because all surgical planes are affected by AVM, resections cause more bleeding than removal of a regional AVM.

Medical Management of AVM

There are limited prospective studies on the medical treatment of AVMs. It is clear that medication has a role in high-risk patients with no other treatment options. With discovery of germline and somatic mutations in AVMs, precision medicine may play a large role in future therapy. In hereditary hemorrhagic telangiectasia (HHT), several medications are being investigated for symptom relief and control of the AVM. These include bevacizumab, tranexamic acid, tamoxifen, propranolol, sirolimus, thalidomide derivatives, and pazopanib [15–17]. Recent discovery of somatic mutations of

MAP2K1 and *KRAS* raises the possibility of treatment with MEK inhibitors and other agents in the *RAS* pathway [3, 4]. Most of these agents are presently used in oncology. Early studies are in development using some of these agents.

Syndromes Associated with AVM

Capillary Malformation-Arteriovenous Malformation (CM-AVM)

This autosomal dominant condition affects 1/100,000 persons and is caused by a mutation in *RASA1 or EPHB4*. Lesions usually are small, multifocal, round, and pinkish-red; 50% are surrounded by a pale halo. One-third of children also have either Parkes Weber syndrome, extracerebral AVM, or intracerebral/spinal AVM. A patient suspected of having CM-AVM should be evaluated for AVMs on physical examination, and MRI of the brain and spine is considered.

Cobb Syndrome

This term previously had been used for a midline capillary malformation of the posterior trunk with an underlying spinal AVM. Patients labeled with "Cobb syndrome" likely have either CLOVES syndrome or CM-AVM. One-fourth of patients with CLOVES syndrome have spinal/paraspinal AVMs, and truncal capillary malformations are common in this condition. *RASA1* mutations have been documented in patients with spinal AVMs and overlying capillary malformations (CM-AVM).

Hereditary Hemorrhagic Telangiectasia (HHT)

This autosomal dominant disease (also referred to as Osler-Weber-Rendu syndrome) affects 1/10,000 persons and is caused by mutations in endoglin *(ENG)*, activin A receptor type II-like 1 *(ACVRL1/ALK1)*, or *SMAD4*. These mutations affect transforming growth factor beta signaling. Clinical findings consist of epistaxis, mucocutaneous telangiectasias, and visceral AVMs. The patient may exhibit upper gastrointestinal bleeding, stroke from pulmonary arteriovenous shunting, cerebral hemorrhage, heart failure, portal hypertension, and/or chronic anemia. Patients undergo genetic testing, echocardiography for pulmonary AVMs, brain MRI, and abdominal ultrasound; endoscopy is indicated for patients with a *SMAD4* mutation to document whether polyps are present.

PTEN-Associated Vascular Anomaly (PTEN-AVA)

The PTEN (phosphatase and tensin homologue) gene encodes a tumor suppressor lipid phosphatase. Patients with PTEN mutations have the autosomal dominant PTEN hamartoma tumor syndrome (previously referred to as Cowden or

Bannayan-Riley-Ruvalcaba syndrome). One-half of individuals have a fast-flow vascular anomaly with arteriovenous shunting, referred to as a PTEN-associated vascular anomaly (PTEN-AVA). Unlike a typical AVM, PTEN-AVAs can be multifocal, are typically intramuscular, contain ectopic adipose tissue, and have disproportionate, segmental dilation of draining veins. Patients exhibit macrocephaly, and males have penile freckling; other features can include developmental delay, thyroid lesions, and gastrointestinal polyps. Surveillance is required particularly for the development of epithelial, endocrine, and gastrointestinal malignancies. PTEN-AVAs are managed similarly to non-syndromic AVMs (i.e., embolization and/or resection).

Wyburn-Mason Syndrome

This rare sporadic condition consists of retinal AVMs with or without brain AVMs and a facial vascular malformation (capillary malformation or AVM). The syndrome also is referred to as Bonnet-Dechaume-Blanc syndrome or retinocephalofacial vascular malformation syndrome [18]. One-third of children do not contain a cutaneous lesion but exhibit AVMs of the retina and have neurological symptoms with or without brain AVMs. One-half of patients have retinal AVMs without cutaneous or brain lesions.

Parkes Weber Syndrome (PWS)

PWS consists of a diffuse AVM of an extremity (typically one leg) causing soft tissue and/or bony overgrowth. The cutaneous stain of the affected limb is warmer than a typical capillary malformation. PWS can be sporadic or familial due to a mutation in *RASA1* (CM-AVM1) or *EPHB4* (CM-AVM2) [19]. Patients have subcutaneous and intramuscular microshunting, often with cardiac volume overload, and can develop congestive heart failure. MRI is obtained to confirm the diagnosis and determine the extent of the malformation. Dilated feeding and draining vessels are illustrated as flow voids. The enlarged limb muscles and bones exhibit abnormal signal and enhancement. Most patients are observed until symptoms necessitate intervention. Children are monitored by an orthopedic surgeon for axial overgrowth. Embolization may be useful for pain, ulceration, or congestive heart failure, in those patients with discrete shunts, but the typical infiltrating small vessel AVM does not respond and may actually worsen with embolization. Occasionally, amputation is necessary [13].

Conclusion

Arteriovenous malformations are complicated vascular anomalies associated with germline and somatic mutations. Overall the natural history favors progression over time and in the most severe patients leads to life-threatening complications. These anomalies need to be treated by skilled practitioners in an interdisciplinary center. In the future, targeted medications will complement the surgical and interventional treatments and improve the overall outcome for these patients.

References

1. Kohout MP, Hansen M, Pribaz JJ, Mulliken JB. Arteriovenous malformations of the head and neck: natural history and management. Plast Reconstr Surg. 1998;102(3):643–54.
2. Lu L, Bischoff J, Mulliken JB, Bielenberg DR, Fishman SJ, Greene AK. Increased endothelial progenitor cells and vasculogenic factors in higher-staged arteriovenous malformations. Plast Reconstr Surg. 2011;128(4):260e–9e.
3. Couto JA, Huang AY, Konczyk DJ, Goss JA, Fishman SJ, Mulliken JB, et al. Somatic MAP2K1 mutations are associated with extracranial arteriovenous malformation. Am J Hum Genet. 2017;100(3):546–54.
4. Nikolaev SI, Fish JE, Radovanovic I. Somatic activating KRAS mutations in arteriovenous malformations of the brain. N Engl J Med. 2018;378(16):1561–2.
5. Burrows PE. Angioarchitecture of hereditary arteriovenous malformations. Semin Intervent Radiol. 2017;34(3):250–7.
6. Razek AA, Gaballa G, Megahed AS, Elmogy E. Time resolved imaging of contrast kinetics (TRICKS) MR angiography of arteriovenous malformations of head and neck. Eur J Radiol. 2013;82(11):1885–91.
7. Cho SK, Do YS, Shin SW, Kim DI, Kim YW, Park KB, et al. Arteriovenous malformations of the body and extremities: analysis of therapeutic outcomes and approaches according to a modified angiographic classification. J Endovasc Ther. 2006;13(4):527–38.
8. Park KB, Do YS, Kim DI, Kim YW, Shin BS, Park HS, et al. Predictive factors for response of peripheral arteriovenous malformations to embolization therapy: analysis of clinical data and imaging findings. J Vasc Interv Radiol. 2012;23(11):1478–86.
9. Houdart E, Gobin YP, Casasco A, Aymard A, Herbreteau D, Merland JJ. A proposed angiographic classification of intracranial arteriovenous fistulae and malformations. Neuroradiology. 1993;35(5):381–5.
10. Liu AS, Mulliken JB, Zurakowski D, Fishman SJ, Greene AK. Extracranial arteriovenous malformations: natural progression and recurrence after treatment. Plast Reconstr Surg. 2010;125(4):1185–94.
11. Berenstein A, Scott J, Choi IS, Persky M. Percutaneous embolization of arteriovenous fistulas of the external carotid artery. AJNR Am J Neuroradiol. 1986;7(5):937–42.
12. Cho SK, Do YS, Kim DI, Kim YW, Shin SW, Park KB, et al. Peripheral arteriovenous malformations with a dominant outflow vein: results of ethanol embolization. Korean J Radiol. 2008;9(3):258–67.
13. Greene AK. Arteriovenous malformation. In: Greene AK, editor. Vascular anomalies: classification, diagnosis and management. St. Louis: Quality Medical Publishing; 2013.
14. Greene AK, Orbach DB. Management of arteriovenous malformations. Clin Plast Surg. 2011;38(1):95–106.
15. Hsu YP, HSU CW, Bai CH, Cheng SW, Cheng C. Medical treatment for epistaxis in hereditary hemorrhagic telangiectasia: a meta-analysis. Otolaryngol Head Neck Surg. 2019;160(1):22–35. https://doi.org/10.1177/0194599818797316. Epub 2018 Sep 11.
16. Parambil JG, Woodard TD, Koc ON. Pazopanib effective for bevacizumb-unresponsive epistaxis in hereditary hemorrhagic telangiectasia. Laryngoscope. 2018;128(10):2234–6. https://doi.org/10.1002/lary.27129.. Epub 2018 Feb 16.

17. Lu J, Anvari R, Wang J, Huang J, Pei S, Xiang Y, Huang J, Yin Z, Chen J, Nelson JS, Tan W. Propranolol as a potentially novel treatment of arteriovenous malformations. JAAD Case Re. 2018;4(4):355–8. https://doi.org/10.1016/j.jdcr.2017.11.005. eCollection 2018 May.
18. Schmidt D, Pache M, Schumacher M. The congenital unilateral retinocephalic vascular malformation syndrome (bonnet-dechaume-blanc syndrome or wyburn-mason syndrome): review of the literature. Surv Ophthalmol. 2008;53:227–49.
19. Amyere M, Revencu N, Helaers R, Pairet E, Baselga E, Cordisco M, et al. Germline loss-of-function mutations in EPHB4 cause a second form of capillary malformation-arteriovenous malformation (CM-AVM2) deregulating RAS-MAPK signaling. Circulation. 2017;136(11):1037–48.

Overgrowth Syndromes Associated with Vascular Anomalies

12

Adrienne M. Hammill, Samantha A. Spencer, and Ahmad Alomari

Abbreviations

AVF	Arteriovenous fistula
AVM	Arteriovenous malformation
BRRS	Bannayan-Riley-Ruvalcaba syndrome
CBC	Complete blood count
CLOVES	Congenital lipomatous overgrowth, vascular anomalies, epidermal nevi, and skeletal and/or spinal anomalies
CM	Capillary malformation
CM-AVM	Capillary malformation-arteriovenous malformation
CRP	C-reactive protein
CTH	Cerebellar tonsillar herniation
EKG	Electrocardiogram
IVC	Inferior vena cava
KTS	Klippel-Trenaunay syndrome
LM	Lymphatic malformation
LMWH	Low-molecular-weight heparin

A. M. Hammill (✉)
Division of Hematology, Hemangioma and Vascular Malformation Center,
University of Cincinnati College of Medicine, Cincinnati Children's Hospital Medical Center,
Cincinnati, OH, USA
e-mail: adrienne.hammill@cchmc.org

S. A. Spencer
Orthopedic Center, Boston Children's Hospital, Harvard Medical School, Boston, MA, USA
e-mail: Samantha.Spencer@childrens.harvard.edu

A. Alomari
Department of Radiology, Boston Children's Hospital, Harvard Medical School,
Boston, MA, USA
e-mail: Ahmad.Alomari@childrens.harvard.edu

C. C. Trenor III, D. M. Adams (eds.), *Vascular Anomalies*,
https://doi.org/10.1007/978-3-030-25624-1_12

M-CM	Macrocephaly-capillary malformation syndrome
MRI	Magnetic resonance imaging
NSAIDs	Nonsteroidal anti-inflammatory drugs
PHTS	PTEN hamartoma tumor syndrome
PKWS	Parkes Weber syndrome
PS	Proteus syndrome
US	Ultrasound
VM	Venous malformation

Introduction

Overgrowth syndromes associated with vascular anomalies present special challenges to the patient and the treatment team. Proper diagnosis and management by a specialized interdisciplinary team are optimal as best outcomes require a thorough understanding of several basic principles and development of individualized treatment plans. Clinical exam remains essential although there is clinical overlap among various syndromes, with variable severity and degrees of overgrowth. In recent years there has been increasing understanding of the genetic basis of these conditions, which has provided improved understanding of the molecular pathways involved and will yield increasing treatment options in the future. It is helpful to differentiate germline from somatic mosaic genetic mutation overgrowth syndromes. Germline inheritance shows autosomal dominant transmission with whole body involvement, while somatic mutation results in limited involvement with only affected parts of the body carrying the mutated gene/overgrowth pathway. Treatment is tailored to each patient's current and potential future problems. Early treatment of lesions may be able to prevent major morbidity, so prompt diagnosis and recognition of potential associated complications are essential.

This chapter will cover major overgrowth syndromes along with diagnosis and current treatment options.

Diagnosis

History and Physical Exam

Each overgrowth syndrome has a pattern of physical findings that enables clinical diagnosis in most cases; however, overlap does occur, and occasionally additional information, such as imaging and pathology, is required to make the diagnosis.

A detailed history should be obtained, including any prenatal and postnatal findings, specifics of the timing of onset and the course of overgrowth. Additional history should focus on skin or visceral changes. Variations in lesions, including increased swelling or change in color or texture with infection, activity, growth spurts, or hormonal changes, should be noted. Associated signs and symptoms, including pain, functional difficulties, and gait changes, are also important. A history of thrombosis, both tender superficial clots and calcified phleboliths, and any more significant clotting history including deep venous thrombosis or pulmonary embolism, are of particular interest. Any bleeding history, particularly hematuria or gastrointestinal bleeding, should also be noted. A complete history should include a developmental history and a family history as well.

Clinical exam is essential. A whole body skin exam should be performed. Skin markings should be noted and palpated for temperature, texture, tenderness, and/or thrill. Superficial capillary malformation often suggests deeper overgrowth or additional venous or lymphatic malformations in the underlying tissues. Capillary staining can also be associated with other anomalies based on its location, such as genitourinary abnormalities or spinal anomalies when located over the central lumbar/sacral area. With involvement of the limb girdle, there is a high rate of pelvic disease which may include the rectosigmoid colon, urinary bladder, and uterus.

Phlebectasia (ectatic veins) should be characterized clinically and with imaging studies. These are often found on the lateral aspect of the limbs and may be found on the seemingly less-affected limb. Abnormal veins can also be found in the chest, axilla, abdomen, and pelvis. Identification of these veins is essential as their larger caliber leads to stagnant blood flow, thereby imparting a higher risk of thromboembolism even in the absence of thrombophilia. Precise mapping of these abnormal veins is essential.

Clinical exam reliably differentiates fast-flow malformations, such as Parkes Weber syndrome (PKWS), from the slow-flow malformation typically noted in Klippel-Trenaunay syndrome (KTS). High-flow lesions are warm or even hot to touch, warmer than the surrounding tissue, and may have an audible bruit or palpable thrill in the area directly overlying the arteriovenous connection.

Any asymmetry should be noted and can include overgrowth on one side of the face or body, as in hemihypertrophy or asymmetric tissue and/or masses. The location of such tissue/masses may be helpful in differentiating between the overgrowth syndromes.

Limb overgrowth can be quantified by using a measuring tape to compare limb lengths and circumferences. Gait abnormalities are commonly seen in the setting of limb length discrepancy, so it is important to observe the patient walk. Musculoskeletal exam should document limb functionality noting contractures, masses, joint mobility, motor skills, and any limb anomalies. Particular attention should be paid to the hands and feet, as these may show unusual spacing between fingers and/or toes.

Laboratory and Additional Studies

Laboratory workup should evaluate thrombotic status whenever there is a venous component, including complete blood count, fibrinogen, and D-dimer. A renal panel should also be obtained to evaluate kidney function in case the patient will require anticoagulation for interventions or procedures in the future. Patients with poor weight gain or failure to thrive require nutritional workup and support. Testing for genetic mutations is useful to guide therapy decisions; most cases will require tissue as many of these syndromes have somatic mosaic mutations which may not be identified by genetic testing of blood.

Cardiac evaluation may be appropriate in some patients. Cardiac arrhythmias have been reported in M-CM; thus early EKG is recommended. Full evaluation, including EKG and echocardiography, should be performed regularly in patients with high-flow lesions (Parkes Weber syndrome and some vascular lesions in the setting of PTEN) to evaluate for cardiac overload or failure.

Imaging

Early imaging for CLOVES and KTS is recommended in the neonatal or early infantile period or at the time of initial presentation. MRI is the modality of choice to characterize the various components of the disorder including overgrowth, vascular malformations, and musculoskeletal, visceral, and/or neural axis anomalies. Basic sequences, including multiplanar T2-weighted imaging with fat saturation, provide the majority of findings. T1-weighted imaging, with both pre- and post-contrast sequences and MR venography, can be helpful to demonstrate ectatic or abnormal veins. Imaging should specifically evaluate for phlebectasia, particularly involving the marginal venous system and subclavian veins, as this can cause life-threatening thromboembolism and is one of the leading causes of mortality in these patients. However, MRI can be less sensitive in depicting compressed large veins or small deep veins.

MRI of the brain should be considered in any patient with macrocephaly or developmental delays. Classic imaging findings include hemimegalencephaly (in some patients with CLOVES) or megalencephaly and/or polymicrogyria (in many patients with M-CM).

Ultrasonography (US) is a practical, dynamic tool which is widely available and can provide immediate information about venous and lymphatic anomalies, as well as readily identifying acute complications such as thrombosis and intralesional bleeding. US is also a major tool for guiding minimally invasive treatment.

Cases of Wilms' tumor have now been reported in M-CM and CLOVES; thus serial renal ultrasound until the age of 7–8 years is recommended [1].

CT scan is reserved for detailed evaluation of the bony part of the limb and pelvis. CT provides quick evaluation in urgent situations such as imaging of pelviabdominal or pulmonary vessels for thromboembolism or phlebectasia.

Plain radiographs can be used to assess osseous changes including bone deformities, flexion contractures, joint degeneration, osteopenia, and leg length discrepancy. Standing leg x-rays can be used to evaluate for leg length discrepancy once patients reach walking age and should be followed serially to determine the appropriate time for intervention.

The use of diversion venography allows for the demonstration of intact deep venous system, whereas conventional venography may fail to illustrate the deep veins due to preferential flow of blood into the large anomalous veins. Angiography is not a primary imaging tool in low-flow lesions, but may be useful in high-flow lesions as in Parkes Weber syndrome or some cases of PTHS.

The Syndromes

Klippel-Trenaunay Syndrome (KTS)

Klippel-Trenaunay syndrome (KTS) (OMIM # 149000) is the prototype of uncommon overgrowth disorders associated with different types of complex vascular anomalies (Fig. 12.1).

The overgrowth in KTS is typically limited to one lower extremity and the limb girdle, although the definition of KTS has sometimes been extended to include involvement of both lower limbs. The affected limb demonstrates lymphatic overgrowth and slow-flow malformations (capillary, lymphatic, and venous) [2]. These vessel components are each associated with different potential complications, such as phlebectasia and possible thromboembolism within the ectatic veins, infection in lymphatic malformations, and leaking of lymphatic fluid from lymphatic vesicles.

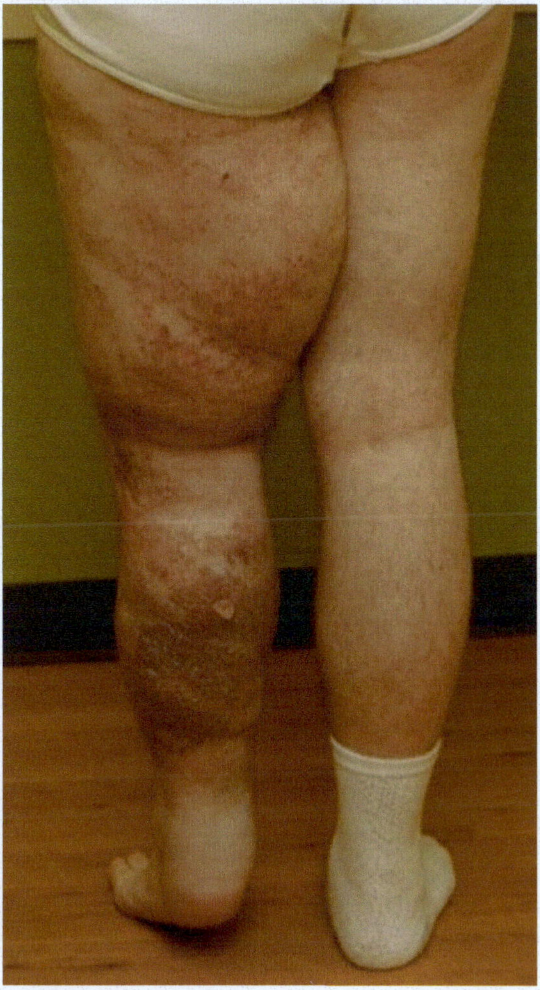

Fig. 12.1 Patient with KTS. Note the capillary lymphatic venous malformation and bulky overgrowth. This patient has previously undergone multiple surgical and interventional procedures

The anomalous venous component in KTS is composed of a complex network of enlarged dysmorphic incompetent veins distributed in the superficial and deep compartments. These dysfunctional vessels attain a considerable size, and an abnormal large communicating tributary network exists within the deep venous system. This venous network may include the marginal vein proper, small saphenous, sciatic, inferior gluteal, and internal iliac veins. Ectasias of the popliteal vein, deep femoral vein, and inferior vena cava (megacava) are common findings [3]. The deep venous system may demonstrate underdevelopment, dilatation, or duplication. Pooling and stagnation of blood in the lower limb cause distention, pain, and, in severe cases, postural hypotension. Thromboembolism remains the most significant complication.

Different forms of lymphatic malformations exist in KTS, including macrocystic and microcystic lymphatic cysts, and cause the majority of the acute symptoms such as recurrent episodes of infections, intralesional bleeds, and pain. Cutaneous manifestations of LM include vesicles and plaques usually concentrated within and around the CM on the lateral aspect of the thigh and calf. These lesions are prone to recurrent bleeding, leakage of lymph, infection, ulceration, and poor healing (Fig. 12.2).

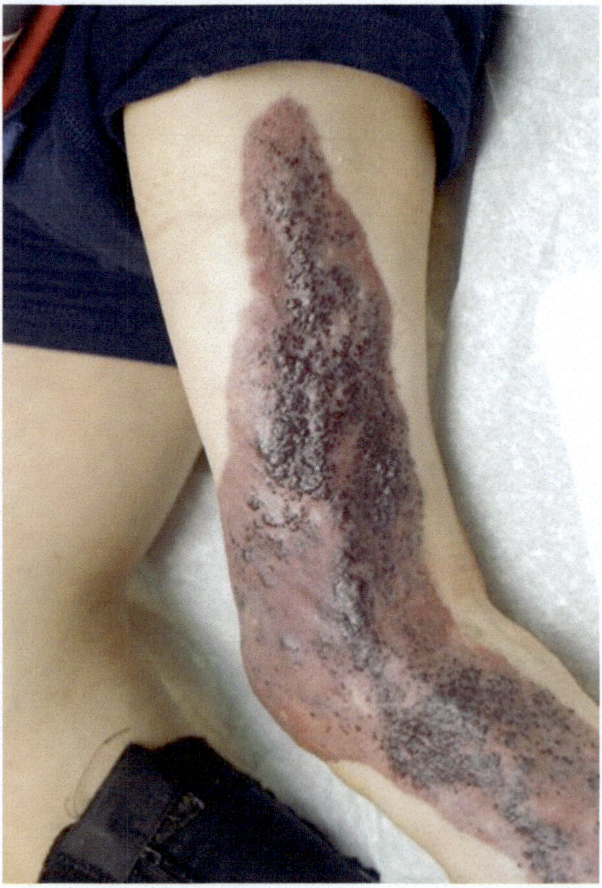

Fig. 12.2 Lymphatic blebs in a KTS patient. They are raised and crusting. Also visible is the dilated marginal vein

Lymphatic macrocysts are often found in the thigh, limb girdle, and pelvis, but are generally less symptomatic than the microcystic type. The latter are typically extensive and affect the fatty extrafascial and intrafascial compartments of the limb. In the pelvis, microcystic LM and fatty overgrowth commonly present as concentric encasement of a thickened anorectum and sigmoid and are often associated with rectal bleeding. The urinary bladder may be elongated with anteroventral displacement. The presence of abnormal superficial venous channels in bladder or urethral mucosa frequently presents as bleeding per urethra.

Clinical Findings

The affected limb is usually diffusely enlarged, both in girth and length. The capillary malformation (CM) is characteristically large and located on the lateral aspect of the thigh and calf. Smaller stains can also be seen in the foot and limb girdle. The CM typically contains lymphatic vesicles and overlies the course of the marginal venous system. Mosaic PIK3CA mutations have been identified in some but not all KTS patients.

CLOVES Syndrome

CLOVES is an acronym for *c*ongenital *l*ipomatous *o*vergrowth, *v*ascular malformations, *e*pidermal nevi, and *s*coliosis/spinal/skeletal anomalies [4]. This syndrome is highly variable as it results from a mosaic *PIK3CA* mutation that occurs early in embryonic development [5]. Thus, parts of the body carry the mutation with variable abnormalities, while unaffected parts of the body do not carry the mutation. Presentation of CLOVES is highly variable depending on where the mutated cells are located.

CLOVES patients have findings similar to that in KTS as discussed above, generally including at least one limb but with more extensive involvement extending into the trunk. Truncal involvement includes fatty lipomatous overgrowth and risk of spinal involvement (Fig. 12.3).

Associated vascular malformations are usually combined capillary venous lymphatic malformations, although high-flow arteriovenous malformations have been reported particularly in the spine. Capillary staining is usually visible overlying affected areas, often patchy and discontiguous. As in KTS, lymphatic blebs impart risk of infection as well as bleeding if overlying a capillary malformation. Venous abnormalities are particularly prominent in these patients, with anomalous veins that can enlarge and lead to thromboses, both deep venous thromboses (DVT) and pulmonary embolism (PE), particularly periprocedurally. Like in KTS, an enlarged lateral marginal leg vein (vein of Servelle) is common; in addition, anomalous truncal and upper extremity systems can be seen in CLOVES.

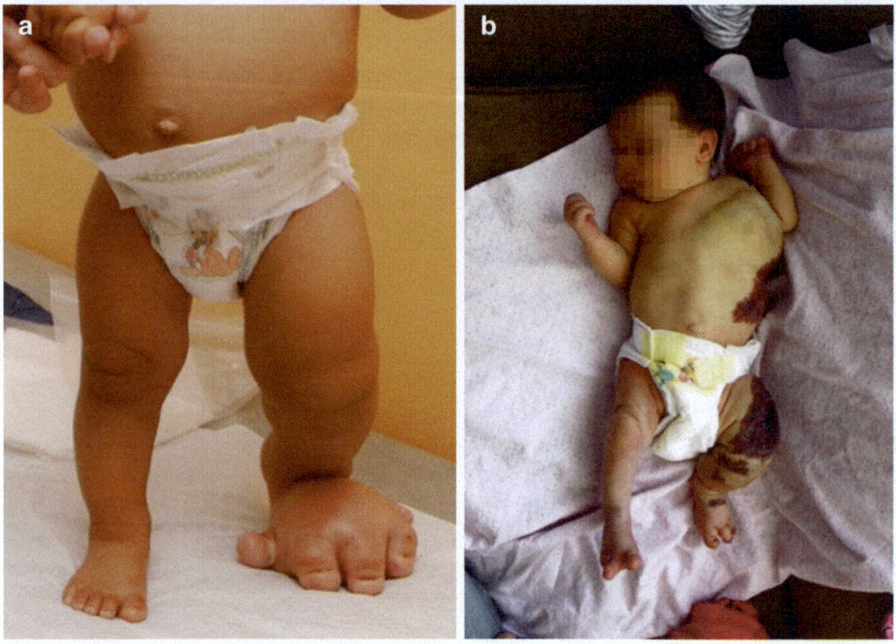

Fig. 12.3 Two patients with CLOVES. Both demonstrate classic foot abnormalities. Patient A has evidence of lipomatous overgrowth of the left leg. Patient B has truncal and leg overgrowth with lipomatosis and capillary venous malformation

Clinical Findings

Large areas of overgrowth consisting of fat, lymphatic malformation, or lymphaticovenous malformation are typical, particularly on the trunk. This growth tends to be progressive and may not cease with skeletal maturity.

Epidermal nevi are often present and can be extensive or more limited in area.

Limb overgrowth, often severe, is frequently present and may affect more than one extremity. As in KTS, this includes both girth and length overgrowth, with significant leg length discrepancy possible. Patients are also noted to have relative wasting (lipoatrophy) of "unaffected" limbs, with frequent concerns for malnutrition without metabolic evidence of calorie deprivation.

Classically, patients have notable foot abnormalities, including sandal gap deformity and other unusual spacing of the digits (Fig. 12.3).

Spinal anomalies along with scoliosis are common, including spinal arterial venous malformations.

Imaging

As for KTS, MRI with contrast is the preferred imaging modality to assess for extent of internal and soft tissue involvement in CLOVES.

Early whole spine MRI is indicated to evaluate for intrathecal anomalies such as tethered cord or vascular malformation.

Unlike KTS patients, CLOVES patients do have increased risk of Wilms' tumor of the kidney (approximately 3%). Children should be screened according to a protocol of serial abdominal ultrasounds every 3 months until age 8.

Macrocephaly-Capillary Malformation (M-CM)

Macrocephaly-capillary malformation (M-CM) is a rare syndrome involving macrocephaly, capillary malformation often with a distinct pattern reminiscent of CMTC, somatic overgrowth, brain abnormalities, and varying degrees of developmental delay (OMIM # 602501). It has been previously called macrocephaly-cutis marmorata telangiectatica congenita (M-CMTC), megalencephaly-cutis marmorata telangiectatica congenita, and megalencephaly-capillary malformation-polymicrogyria (MCAP). Recently, many patients with this syndrome have been found to carry PIK3CA mutations in affected tissues [6].

The syndrome was first described in 1997 as consisting of vascular birthmark, macrocephaly, and early overgrowth (including prenatally, manifested by high birthweight and very large head circumference), resulting in developmental delays and localized skeletal defects including asymmetric overgrowth and toe syndactyly [7, 8]. Neurologic issues include hypotonia and cognitive impairments and nonobstructive hydrocephalus. Clinical diagnostic criteria have been proposed independently by two groups, but neither has been widely adopted as definitive [9, 10].

Physical Findings

Craniofacial findings are often most striking including occipito-frontal head circumference several standard deviations above the mean. This measurement is often increased at birth, but increases markedly during infancy. Frontal bossing may be present. Capillary malformation is often present on the face, most commonly involving the philtrum and/or nose.

A more reticulated pattern of capillary malformation may be seen on the body, and asymmetric overgrowth may be visible (Fig. 12.4). Skeletal abnormalities include syndactyly and polydactyly, as well as sandal gap deformity.

Neuroimaging and Neuropathology

Neuroimaging is usually abnormal [11]. Patients commonly show ventriculomegaly (obstructive or nonobstructive). Patients often show evidence of cortical dysgenesis, including focal cortical dysplasia and polymicrogyria, often in a perisylvian distribution. White matter abnormalities are frequently observed, attributed to delayed myelination or dysmyelination. Brain asymmetry is also common and tends to correlate with ipsilateral facial hemihyperplasia. Posterior fossa crowding is seen in a

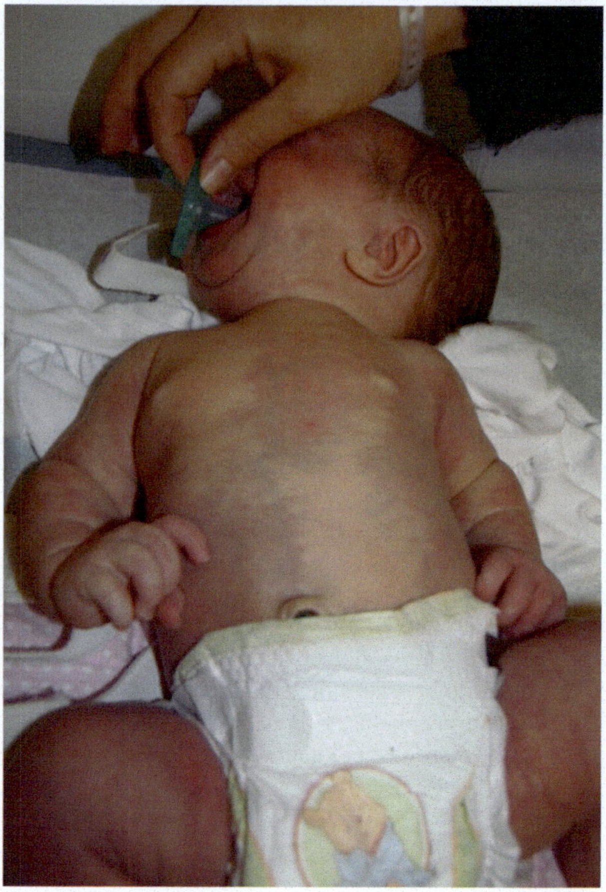

Fig. 12.4 Patient with M-CM and macrocephaly. Notice the faint capillary malformation and overgrowth

majority of cases. Cerebellar tonsillar herniation (CTH) occurs frequently in M-CM, in up to 70% of patients in two studies, often developing during infancy rather than as a congenital process [11, 12]. The postnatal development of herniation suggests that rapid excessive brain growth in the first few months to year of life may be responsible for the CTH. CTH, with potential for brainstem compression, has been implicated in several sudden deaths, and posterior fossa decompression should be considered in patients with evidence of CTH. While many patients have ventriculomegaly, ventricular shunting has not been shown to improve macrocephaly in M-CM patients, so may not be sufficient alone to decrease the risk of CTH and brainstem compression.

Given the progressive brain changes that can occur during infancy and early childhood, MRI of the brain is recommended at the time of diagnosis and every 6 months until the age of 2 years, with a follow-up at 3 years of age. Brain growth is generally complete by age 3, and it is expected that imaging should become stable at that time.

Neuropathology has not been studied extensively to date. Microscopic evaluation of brains from two affected individuals revealed extensive neuromigration defects – including polymicrogyria and heterotopia [11].

Parkes Weber Syndrome (PKWS)

Parkes Weber syndrome (PKWS), first described in 1907, is characterized by bone and soft tissue hypertrophy of an extremity in association with capillary malformation and high-flow vascular lesion(s), generally multiple arteriovenous fistulas (AVFs) or microfistulas (OMIM #608355). The affected limbs show increasing overgrowth over time, with both increased girth and length, resulting in limb length discrepancy. Skin changes are also progressive over time, with increasing color change and even ischemia leading to ulceration and pain in the distal extremity. Venous dilatation gradually occurs as a result of high pressure in the venous system through communication with the arterial system and tends to extend proximally over time. Long-term, the high flow through the AVM/AVFs and the extensive network of ectatic draining veins can lead to high output heart failure and cardiac dysfunction.

A subset of patients with Parkes Weber syndrome develop PKWS as a part of a familial syndrome, called capillary malformation-arteriovenous malformation (CM-AVM). Many families with CM-AVM have been shown to have a mutation in RASA1 [13, 14], with additional families recently shown to have mutation in EPHB4 [15]. These patients have multiple capillary malformations, often with a small surrounding halo suggesting steal, on their skin. Some will have associated AVMs of the brain and spinal cord.

Physical Findings

On exam, the affected limb is larger and longer than the unaffected side. The overlying capillary malformations are warm or even hot to touch and often have palpable thrill or audible bruit. Distended draining veins are usually prominent and may be traced proximally toward the heart. There may be ulceration of the digits or proximal extremity (Fig. 12.5). Lymphedema is often present within the affected limb.

Imaging and Other Studies

MRI is useful in characterizing the soft tissue changes, but angiography is necessary to map the abnormal connections between arteries and veins in order to consider intervention.

Echocardiogram and EKG are recommended to follow cardiac function at regular intervals.

PTEN Hamartoma Tumor Syndrome (PHTS)

PTEN is an important tumor suppressor gene located on chromosome 10q22–23, responsible for downregulation of the PI3K/Akt/mTOR pathway via its phosphatase activity (OMIM #601728). Loss of negative regulation allows for increased growth and inappropriate cell survival and has been implicated in multiple cancers.

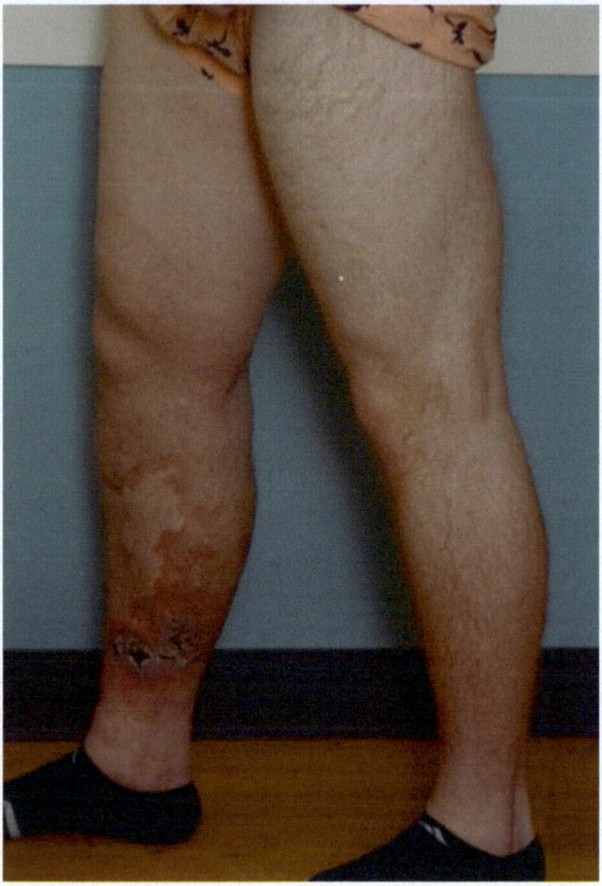

Fig. 12.5 Patient with PKWS in the setting of familial CM-AVM. Notice the faint capillary malformation, warm to touch. This lesion was complicated by a non-healing ulcer

Inheritance is autosomal dominant in fashion, although the majority of germline mutations occur *de novo*. Patients with PTEN hamartoma tumor syndromes (PHTS) are at significantly increased lifetime risk for multiple neoplasms both benign and malignant, particularly in breast, thyroid, renal, and endometrial tissues.

The PTEN hamartoma tumor syndrome encompasses Cowden syndrome, Bannayan-Riley-Ruvalcaba syndrome (BRRS), PTEN-related Proteus syndrome (PS), and Proteus-like syndrome [16]. While initially only Cowden syndrome was identified as having an increased risk of cancer, all of these "PTENopathy" phenotypes are now considered to carry the same increased risks for cancer development and are recommended for the same screening on the basis of their genetics [17].

The PI-3-kinase:AKT:PTEN pathway has been implicated in cell growth and proliferation phenotypes, including a number of vascular anomalies [18], and not surprisingly patients with PHTS may have vascular malformations as part of their phenotype. In fact, this was added as a minor diagnostic criterion for PTENopathies in 2013 [19]. The vascular malformations in patients with PTEN vary widely and include high-flow AVM type lesions as well as mixed- and low-flow lesions, often with ectopic fat [20]. A subset of these lesions, collectively designated PTEN hamartoma of soft tissue (PHOST), tend to be intramuscular and painful and have a distinctive microscopic appearance [21]. Histopathology reveals increased fat and myxoid fibrous tissue, intermixed with abnormal vascular channels.

However, clinically there is overlap with PIK3CA and AKT mutations. In one study of patients meeting criteria for PTEN based on Cleveland Clinic's risk calculator (http://www.lerner.ccf.org/gmi/ccscore) but without an identifiable mutation, 11% of patients were found to have germline PIK3CA or AKT mutations [22].

Clinical Exam

Classic findings typically noted in patients with PTEN hamartoma tumor syndrome (PHTS) include macrocephaly and penile freckling. Patients with PTEN mutations frequently have benign overgrowth, including lipomas, papillomas, and tricholemmomas. Vascular masses are often fatty, may be warm, and may have overlying vascular discoloration or internal vascularity (Fig. 12.6). In addition, patients frequently have some developmental delays and have an increased risk of autism.

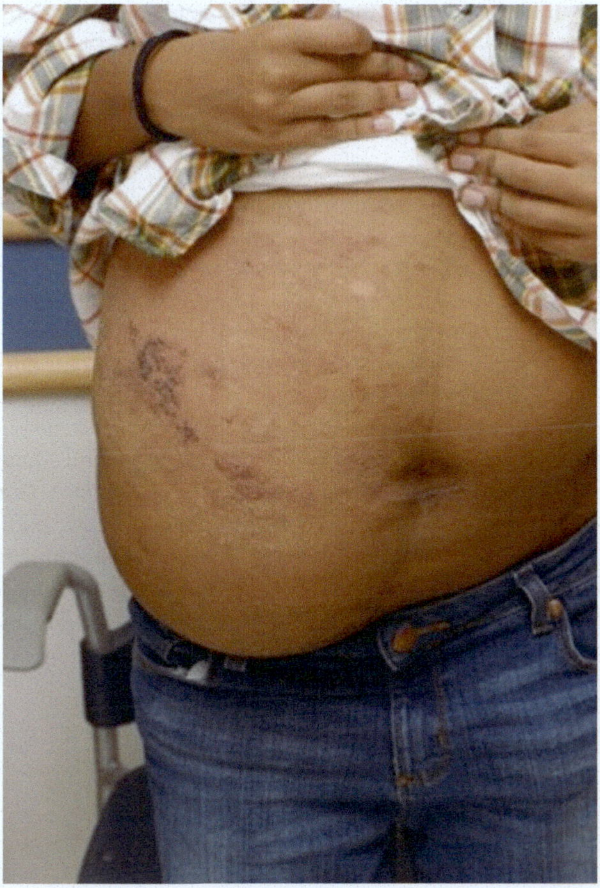

Fig. 12.6 Patient with PHTS and large abdominal wall hamartoma with lymphatic component and visible superficial lymphatic vessels

Imaging

In addition to imaging of the affected areas, patients with PHTS may require imaging of the CNS and tumor surveillance of the thyroid, breast, and kidneys. This can be best done in a Cancer Predisposition Clinic or by a geneticist as part of a comprehensive screening program [15].

Summary (Table 12.1)

Treatment Principles

General

For each of these overgrowth syndromes, it is important to understand the natural history of the condition in order to anticipate problems relevant to the patient. For example, in M-CM developmental delays with low muscle tone and fatigue are prevalent, while in PTEN autism spectrum disorder is often seen concomitantly. These are lifelong and not progressive and have established treatments, which should be applied as they are in the general population affected by the same problems. In contrast, limb length discrepancy and overgrowth generally progress and should be treated if the discrepancy is over 2 cm/1 inch.

Another issue is the rapid pace of changing knowledge in the field. The patient and family should be counseled about the variety of treatment options at present and advised that these will likely change in the coming years. Thus, any treatment plan must weigh risks and benefits now against the possibility that a better treatment will exist in the near future. For disorders with aberrant veins (KTS/CLOVES), these must be closed prior to invasive surgical procedures due to risk of thromboembolism with immobility. A hematology consult for evaluation of thrombosis risk and anticoagulation planning should also be completed prior to any treatment. High-risk patients may need perioperative anticoagulation (usually with Lovenox) as well as an IVC filter in certain cases.

Symptoms caused by the vascular components can be acute (such as pain, thromboembolism, or infection) or chronic (such as bleeding from intestinal, genitourinary, or cutaneous lesions or venous hypertension). Limb overgrowth may lead to various degrees of dysfunction, chronic disability, and lowered quality of life.

Early diagnosis and timely approach are paramount to treat symptoms and prevent high-risk morbidity. Coordinated management by a specialized interdisciplinary team prevents fragmentation or delay of care. The major therapeutic options for these overgrowth syndromes include the combination of conservative, medical, minimally invasive, and surgical.

Table 12.1 Summary table of characteristics of each overgrowth syndrome

Overgrowth syndrome	Gene(s)	Inheritance pattern	Overgrowth pattern	Vascular malformation	Other findings
Klippel-Trenaunay syndrome (KTS)	PIK3CA	Somatic mosaic	Usually limited to the limb girdle and one lower extremity – Girth and length	Capillary Lymphatic Venous	Phlebectasia Risk of thromboembolism Leaking of lymphatic fluid from vesicles/blebs Recurrent infections in lymphatic malformation
Congenital Lipomatous overgrowth, vascular anomalies, epidermal nevi, and skeletal/spinal anomalies (CLOVES)	PIK3CA	Somatic mosaic	Lipomatous overgrowth of trunk often with wasting of unaffected limbs	Capillary venous ectasias Lymphatic Rarely high-flow spinal lesion	KTS findings, above Sandal-gap deformity and/or syndactyly of toes Spinal anomalies, including tethered cord
Macrocephaly-capillary malformation (M-CM)	PIK3CA	Somatic mosaic	Somatic overgrowth usually involving brain and face and may involve body as well	Capillary malformation (usually face), often in a reticular pattern reminiscent of CMTC	Brain overgrowth-megalencephaly Frequent cortical dysplasia – polymicrogyria High risk of cerebellar tonsillar herniation
Parkes Weber syndrome (PKWS)	RASA-1 EPHB4	Germline	Limited to single limb, secondary to high flow	Capillary + arteriovenous malformations or (micro) fistulas	Frequently progressive risk of heart failure
PTEN hamartoma tumor syndrome (PTHS)	PTEN	Autosomal dominant	Lipomatous masses (PHOST histology)	Capillary or venous or lymphatic or combined May even be high-flow (AVM) though usually atypical	Macrocephaly Penile freckling Autism Family history cancers (thyroid, breast, renal, endometrial)

Conservative Management

Conservative management of patients with these overgrowth syndromes may include elastic compression stockings, physical therapy, proper skin care and hygiene practices, pain management, and psychosocial support. Shoe lifts may help patients with mild leg length discrepancy or even more severe discrepancies until definitive surgical intervention can be performed.

Education of the patients and their families and regular follow-up with an interdisciplinary team are crucial for proper care of these patients.

Interventional (Minimally Invasive) Management

Closure of dilated veins reduces the risk of thromboembolism and venous distension. This should be performed early in childhood if possible and particularly prior to surgical procedures. We recommend closing specific dilated veins (lower limb and truncal marginal veins, axillary-subclavian, sciatic, and short saphenous veins) early in life. Later in life, these enlarged veins must be identified prior to any procedures and treated if possible.

Diversion and selective venography are used to demonstrate the small deep venous system of the affected limb. Ectatic anomalous veins are disconnected from the normal veins to prevent migration of clots caudally. Minimally invasive techniques such as embolization and endovenous laser treatment can be safely used to permanently close these veins. In addition, phlebectomy and ligation of the superficial segments of the anomalous veins can be performed through small incision(s) along the course of the vein.

Lymphatic macrocysts are amenable to percutaneous aspiration and sclerotherapy. Carbon dioxide laser can be used to evaporate lymphatic vesicles and plaques.

Embolization may be used in high-flow lesions, including those in Parkes Weber, a subset of PTHS lesions, and small number of CLOVES patients.

The color of CM can be diminished with the use of pulsed dye laser, although is generally less effective on extremities than on the face.

Surgical Management

Patients who are seriously disabled by the massive size of the affected limb, as with significant bulky circumferential limb overgrowth, may benefit from surgical debulking. This lightens the load on the limb but carries significant morbidity. This can be extrafascial lymphaticovenous debulking in Klippel-Trenaunay or removal of large fatty growths in CLOVES. Liposuction can only be used for isolated fatty overgrowth in selected cases and is not appropriate for areas with vascular malformations.

Preoperative imaging and closure of anomalous veins should be completed prior to any surgical procedures in order to reduce the morbidity from perioperative thromboembolism.

Endorectal pull-through procedure should be considered for patients who are transfusion-dependent due to severe chronic gastrointestinal hemorrhage.

Orthopedic Treatments

The goal of orthopedic management is to maintain a balanced pelvis and spine with functional limbs and plantigrade shoeable feet that allow independent ambulation. With multidisciplinary management, this can be accomplished in most patients.

Leg length discrepancy is common in Klippel-Trenaunay and CLOVES. This should be assessed clinically and shoe lift prescribed for any limp with definitive limb length equalization planned for discrepancies that imbalance the pelvis by more than 2 cm/1 inch at maturity. Equalization is usually accomplished by selective physeal ablation of the proximal tibia and/or distal femur (epiphysiodesis) around the age of puberty (10–11 in girls, 13–14 in boys in most cases). Epiphysiodesis is a minor procedure which takes approximately 1 hour, with the physis closed either by percutaneous drilling/curettage or transphyseal screw placement. Excellent predictive growth charts and models exist to determine appropriate timing. This method is best for discrepancies in the range of 2–6 cm/1–3 inches. Guided growth can be used for angular deformities and is minimally invasive. A small tethering device or partial physeal closure is implanted on the side of deformity, and correction is obtained with further physeal growth gradually correcting the deformity (Fig. 12.7).

Intra-articular disease can lead to limb contractures. Early contracture can be managed with physical therapy and night extension bracing but will likely progress. In some cases, tendon lengthening is possible. Intra-articular venous malformation can be managed with combined sclerotherapy followed by synovectomy. However, there is a high rate of recurrence, so multiple procedures may be needed to avoid end-stage arthritis. Few patients with end-stage arthritis and severe vascular

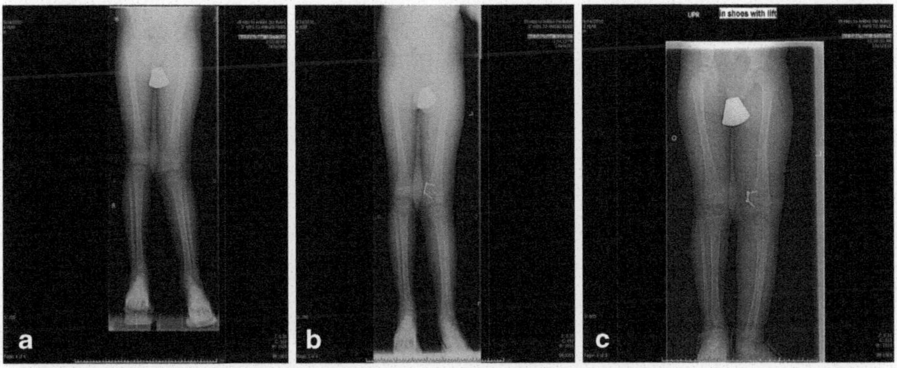

Fig. 12.7 Guided growth can also be used for angular deformities and is minimally invasive. A small tethering device or partial physeal closure is implanted on the side of deformity and correction is obtained with further physeal growth gradually correcting the deformity

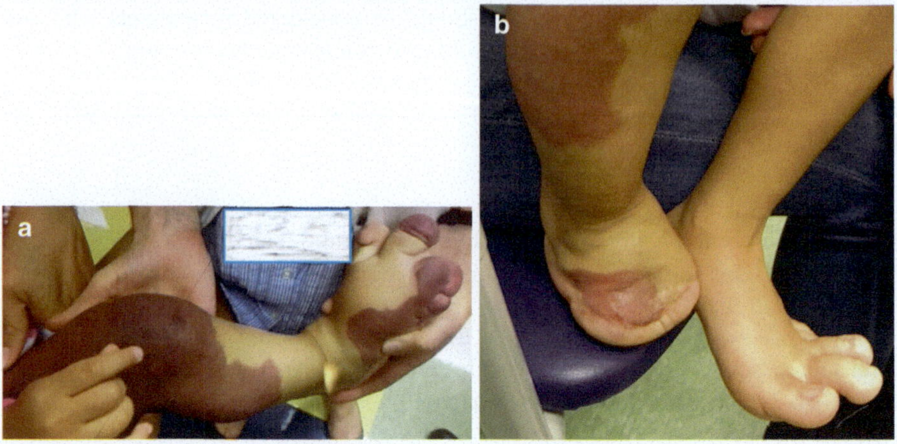

Fig 12.8 (**a**) A patient pre and post surgical amputation of the forefoot. (**b**) A patient pre and post surgical amputation with improvment in the functionality of the foot

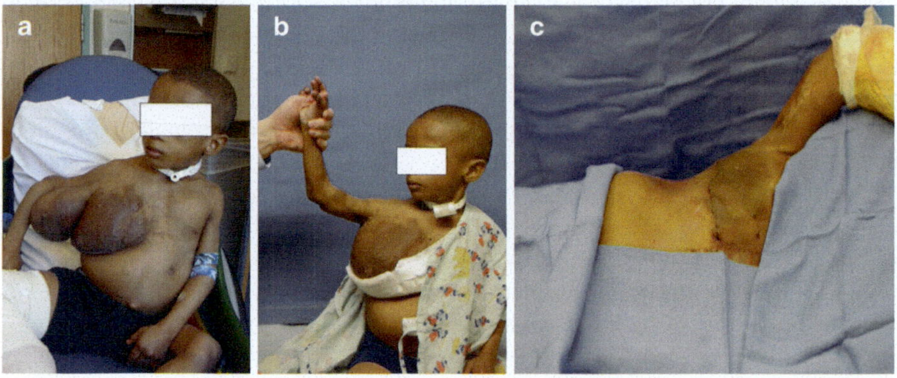

Fig. 12.9 Staged debulking procedures with the final result improving the funtionality of the upper extremity

malformation involving the limb are eligible for joint replacements due to the poor soft tissue and/or bone quality and the resulting high-risk of bleeding, wound complication, and infection.

Severely enlarged hands and feet with macrodactyly may be best served by ray resection or amputation of the forefoot (Fig. 12.8). Focal overgrowth can be debulked with significant improvement (Fig. 12.9). Thus, this is used in severe overgrowth to facilitate the ability to wear clothes and shoes off the shelf. In cases of truly massive parasitic limbs that have little to no function, amputation may be the best option. In cases of high-flow lesions that show signs of impending heart failure, amputation can be considered on a case-by-case basis.

Scoliosis is often atypical and does not respond well to bracing. Progressive curves >50 degrees may require neurosurgical intervention.

Neurosurgical Treatments

Spinal deformity and involvement is commonly seen in CLOVES. MRI is essential to facilitate appropriate neurosurgical treatment of tethered spinal cord or compressive lesions. Preoperative sclerotherapy may be needed for paraspinal malformations to minimize bleeding risk. Progressive scoliosis rarely responds to bracing and is treated with instrumented spinal fusion.

Patients with M-CM may experience ventriculomegaly (+/− increased pressure) and cerebellar tonsillar herniation. Such patients may require posterior decompression and/or ventricular shunting to prevent brain stem herniation.

Medical Therapies

Patients with a lymphatic component, particularly with leaking or bleeding blebs, may experience infections within their lesions. This can be a local cellulitis or a more complicated infection with bacteremia and sepsis. Education of families is crucial to help distinguish signs of cellulitis (erythema, swelling, warmth, pain, and fever) from those of superficial phlebitis. Patients should not delay treatment and should be evaluated promptly by a medical provider. If cellulitis is suspected, antibiotics should be started immediately after blood work is obtained, which should include a complete blood count (CBC) with differential, markers of inflammation such as C-reactive protein (CRP), and blood culture given the rapid rate at which these can progress from localized to systemic. Antibiotics may need to be administered intravenously and for a longer course than is usual for patients without underlying syndromes. Documentation of the number and severity of infections can be helpful in determining if prophylactic antibiotics should be implemented for individual patients. A care plan that includes a personalized problem list and suggestions for treatment options in case of acute illness can be a valuable tool for patients.

Patients with a significant venous component, particularly patients with KTS, are likely to have a coagulopathy (elevated D-dimer +/− low fibrinogen). The coagulopathy may need to be treated with anticoagulation prior to procedures to prevent bleeding and following procedures to prevent thrombosis. Low-molecular-weight heparin (LMWH) has been the treatment of choice, as new oral Xa inhibitors have not yet been evaluated for this indication. Once a patient has had a deep venous thrombosis, a chronic course of anticoagulation may be needed. Inferior vena cava (IVC) filter placement should also be considered with the interdisciplinary team on an individual patient basis.

Some patients have reported improvement in pain during perioperative courses of LMWH. For some with very significant clotting (frequent tender clots or phleboliths), LMWH may be used to manage this clotting and pain. NSAIDs are frequently recommended in short courses (scheduled dosing for 3–7 days) to decrease the inflammation associated with occasional clots. Some patients may benefit from chronic anti-inflammatory medications, such as celecoxib.

Until fairly recently, there was little medical intervention available for patients with these overgrowth syndromes. However, with the identification of more genes causing vascular anomalies, it has become clear that the PI-3-kinase/AKT/mTOR pathway is crucial to regulate growth. Loss of negative regulation, as in inactivating mutations of PTEN or TSC1/TSC2, or upregulation of pro-growth proteins through activating mutations, as in PIK3CA or AKT, result in loss of homeostasis and overgrowth of affected tissues. mTOR serves to integrate all of these incoming signals, and inhibition of mTOR using rapamycin (sirolimus) and its rapalogs has proven to be a valuable tool in the treatment of these patients [23].

A recent Phase II study investigated the use of sirolimus for the treatment of patients with complicated vascular malformations, including several with overgrowth syndromes [24]. The study included 13 patients with capillary venous lymphatic malformations (including many meeting criteria for Klippel-Trenaunay and CLOVES), as well as 6 patients with known PTEN mutations and vascular anomaly. At the end of the study, of the 11 evaluable patients with CLVM and the 4 evaluable patients with PTEN-related vascular malformations, all 15 experienced a partial response to sirolimus therapy. These partial responses included improved quality of life, decreased pain, and improvement in function. In addition, none of these 15 patients experienced further growth of their malformations while on sirolimus. Much more remains to be learned about the use of mTOR inhibition for these patients, including length of treatment required, trough levels of drug required for efficacy, and potential long-term complications. Monitoring is ongoing in the Phase II study, with patients being monitored for 5 years following their completion of the study.

Newer options, also related to the PIK3CA/AKT/mTOR and RAS/MAPK/MEK pathways, are now becoming available (see Chap. 4). Venot et al. recently treated 19 patients having a diagnosis of PROS (4 adults and 15 children) with a PIK3CA inhibitor under a compassionate use protocol, with all patients noting improvement (radiologically and clinically) with minimal side effects [25]. In addition, there is an open AKT inhibitor study for patients with PIK3CA-related overgrowth syndromes (ClinicalTrials.gov Identifier: NCT03094832).

Conclusions

Proper diagnosis is critical and should involve a careful history, complete physical exam, laboratory studies, and pathology and imaging as appropriate. Correct diagnosis will inform potential complications and drive follow-up and interventions necessary to optimize function and quality of life for the patient. Genetic causes have recently been identified in many of these overgrowth syndromes, but may be somatic and are therefore not necessarily detected by genetic testing of blood, though should be present in affected tissues.

Optimal treatment plans will include a multidisciplinary team providing coordinated care, as most patients will require surgical interventions, interventional procedures, and/or medical therapies at some point in their lives for maximal function and quality of life.

References

1. Peterman CM, Fevurly RD, Alomari AI, Trenor CC 3rd, Adams D, Vadeboncoeur S, Liang M, Greene AK, Mulliken JB, Fishman SJ. Sonographic screening for Wilms tumor in children with CLOVES syndrome. Pediatr Blood Cancer. 2017;64(12) https://doi.org/10.1002/pbc.26684. Epub 2017 Jun 19. PubMed PMID: 28627003.
2. Jacob AG, et al. Klippel-Trenaunay syndrome: spectrum and management. Mayo Clin Proc. 1998;73(1):28–36.
3. Oduber CE, et al. The persistent embryonic vein in Klippel-Trenaunay syndrome. Vasc Med. 2013;18(4):185–91.
4. Sapp JC, et al. Newly delineated syndrome of congenital lipomatous overgrowth, vascular malformations, and epidermal nevi (CLOVE syndrome) in seven patients. Am J Med Genet A. 2007;143A(24):2944–58.
5. Kurek KC, et al. Somatic mosaic activating mutations in PIK3CA cause CLOVES syndrome. Am J Hum Genet. 2012;90(6):1108–15.
6. Lee JH, et al. De novo somatic mutations in components of the PI3K-AKT3-mTOR pathway cause hemimegalencephaly. Nat Genet. 2012;44(8):941–5.
7. Moore CA, et al. Macrocephaly-cutis marmorata telangiectatica congenita: a distinct disorder with developmental delay and connective tissue abnormalities. Am J Med Genet. 1997;70(1):67–73.
8. Clayton-Smith J, et al. Macrocephaly with cutis marmorata, haemangioma and syndactyly–a distinctive overgrowth syndrome. Clin Dysmorphol. 1997;6(4):291–302.
9. Robertson SP, et al. Macrocephaly–cutis marmorata telangiectatica congenita: report of five patients and a review of the literature. Clin Dysmorphol. 2000;9(1):1–9.
10. Franceschini P, et al. Macrocephaly-cutis marmorata telangiectatica congenita without cutis marmorata? Am J Med Genet. 2000;90(4):265–9.
11. Conway RL, et al. Neuroimaging findings in macrocephaly-capillary malformation: a longitudinal study of 17 patients. Am J Med Genet A. 2007;143A(24):2981–3008.
12. Garavelli L, et al. MRI and neurological findings in macrocephaly-cutis marmorata telangiectatica congenita syndrome: report of ten cases and review of the literature. Genet Couns. 2005;16(2):117–28.
13. Eerola I, et al. Capillary malformation-arteriovenous malformation, a new clinical and genetic disorder caused by RASA1 mutations. Am J Hum Genet. 2003;73(6):1240–9.
14. Revencu N, et al. RASA1 mutations and associated phenotypes in 68 families with capillary malformation-arteriovenous malformation. Hum Mutat. 2013;34(12):1632–41.
15. Amyere M, et al. Germline loss-of-function mutations in EPHB4 cause a second form of Capillary Malformation-Arteriovenous Malformation (CM-AVM2) deregulating RAS-MAPK signaling. Circulation. 2017;136(11):1037–48.
16. Eng C. PTEN Hamartoma tumor syndrome. In: Adam MP, Ardinger HH, Pagon RA, editors. GeneReviews® [Internet]. Seattle: University of Washington, Seattle; 1993–2017.
17. Mester J, Eng C. When overgrowth bumps into cancer: the PTEN-Opathies. Am J Med Genet C Semin Med Genet. 2013;163C(2):114–21.
18. Hammill AM, et al. Sirolimus for the treatment of complicated vascular anomalies in children. Pediatr Blood Cancer. 2011;57(6):1018–24.
19. Pilarski R, et al. Cowden syndrome and the PTEN hamartoma tumor syndrome: systematic review and revised diagnostic criteria. J Natl Cancer Inst. 2013;105(21):1607–16.
20. Tan WH, et al. The spectrum of vascular anomalies in patients with PTEN mutations: implications for diagnosis and management. J Med Genet. 2007;44(9):594–602.
21. Kurek KC, et al. PTEN hamartoma of soft tissue: a distinctive lesion in PTEN syndromes. Am J Surg Pathol. 2012;36(5):671–87.
22. Orloff MS, et al. Germline PIK3CA and AKT1 mutations in Cowden and Cowden-like syndromes. Am J Hum Genet. 2013;92(1):76–80.

23. Yap TA, et al. Targeting the PI3K-AKT-mTOR pathway: progress, pitfalls, and promises. Curr Opin Pharmacol. 2008;8(4):393–412.
24. Adams DM, et al. Efficacy and safety of Sirolimus in the treatment of complicated vascular anomalies. Pediatrics. 2016;137(2):e20153257.
25. Barclay SF, Inman KW, Luks VL, et al. A somatic activating NRAS variant associated with kaposiform lymphangiomatosis. Genet Med. 2018;21(7):1517–24. https://doi.org/10.1038/s41436-018-0390-0.. [Epub ahead of print

Hemostasis/Thrombosis Considerations in Vascular Anomalies

13

Leonardo R. Brandão and Clifford M. Takemoto

Introduction

Vascular anomalies represent a heterogeneous group of lesions and conditions formerly identified as vascular birthmarks. Since many of these lesions are recognized early in life, it was common for pediatricians to be involved in the care of such patients. Nowadays, vascular anomalies represent an emerging field of medicine in which pediatric hematologists and oncologists play an important role. In addition to diagnosing and managing systemic therapies to treat children diagnosed with vascular anomalies, expertise is also needed to manage coagulation-related problems [1]. There has been an increased recognition of coagulopathy with both vascular malformations and vascular tumors which has resulted in an expanding role of hematologists in the management of these patients.

The International Society for the Study of Vascular Anomalies (ISSVA) classification of vascular anomalies has provided a framework to differentiate clinical entities (Chap. 1). Since the 2014 edition, the addition of genetic mutations that further characterizes these anomalies (Chap. 3) has allowed clinicians to start to unravel their different phenotypic expressions and to look for potential therapeutic targets [2]. Conversely, despite progress in understanding the association between vascular anomalies with their correspondent coagulopathy, a paucity of published literature to clarify the pathophysiology and to guide diagnosis and management of bleeding and thrombotic risks in this population remains.

In light of these challenges, this chapter will review the coagulation complications in patients with vascular anomalies. The distinct coagulation-related clinical scenarios relevant to the vascular anomaly subtypes will be addressed

L. R. Brandão (✉)
Division of Haematology/Oncology, The Hospital for Sick Children, Toronto, ON, Canada
e-mail: leonardo.brandao@sickkids.ca

C. M. Takemoto
Department of Hematology, St. Jude Children's Research Hospital, Memphis, TN, USA

C. C. Trenor III, D. M. Adams (eds.), *Vascular Anomalies*,
https://doi.org/10.1007/978-3-030-25624-1_13

with discussions of the current knowledge of pathophysiology, clinical, laboratory, and imaging diagnostic features. Severe complications pertaining to the main types of coagulopathy (e.g., severe bleeding during procedures, deep vein thrombosis (DVT), pulmonary embolism (PE)) will be highlighted. In addition, management algorithms for bleeding and thrombotic risks will be suggested.

Coagulopathy

Consumptive Coagulopathy Disseminated intravascular coagulation (DIC) is a clinical condition that arises from unregulated activation of the coagulation system leading to deposition of fibrin in the intravascular compartment [3]. Depending on the magnitude of fibrin deposition, the occlusion of small and midsized vessels that may ensue can lead to organ dysfunction and significant morbidity and mortality. It is not a single disease but rather a dysregulated physiologic response to a number of processes. Common to many triggers of DIC is the initiation of coagulation activation by tissue factor and inadequate dampening of downstream thrombin activation (Fig. 13.1).

In general, consumptive coagulopathy is thought to be a common mechanism for thrombocytopenia and for coagulation factor derangement associated with vascular lesions. Historically, there has been significant confusion on the terminology used to describe coagulopathies associated to vascular anomalies. For example, the coagulopathy originally described in an infant with severe thrombocytopenia associated to a rapidly growing “hemangioma” was later termed the Kasabach-Merritt phenomenon (KMP). This name became a synonym for any coagulopathy indistinctly associated with superficial or visceral vascular lesions [4, 5]. It was only after the taxonomy of vascular anomalies evolved to two distinct categories based on the biology of their endothelial cells, that is, vascular malformations and vascular tumors, that a proper differentiation of their respective coagulation disturbances commenced [6, 7].

Important differences of the coagulopathies encountered in patients with vascular malformations and vascular tumors should be pointed out, as distinct therapies are required to prevent their progression. The activation of coagulation seen with vascular malformations is relatively mild and is initiated and confined primarily within the vascular lesion; it is known as localized intravascular coagulopathy (LIC). In contrast, the more severe coagulopathy associated with vascular tumors is designated as KMP. Although KMP is triggered locally and is due to intra-tumoral platelet trapping, it usually becomes widespread and life-threatening. Severe thrombocytopenia, hemolytic anemia, and hypofibrinogenemia are common, and the blood smear demonstrates microangiopathy (Fig. 13.4). KMP is one of the several vascular malformation-associated thrombocytopenias. A detailed discussion of these two main types of coagulopathies, LIC and thrombocytopenias (with less emphasis on KMP which is described in Chap. 6), will follow.

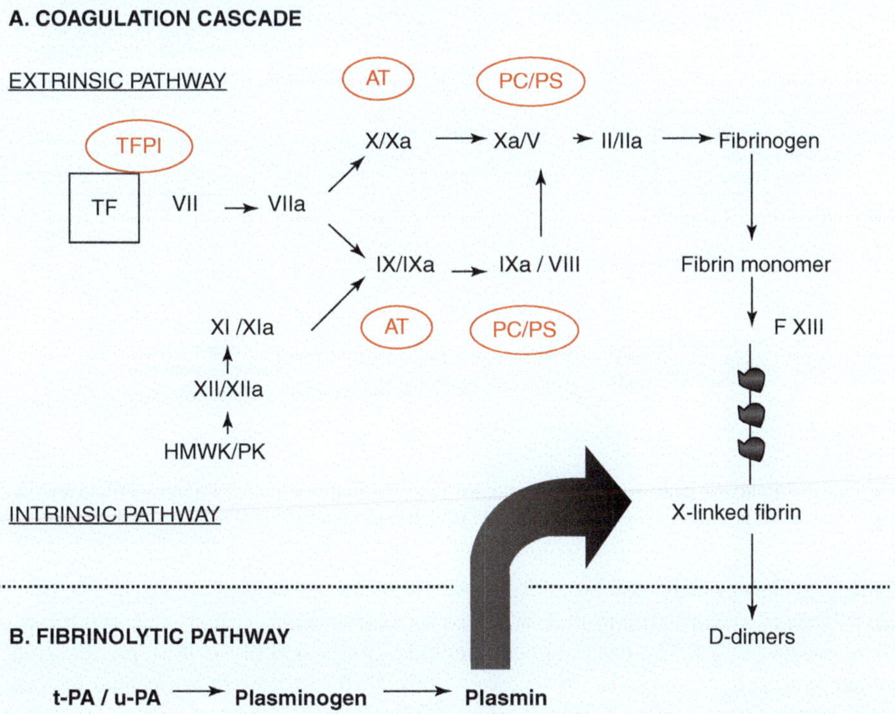

Fig. 13.1 The simplified coagulation cascade and the fibrinolytic pathway. Legends: Red circles, natural coagulation inhibitors; black, procoagulant system. Arrows indicate subsequent step of activation of the coagulation factors in the coagulation cascade. Bold: fibrinolytic pathway. Abbreviations: PC, protein C; PS, protein S; AT, antithrombin; TFPI, tissue factor pathway inhibitor; TF, tissue factor; VII, factor VII; VIIa, activated factor VII; X, factor X; Xa, activated factor X; V, factor V; II, prothrombin; IIa, activated thrombin; IX, factor IX; IXa, activated factor IX; FXIII, factor XIII; XII, factor XII; XIIa, activated factor XII; HMWK, high molecular weight kininogen; PK, prekallikrein; t-PA, tissue plasminogen activation; u-PA, urokinase

Localized Intravascular Coagulopathy

As mentioned above, the term LIC has been coined to describe activation of the coagulation system associated with venous malformations and to be distinguished from KMP [8]. The original report in the literature of pediatric patients with LIC included cases with a spectrum of laboratory findings ranging from D-dimer elevation alone to hypofibrinogenemia, thrombocytopenia and prothrombin (PT)/activated partial thromboplastin time (aPTT) prolongation, referred as venous malformation associated DIC (VM-DIC). Clinically, LIC/VM-DIC occurs in patients with slow-flow vascular malformations including capillary (CM, Chap. 8), VM (Chap. 9), lymphatic (LM, Chap. 10), or combined lesions (i.e., CVM), in addition to malformations associated with other nonvascular anomalies (Chap. 12). Its hallmark is the elevation of fibrin degradation products in the circulation (i.e., D-dimer), a likely more specific finding to VM than to lesions involving other histopathological vascular malformation variants [9].

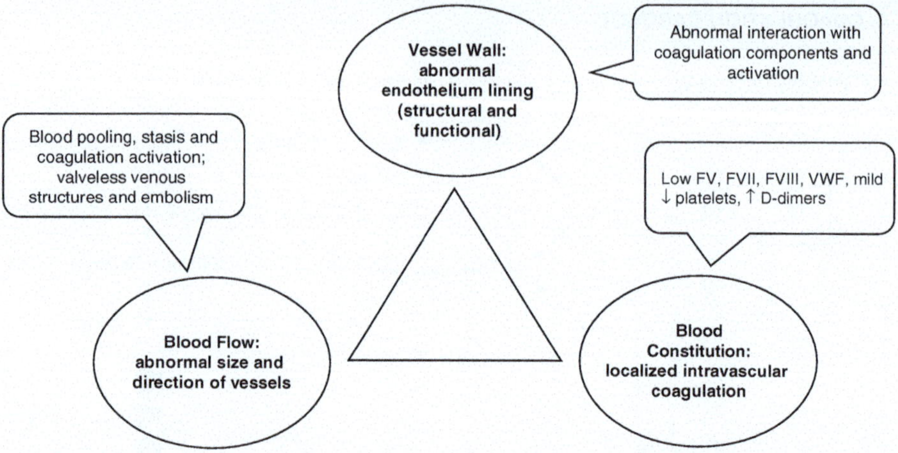

Fig. 13.2 Virchow's triad applied to low-flow vascular malformations. Legends: FV, factor V; FVII, factor VII; FVIII, factor VIII; VWF, von Willebrand factor; FSP, fibrinogen split products

Pathophysiology LIC can be understood within the framework of Virchow's triad, hypothesized to explain abnormal thrombus formation in the context of venous thrombotic events (VTE). The triad elements include diminished blood flow, an abnormal vessel wall, and an excessive blood coagulability [10]. In slow-flow vascular lesions, stasis of blood through anatomically distorted vessels and contact with an abnormal endothelium lining result in an unbalanced equilibrium between thrombus formation and fibrinolysis; this provides a hypercoagulable milieu conducive to thrombin formation and LIC. Stagnant blood leads to the production of thrombin and subsequent conversion of fibrinogen to fibrin. Moreover, fibrinolysis of the excessively formed fibrin results in increased circulating levels of cross-linked fibrin fragments (e.g., D-dimers) (Fig. 13.2). Although the term LIC suggests a localized phenomenon, the findings of D-dimer elevation and other markers of mild consumptive coagulopathy in peripheral blood demonstrate the systemic nature of this process. Older case reports had already highlighted instances where LIC progressed to VM-DIC characterized by systemic consumption of coagulation factors V (FV), FVII, FVIII, and fibrinogen, to PT prolongation, and, ultimately, to the activation of the entire coagulation process with additional mild thrombocytopenia and hyperfibrinolysis [11, 12].

More recently, investigators studied LIC in patients with objectively confirmed extensive VM using thromboelastometry (e.g., ROTEM®), a global hemostatic assay that evaluates the mechanical properties of a thrombus. Those patients exhibited increased fibrinolysis, FXIII consumption, and higher LIC severity [13]. In addition, patients with extensive lesions express elevated circulating levels of angiogenic markers such as angiopoietin-2 (Ang-2) and endothelial receptor tyrosine kinase TIE-2, either in direct or indirect correlation with their fibrinogen, D-dimer, or plasminogen activator inhibitor-1 (PAI-1) levels. The unbalanced Ang-TIE-2 findings in association to a deranged thrombin formation and fibrinolysis suggest an expanded role of the coagulation process, in that thrombin and plasmin may regulate angiogenesis and mediate the enzymatic degradation of the basal membrane of newly formed abnormal vessels within the malformation in a crosstalk between angiogenesis and coagulation [14].

In addition, the coagulation laboratory profile of patients diagnosed with capillary lymphovenous malformation (CLVM), a form of VM with increased risk for thrombotic complications, revealed a potential prothrombotic state. Specifically, when patients with two different degrees of LIC severity identified by D-dimer abnormality stratification (i.e., highest D-dimer tertile vs. lowest tertile) were compared, patients with higher D-dimer levels had lower circulating levels of the natural anticoagulant protein C (PC) (adults) or both proteins C and S (PS) (children) in comparison to healthy individuals. While statistically significant lower levels were noted, their absolute values did not correspond to levels compatible with PC or PS deficiency, raising questions about their clinical significance. Furthermore, in the adult cohort where thrombotic complications were more pronounced, the endogenous thrombin potential was surprisingly not elevated in comparison to adult controls. Conversely, those patients had an exacerbated fibrinolysis which, in combination to the local coagulation consumption and abnormal blood flow, was likely responsible for the LIC-related laboratory and clinical findings [15].

Clinical Manifestations An ad hoc review of the pediatric literature disclosed a prevalence of LIC in children from 1% to 88% (Table 13.1). This wide range reflects the different study designs, characteristics, and referral patterns of the centers, lack of universal screening, heterogeneity of LIC diagnostic criteria, and variability of the laboratory methods utilized. Patients with milder LIC are usually asymptomatic, as mild/moderate D-dimer elevation represents their sole laboratory finding. In multifocal or diffuse VM, where lesions are larger or deeper, a more severe D-dimer elevation accompanied by severe hypofibrinogenemia (<100 mg/dL) and mild thrombocytopenia may occur.

Table 13.1 Prevalence of localized intravascular coagulation (LIC) in pediatric patients with venous malformation (VM)

Author	Study design	Patient numbers	Age	Outcome
Enjolras et al. [8]	RC	27	Birth – 16 years	88% LIC[a]
Hein et al. [46]	RC	176	Birth – 18 years	1% LIC 7% bleeding
Mazoyer et al. [7]	PC	24	N/A	~80% LIC[a] 12.5% bleeding
Mazoyer et al. [22]	PC	26	2–15 years	60% D-dimer (+) 12% type I VWD
McRae et al. [65]	RC	13	0–17 years	54% D-dimer (+) 23% VTE
Hung et al. [66]	RC	24	0–12 years	33% D-dimer (+)
Leung et al. [67]	PC	18	0–18 years	44% D-dimer (+)
Overall		308	Birth – 18 years	1–88% LIC 7–12.5% bleeds

[a]LIC correlates with VM extension and a VM severity score, but not with its location

When LIC progresses, special attention is required to patients with intra-articular VM or within the genitourinary or gastrointestinal tract, due to the risk of hemarthrosis, hematuria, or melena/hematochezia and chronic anemia, respectively. Of interest, known exacerbators include local injuries (bone fractures), sclerosing agents (e.g., alcohol-based agents or sodium tetradecyl sulfate), pregnancy, infection, puberty, or surgery [16–19]. Additional clinical findings in patients with a more chronic form of LIC are recurrent peripheral superficial thrombi that calcify (phleboliths), leading to symptomatic inflammation associated with mild laboratory findings such as D-dimer elevation and pain (Fig. 13.3) [1, 6]. Peripheral blood smears in patients with VM and coagulopathy often show

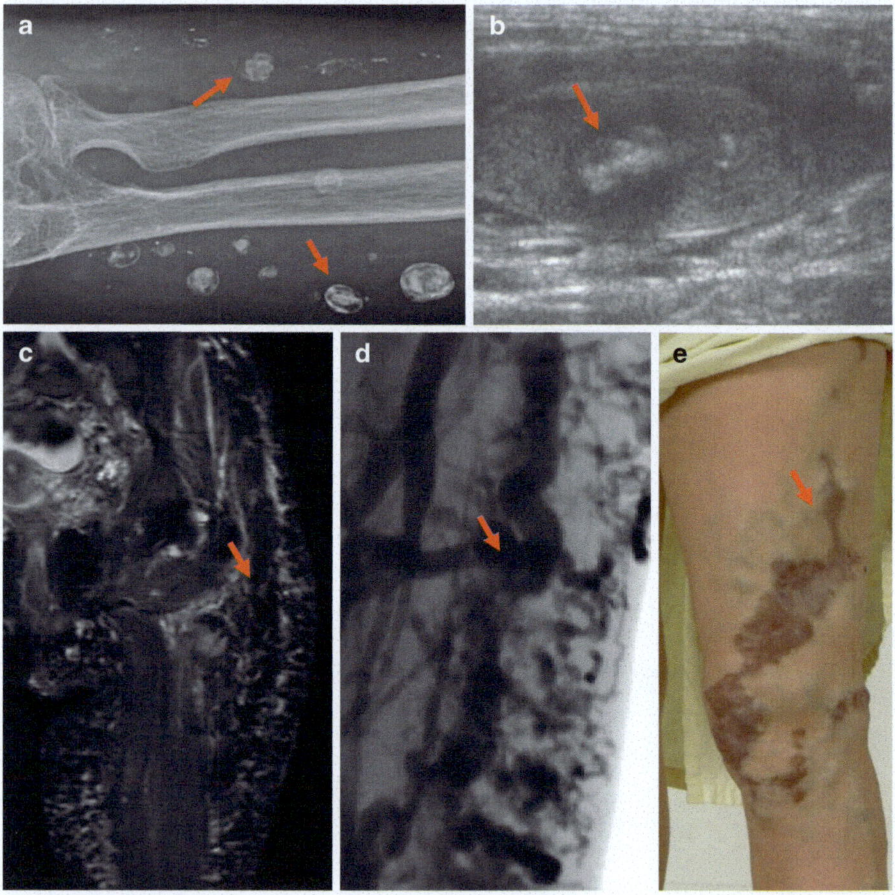

Fig. 13.3 Radiological imaging findings related to localized intravascular coagulation (LIC). *Legends*: Phleboliths (arrows) in patient with extensive upper extremity venous malformation identified by X-ray (**a**) and ultrasound (**b**). *Legends*: Persistent embryonic vein (i.e., lateral margin vein of Servelle depicted by arrows) identified by magnetic resonance imaging (**c**), venogram (**d**), and physical exam (**e**). (Pictures: courtesy of Dr. Philip John, Interventional Radiologist, The Hospital for Sick Children)

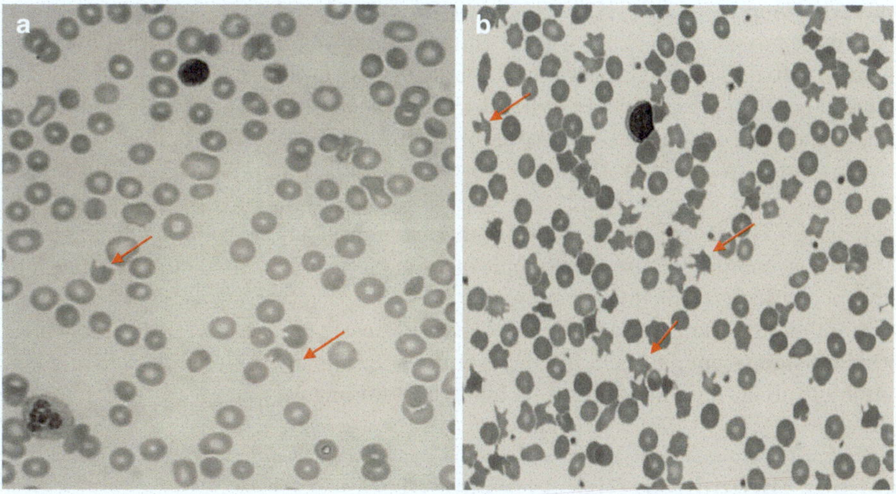

Fig. 13.4 Peripheral blood smear comparison. (A) Kaposiform hemangioendothelioma. (B) Venous malformation after sclerotherapy. *Figure*: Peripheral blood smears of patients with coagulopathy and vascular malformations. (**a**) Microangiopathic changes in patient with KHE. Note the absence of platelets. Arrows depict schistocytes. (**b**) Poikilocytes ("animal cracker" cells) in patient with extensive venous malformations after sclerotherapy, depicted by arrows

the presence of bizarre poikilocytes; some hematologists have coined these as "animal cracker" cells; this is in contrast to the findings of microangiopathy seen with KMP (Fig. 13.4).

Management The use of heparin has long been reported in children with coagulopathy associated with vascular lesions [20, 21]. However, there is paucity of data to guide the management of LIC. As such, there is no consensus for the management of the coagulopathy associated with slow-flow lesions. Low molecular weight heparin (LMWH) effectively decreases thrombin activation in patients with LIC associated with VM and results in reduction of D-dimer (Fig. 13.6) [22, 23]. Patients with pain also report improvement with LMWH, in part due to reduction in superficial thrombotic events within these lesions.

LMWH is commonly used to manage periprocedural coagulopathy although no evidence-based guidelines exist. Different regimens varying in intensity or duration have been suggested. An online poll of members of the American Society of Pediatric Hematology/Oncology (ASPHO) showed that recommendations for anticoagulation treatment were dependent on the LIC severity and perceived bleeding and thrombosis risk. For asymptomatic patients with isolated D-dimer elevation, 20% of respondents would favor LMWH; for patients with D-dimer elevation and painful phleboliths, 58% would use LMWH; and for pre-procedure management of patients with CLVM and hypofibrinogenemia, 63% would favor LMWH [24]. Following this survey, a subsequent meeting of the Vascular Anomaly Special

Interest Group from ASPHO was held in Toronto, Canada, 2016, where members were polled to generate consensus recommendations about periprocedural management of LIC [25]. Practitioners used the degree of D-dimer elevation, fibrinogen depression, thrombocytopenia, type of treatment, and type of vascular malformation in their decision to use periprocedural anticoagulation. The regimen proposed was to start enoxaparin at 0.5 mg/kg/dose twice daily, administering it 10–14 days prior and after the procedure. Chronic anticoagulation may be considered for patients who have had a history of thrombotic complications or have chronic pain. LMWH is commonly used, although other anticoagulants or antiplatelet agents have been used (see the next section).

Another important therapeutic option is the use of compression garments, which provides significant pain relief in the event of symptomatic phleboliths and amelioration or full correction of mild LIC laboratory findings [1, 7].

Venous Thrombosis Risk Assessment

Both bleeding and thrombotic complications can be seen with the coagulopathy associated with slow-flow lesions. However, there appears to be a significantly increased risk of VTE associated with overgrowth syndromes. Frequencies between 4% and 11% of both DVT and PE have been described in Proteus syndrome [26–28], Klippel-Trenaunay syndrome (CLVM) [29], and CLOVES syndrome [30, 31]. The underlying risks for thrombotic complications in these syndromes are likely multifactorial and include venous stasis due to venous malformations and venous ectasias (thorax or limbs), thrombin activation with LIC, and frequent exposure to surgical procedures and sclerotherapy. There is phenotypic heterogeneity in this patient population and persistent embryonic veins (i.e., lateral marginal vein and sciatic vein in the lower limbs), a potential source of embolism, may appear in as many as 65% of patients with CLVM [31, 32]. These vascular lesions can be associated with mutations in the PI3K-AKT pathway; the role that abnormal signaling may play in thrombotic risk through regulation of endothelial function or platelet activation is yet to be elucidated.

Pre-procedural LMWH has been used to manage the coagulopathy associated with venous malformations; however, it is also important to consider the post-procedure VTE risk in patients with these lesions; accurate identification of those at high risk of VTE and administration of prophylaxis with heparin may reduce the morbidity and mortality risk associated with VTE. The paucity of evidence to guide VTE prophylaxis recommendations presents challenges in the pediatric population. General approaches to risk assessment include the identification of VTE risks such as immobility, surgery, inflammation, estrogens, and older age [33]. The presence of ectatic vessels presents additional risks during sclerotherapy, as these procedures will induce thrombus within the venous malformations. Extension of the thrombi to the deep venous system can result in PE. These authors would consider the presence of venous malformations in association with an older patient with an overgrowth syndrome to present a higher risk of VTE with surgery or sclerotherapy and strong consideration of heparin prophylaxis in the absence of bleeding contraindications. Similarly, non-operative management for ectatic or for persistent embryonic veins with endovenous laser ablation has been recommended [34, 35].

The management of acute DVT or PE in association with vascular malformations should follow standard approaches to treatment [36]. In most cases of a provoked VTE, a common duration of treatment with anticoagulation is for 3 months. However, those with recurrent VTE or persistent significant VTE risks (i.e., overgrowth syndromes) may warrant extended duration of treatment. Modification of risks would be recommended if possible, such as the use of progestins instead of estrogens for females and the encouragement of ambulation.

Thrombocytopenias

Thrombocytopenia may be seen with vascular lesions, in association with a consumptive coagulopathy or in isolation. As stated above, the thrombocytopenia tends to be severe with KMP. Profound thrombocytopenia can also be seen with congenital hemangiomas; however, infantile hemangiomas are not accompanied by thrombocytopenia. The presence and degree of thrombocytopenia and associated coagulopathy with the presentation of a presumed vascular lesion can help guide the differential diagnosis of the lesion (Table 13.2).

Table 13.2 Thrombocytopenia among different vascular anomalies

Features	KHE with KMP	VM/LM/CLVM	NICH	KLA
Platelets	Severe thrombocytopenia	Normal or mild thrombocytopenia Moderate	Usually normal or mild thrombocytopenia; can be severe	Moderate to severe thrombocytopenia
Fibrinogen	Severely low	Normal to low	Normal to low	Can be severely low
PT/aPTT	Prolonged	Normal or prolonged	Normal	Prolonged
D-dimer	Increased	Increased	Mild increase	Increased
Pathogenesis	Platelet trapping; consumption of fibrinogen	Venous stasis and activation of thrombin	Platelet sequestration	Platelet trapping; consumption of fibrinogen
Clinic course	Persistent coagulopathy until tumor treated	Chronic with exacerbations (i.e., inflammation, trauma)	Resolution over several months	Persistent coagulopathy until tumor treated
Management	VCR, steroids, sirolimus	Sclerotherapy, heparin, LMWH	Observation	VCR, steroids, sirolimus

Abbreviations: *KHE* kaposiform hemangioendothelioma, *KMP* Kasabach-Merritt phenomenon, *VM* venous malformation, *LM* lymphatic malformation, *CLVM* capillary lymphovenous malformation, *NICH* non-involuting congenital hemangioma, *KLA* kaposiform lymphangiomatosis, *PT* prothrombin time, *aPTT* activated partial thromboplastin time, *VCR* vincristine, *LMWH* low molecular weight heparin

Kaposiform Hemangioendotheliomas (KHE) and Tufted Angiomas (TA) These two vascular tumors are associated with KMP. Histopathology of these tumors demonstrates platelet trapping and thrombi within glomeruloid areas [37]. While the presence of schistocytes on peripheral blood smear review is consistent with a microangiopathy (Fig. 13.4), von Willebrand factor is not increased in tumors suggesting that the pathogenesis differs from thrombotic thrombocytopenia purpura. Potential mechanisms contributing to thrombocytopenia include platelet activation secondary to yet undefined interactions with tumor endothelium or turbulence within abnormal capillaries. In addition, other concepts about mechanisms of thrombocytopenia have emerged, such as platelet receptor-mediated clearance and NETosis (extracellular chromatin from neutrophils that mediate platelet trapping); these are yet to be explored.

Congenital Hemangiomas Infants with rapidly involuting congenital hemangioma (RICH) can present with profound thrombocytopenia and coagulopathy similar to patients with KMP. However, the clinical presentation of thrombocytopenia and coagulopathy differs from that of DIC seen with KHE and TA. The D-dimer tends not to be as elevated, although thrombocytopenia can be severe. In contrast to KMP, these abnormal laboratory findings are self-limited and are usually not complicated by bleeding problems. A case series of seven patients with RICH showed features of consumptive coagulopathy [38]. In contrast to KMP, platelet counts started to increase at >2 weeks of age and the coagulopathy resolved. Other case reports of RICH with coagulopathy show similar outcome [39–41]. The non-involuting congenital hemangioma (NICH) and RICH lesions with coagulopathy tend to be large and in the extremities. Splenic lesions are described. The pathology of the thrombocytopenia may be secondary to thrombosis and platelet accumulation within the involuting lesions.

LM/CLVM Thrombocytopenia and coagulopathy may be seen in mixed lesions of VM with lymphatic or capillary malformations. Pure lymphatic or capillary malformations are not commonly associated with coagulopathy. Thrombocytopenia, when present, is usually mild. The mechanisms underlying this process are not elucidated, but venous stasis within the lesions is a likely contributor to activation of coagulation. There is no evidence of significant microangiopathy, as schistocytes are uncommon; however, other red cell changes resulting poikilocytes or "animal cracker" shapes are often noted (Fig. 13.4). Blue rubber bleb nevus syndrome (BRBNS) is characterized by multifocal discrete venous lesions on the skin and in the gastrointestinal tract. In addition to coagulopathy, this syndrome can be associated with significant GI hemorrhage and chronic iron deficiency anemia. Coagulopathy can also be associated in combined vascular malformations with lymphatic component. In these conditions, mild thrombocytopenia with elevated fibrin split products is often seen. Mouse models to study lymphangiogenesis have identified platelet disturbances mediated by podoplanin, potentially leading to DIC and providing an alternative explanation for such findings [42].

Kaposiform Lymphangiomatosis (KLA) Hemostatic abnormalities with thrombocytopenia, hypofibrinogenemia, and prolongation of PT/PTT with bleeding are described in 50% of patients with KLA. However, the thrombocytopenia tends to be less severe than that seen with KMP [43, 44]. The pathology of the lesions in KLA and KHE is similar. However, in KLA, spindled cells are found dispersed in clusters. In contrast, the spindled cells in KHE lesions are found in confluent nodules, and microthrombi are more prominent. The mechanisms of thrombocytopenia in KLA are not well defined, but platelet adherence to abnormal lymphatic endothelium is postulated, given the pathologic similarities in KHE and KLA.

Other Vascular Malformations with Thrombocytopenia and Coagulopathy Lesions other than tufted angioma and KHE can result in a consumptive coagulopathy, including congenital fibrosarcomas, hemangiopericytomas, papillary angioendotheliomas, and infantile myofibroma. In other vascular lesions, such as arteriovenous malformations (AVMs), coagulopathy is not common. In patients with AVMs associated with hereditary hemorrhagic telangiectasia, iron deficiency anemia is common due to epistaxis and GI bleeding. Angiodysplasia in the gastrointestinal tract has been described in association with acquired von Willebrand disease and prosthetic heart valves and high-shear states. However, this does not appear to be common with potential high-flow vascular lesions.

Other Therapies

Coagulopathy and pain associated with slow-flow venous and veno-lymphatic lesions usually improve with sclerotherapy administered by interventional radiology approaches. LMWH is also frequently used to reduce superficial and deep thrombotic complications and can also improve the coagulopathy and pain that can be seen with these lesions. Reduction of thrombin activation with heparin treatment may be a central pathway to improvement in the coagulopathy associated with slow-flow lesions. In addition to LMWH, other anticoagulant therapies such as vitamin K antagonists and the direct oral anticoagulants (DOACs) may also be effective (Fig. 13.5). However, there is a paucity of published experience with these agents. The potential role of antiplatelet agents and mammalian target of rapamycin (mTOR) inhibitors will also be discussed (Table 13.3).

Aspirin The use of aspirin is largely anecdotal with a paucity of published experience with its use [45, 46]. There may be benefit in the treatment of vascular tumors with KMP, in which platelet trapping can occur. Several cases of the use of antiplatelet agents (aspirin or aspirin with ticlopidine) for successful treatment of coagulopathy associated with tufted angiomas have been reported [47–49]. Antiplatelet agents have also been used in combination with vincristine for treatment of KMP [50]. In slow-flow lesions, the use of aspirin may be beneficial for treatment of pain, but there is less support for its use for coagulopathy in these lesions. A survey

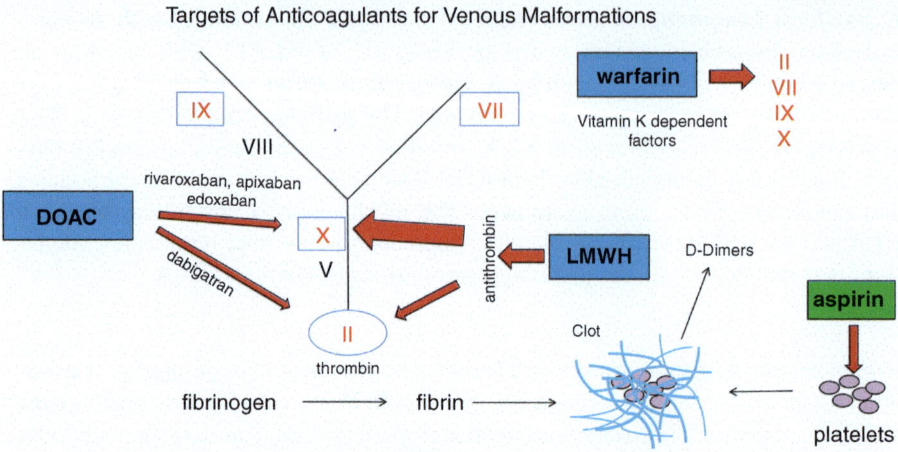

Fig. 13.5 Mechanism of action of anticoagulants for prevention of localized intravascular coagulation (LIC)

Table 13.3 Comparison of therapeutic options for patients with vascular anomalies complicated by LIC

	Vascular lesions	Clinical indications	Target
Acetyl salicylic acid (aspirin)	VM, TA, Sturge-Weber syndrome	Pain	Irreversible inhibition of cyclooxygenases 1 and 2 leading to platelet inhibition for the entire platelet lifespan (7–10 days)
LMWH	VM, VM/LM	Pain, coagulopathy, DVT	Indirect FXa and FIIa inhibition through antithrombin; anti-inflammatory activity
Warfarin	VM, VM/LM	Pain, coagulopathy, DVT	Inhibit gamma carboxylation of vitamin K-dependent factors FIIa, FVIIa, FIXa, FXa, PC, PS
DOAC	VM	Coagulopathy	Dabigatran: FIIa direct inhibition Rivaroxaban: FX direct inhibition Apixaban: FX direct inhibition Edoxaban: FX direct inhibition
Sirolimus	VM/LM, VM, KHE, KLA	Pain, coagulopathy	mTOR pathway inhibition in lymphatics; inhibition of lymphocyte function

Abbreviations: *VM* venous malformation, *TA* tufted angioma, *LMWH* low molecular weight heparin, *VM/LM* venous malformation lymphatic malformation, *DVT* deep vein thrombosis, *FXa* activated factor X, *FIIa* activated factor II, *AT* antithrombin, *FVIIa* activated factor VII, *FIXa* activated factor IX, *PC* protein C, *PS* protein S, *DOAC* direct oral anticoagulant, *FX* factor X, *KHE/KLA* kaposiform hemangioendothelioma, *mTOR* mammalian target of rapamycin

conducted at the University of California San Francisco (UCSF) showed that the use of low-dose aspirin at 5–10 mg/kg/d in patients with VM was associated with benefit and recurrence of pain after discontinuation in some [51]. Aspirin has also been used in capillary malformations such as Sturge-Weber syndrome with improvement in neurodevelopmental outcome [52].

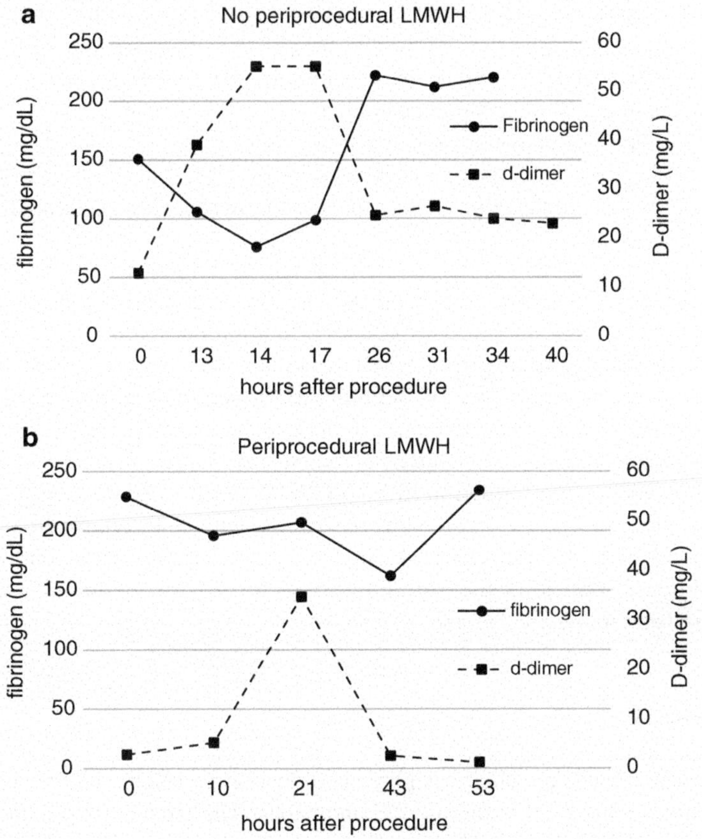

Fig. 13.6 Perioperative coagulation laboratory profile according to low molecular weight heparin (LMWH) use. Figure: Peri-procedural LMWH reduces a D-dimer and decreases hypofibrinogenemia associated with sclerotherapy. (**a**) No pre-treatment with LMWH prior to sclerotherapy. D-dimer is high prior to procedure (13 mg/L) with significant D-dimer elevation and hypofibrinogenemia (nadir of 76 mg/dL) after the procedure. (**b**) Pre-treatment with LMWH for 2 weeks prior and after sclerotherapy. D-dimer is lower prior to procedure (2.8 m/L), and fibrinogen nadir is 162 mg/dL

Vitamin K Antagonists Vitamin K antagonists (i.e., warfarin) are a standard option for treatment of thrombosis. These agents reduce thrombin generation through inhibition of gamma-carboxylation of vitamin K-dependent factors and thus have benefit for treatment of coagulopathy with vascular malformations. There is limited published literature to support the value of these compounds to treat LIC. In the past, their use was not seen favorably [53]. More recently, Mazereeuw-Hautier reported a case series of six patients with severe coagulopathy associated with slow-flow lymphatic/venous malformation. These patients had complications of bleeding and thrombosis, and three were treated with vitamin K antagonists with improvement of coagulopathy [54]. While the published experience for its use is small, vitamin K antagonists may have a role for the treatment of chronic coagulopathy with venous and veno-lymphatic malformations.

Direct Oral Anticoagulants (DOACs) LMWH have been used for the coagulopathy with venous malformations. However, for chronic coagulopathy, or for chronic symptoms such as pain, long-term treatment with subcutaneous injections is challenging. More recently, there have been case reports of the use of DOACs. Dabigatran was found to be as effective as enoxaparin for long-term treatment of hypofibrinogenemia and thrombocytopenia associated with VM, but D-dimers were not decreased [55]. Rivaroxaban has been reported to improve the coagulopathy in several patients [56–58].

mTOR Inhibitors Sirolimus has been shown to be effective for treatment complications of lymphatic malformations [59, 60]. In addition, there is growing experience for the use of sirolimus to treat KMP associated with KHE (Chap. 6). Sirolimus may also reduce the coagulopathy and pain associated with slow-flow venous and veno-lymphatic lesions; however, the published literature to support its use is yet sparse. Boon and colleagues recently published that sirolimus may be effective for treatment of venous malformation in both animal models and humans [61]. There are also several reports of coagulopathy associated with veno-lymphatic malformations responding to sirolimus [62, 63], including blue rubber bleb nevus syndrome [64]. Additional studies for the use of sirolimus to treat coagulopathy and pain of venous malformations are needed.

Conclusions

Pediatric hematologist/oncologist is playing an increasing role in the management of coagulopathies associated with vascular anomalies. The clinical presentation pathogenesis of the coagulopathy differs based on the vascular lesion. The severe DIC seen with KMP is usually distinct from that of the VM-DIC or LIC; however, there can be an overlap in clinical severity. The slow-flow coagulopathy seen with venous malformations (LIC or VM-DIC) is usually asymptomatic but can result in bleeding or thrombosis in particular with surgery or sclerotherapy. LMWH has been used most commonly to manage the coagulopathy with slow-flow lesions; however, there are small published experiences demonstrating efficacy with other anticoagulants. In addition to bleeding risk, individuals with vascular malformations can be at risk for thrombotic complications, in particular those with overgrowth syndromes. Careful VTE risk assessment and appropriate VTE prophylaxis in this population are warranted.

References

1. Adams DM, Wentzel MS. The role of the hematologist/oncologist in the care of patients with vascular anomalies. Pediatr Clin North Am. 2008;55:339–55, viii.
2. ISSVA Classification for Vascular Anomalies. Accessed 9/3/2018. http://www.issva.org/classification.
3. Gando S, Levi M, Toh CH. Disseminated intravascular coagulation. Nat Rev Dis Primers. 2016;2:16037.

4. Kasabach KK, Merritt KK. Capillary hemagioma with extensive purpura. Am J Dis Child. 1940;59(5):1063–70.
5. Hillman RS, Phillips LL. Clotting-fibrinolysis in a cavernous hemangioma. Am J Dis Child. 1967;113:649–53.
6. Mulliken JB, Glowacki J. Hemangiomas and vascular malformations in infants and children: a classification based on endothelial characteristics. Plast Reconstr Surg. 1982;69:412–22.
7. Mazoyer E, Enjolras O, Laurian C, Houdart E, Drouet L. Coagulation abnormalities associated with extensive venous malformations of the limbs: differentiation from Kasabach-Merritt syndrome. Clin Lab Haematol. 2002;24:243–51.
8. Enjolras O, Ciabrini D, Mazoyer E, Laurian C, Herbreteau D. Extensive pure venous malformations in the upper or lower limb: a review of 27 cases. J Am Acad Dermatol. 1997;36:219–25.
9. Dompmartin A, Ballieux F, Thibon P, Lequerrec A, Hermans C, Clapuyt P, Barrellier MT, Hammer F, Labbe D, Vikkula M, Boon LM. Elevated D-dimer level in the differential diagnosis of venous malformations. Arch Dermatol. 2009;145:1239–44.
10. Virchow RLK. Gesammelte Abhandlungen zur Wissenschaftlichen Medzin 219; 1856.
11. D'Amico JA, Hoffman GC, Dyment PG. Klippel-Trenaunay syndrome associated with chronic disseminated intravascular coagulation and massive osteolysis. Cleve Clin Q. 1977;44:181–8.
12. Neubert AG, Golden MA, Rose NC. Kasabach-Merritt coagulopathy complicating Klippel-Trenaunay-Weber syndrome in pregnancy. Obstet Gynecol. 1995;85:831–3.
13. Baraldini V, Copp G, Samprietro F, Della V, Riccipetitoni F, D'Angelo A. Physiopathology of localized intravascular coagulopathy (LIC) associated to segmental venous malformations (VM): hyperfibrinolysis, hypocoagulability, and presence of activated clotting factors. 19th International Society for the Study of Vascular Anomalies, June 16–19; Malmo, SE; 2012.
14. Redondo P, Aguado L, Marquina M, Paramo JA, Sierra A, Sanchez-Ibarrola A, Martinez-Cuesta A, Cabrera J. Angiogenic and prothrombotic markers in extensive slow-flow vascular malformations: implications for antiangiogenic/antithrombotic strategies. Br J Dermatol. 2010;162:350–6.
15. Oduber CE, van Beers EJ, Bresser P, van der Horst CM, Meijers JC, Gerdes VE. Venous thromboembolism and prothrombotic parameters in Klippel-Trenaunay syndrome. NethJMed. 2013;71:246–52.
16. Lee JH Jr, Kirk RF. Pregnancy associated with giant hemangiomata, thrombocytopenia, and fibrinogenopenia (Kasabach-Merritt syndrome). Report of a case. Obstet Gynecol. 1967;29:24–9.
17. Lang PG, Dubin HV. Hemangioma-thrombocytopenia syndrome; a disseminated intravascular coagulopathy. Arch Dermatol. 1975;111:105–7.
18. Mason KP, Neufeld EJ, Karian VE, Zurakowski D, Koka BV, Burrows PE. Coagulation abnormalities in pediatric and adult patients after sclerotherapy or embolization of vascular anomalies. AJR Am J Roentgenol. 2001;177:1359–63.
19. Hassanein AH, Mulliken JB, Fishman SJ, Alomari AI, Zurakowski D, Greene AK. Venous malformation: risk of progression during childhood and adolescence. Ann Plast Surg. 2012;68:198–201.
20. Kelly GL. Heparin therapy for bleeding associated with hemangioma. Surgery. 1969;65:894.
21. Lo SS, Hitzig WH, Frick PG. Clinical experience with anticoagulant therapy in the management of disseminated intravascular coagulation in children. Acta Haematol. 1971;45:1–16.
22. Mazoyer E, Enjolras O, Bisdorff A, Perdu J, Wassef M, Drouet L. Coagulation disorders in patients with venous malformation of the limbs and trunk: a case series of 118 patients. Arch Dermatol. 2008;144:861–7.
23. Dompmartin A, Acher A, Thibon P, Tourbach S, Hermans C, Deneys V, Pocock B, Lequerrec A, Labbe D, Barrellier MT, Vanwijck R, Vikkula M, Boon LM. Association of localized intravascular coagulopathy with venous malformations. Arch Dermatol. 2008;144:873–7.
24. Brandão LR, Hopper E, Raffini L, Lee M. Coagulation Management in Children with vascular malformations (VMs): practice heterogeneity among members of the American Society of Pediatric Hematology-oncology (ASPHO) Special Interest Group (SIG) Vascular Anomalies (VA). Ped Blood Cancer. 2016;63 S1, S23.

25. Avila ML, Lumia CM, Montoya MI, Trenor CC, Adams D, Blei F, Feldman B, Brandão LR. Towards a consensus for standardized assessment of pediatric patients with vascular malformations (VM) at risk for coagulopathy. Res Pract Thromb Haemost. 2018;2(S1):298.
26. Slavotinek AM, Vacha SJ, Peters KF, Biesecker LG. Sudden death caused by pulmonary thromboembolism in Proteus syndrome. Clin Genet. 2000;58:386–9.
27. Eberhard DA. Two-year-old boy with Proteus syndrome and fatal pulmonary thromboembolism. Pediatr Pathol. 1994;14:771–9.
28. Keppler-Noreuil KM, Lozier JN, Sapp JC, Biesecker LG. Characterization of thrombosis in patients with Proteus syndrome. Am J Med Genet A. 2017;173(9):2359–65.
29. Huiras EE, Barnes CJ, Eichenfield LF, Pelech AN, Drolet BA. Pulmonary thromboembolism associated with Klippel-Trenaunay syndrome. Pediatrics. 2005;116:e596–600.
30. Keppler-Noreuil KM, Rios JJ, Parker VE, Semple RK, Lindhurst MJ, Sapp JC, Alomari A, Ezaki M, Dobyns W, Biesecker LG. PIK3CA-related overgrowth spectrum (PROS): diagnostic and testing eligibility criteria, differential diagnosis, and evaluation. Am J Med Genet A. 2015;167A:287–95.
31. Jacob AG, Driscoll DJ, Shaughnessy WJ, Stanson AW, Clay RP, Gloviczki P. Klippel-Trenaunay syndrome: spectrum and management. Mayo Clin Proc. 1998;73:28–36.
32. Gloviczki P, Hollier LH, Telander RL, Kaufman B, Bianco AJ, Stickler GB. Surgical implications of Klippel-Trenaunay syndrome. Ann Surg. 1983;197:353–62.
33. Mahajerin A, Branchford BR, Amankwah EK, Raffini L, Chalmers E, van Ommen CH, Goldenberg NA. Hospital-associated venous thromboembolism in pediatrics: a systematic review and meta-analysis of risk factors and risk-assessment models. Haematologica. 2015;100:1045–50.
34. Gonzalez-Zeh R, Armisen R, Barahona S. Endovenous laser and echo-guided foam ablation in great saphenous vein reflux: one-year follow-up results. J Vasc Surg. 2008;48:940–6.
35. Patel PA, Barnacle AM, Stuart S, Amaral JG, John PR. Endovenous laser ablation therapy in children: applications and outcomes. Pediatr Radiol. 2017;47:1353–63.
36. Monagle P, Chan AK, Goldenberg NA, Ichord RN, Journeycake JM, Nowak-Gottl U, Vesely SK. Antithrombotic therapy in neonates and children: antithrombotic therapy and prevention of thrombosis, 9th ed: American College of Chest Physicians Evidence-Based Clinical Practice Guidelines. Chest. 2012;141:e737S–801S.
37. Lyons LL, North PE, Mac-Moune Lai F, Stoler MH, Folpe AL, Weiss SW. Kaposiform hemangioendothelioma: a study of 33 cases emphasizing its pathologic, immunophenotypic, and biologic uniqueness from juvenile hemangioma. Am J Surg Pathol. 2004;28:559–68.
38. Baselga E, Cordisco MR, Garzon M, Lee MT, Alomar A, Blei F. Rapidly involuting congenital haemangioma associated with transient thrombocytopenia and coagulopathy: a case series. Br J Dermatol. 2008;158:1363–70.
39. Rangwala S, Wysong A, Tollefson MM, Khuu P, Benjamin LT, Bruckner AL. Rapidly involuting congenital hemangioma associated with profound, transient thrombocytopenia. Pediatr Dermatol. 2014;31:402–4.
40. Andreu-Barasoain M, Naz E, Diaz M, Lopez-Estebaranz JL. Rapidly involuting congenital hemangioma associated with transient anemia and thrombocytopenia. Int J Dermatol. 2013;52:1025–6.
41. Hosono S, Ohno T, Kimoto H, Nagoshi R, Shimizu M, Nozawa M, Fuyama Y, Kaneda T, Moritani T, Aihara T. Successful transcutaneous arterial embolization of a giant hemangioma associated with high-output cardiac failure and Kasabach-Merritt syndrome in a neonate: a case report. J Perinat Med. 1999;27:399–403.
42. Cueni LN, Chen L, Zhang H, Marino D, Huggenberger R, Alitalo A, Bianchi R, Detmar M. Podoplanin-Fc reduces lymphatic vessel formation in vitro and in vivo and causes disseminated intravascular coagulation when transgenically expressed in the skin. Blood. 2010;116:4376–84.
43. Croteau SE, Kozakewich HP, Perez-Atayde AR, Fishman SJ, Alomari AI, Chaudry G, Mulliken JB, Trenor CC 3rd. Kaposiform lymphangiomatosis: a distinct aggressive lymphatic anomaly. J Pediatr. 2014;164:383–8.

44. Fernandes VM, Fargo JH, Saini S, Guerrera MF, Marcus L, Luchtman-Jones L, Adams D, Meier ER. Kaposiform lymphangiomatosis: unifying features of a heterogeneous disorder. Pediatr Blood Cancer. 2015;62:901–4.
45. Mathes EF, Haggstrom AN, Dowd C, Hoffman WY, Frieden IJ. Clinical characteristics and management of vascular anomalies: findings of a multidisciplinary vascular anomalies clinic. Arch Dermatol. 2004;140:979–83.
46. Hein KD, Mulliken JB, Kozakewich HP, Upton J, Burrows PE. Venous malformations of skeletal muscle. Plast Reconstr Surg. 2002;110:1625–35.
47. Javvaji S, Frieden IJ. Response of tufted angiomas to low-dose aspirin. Pediatr Dermatol. 2013;30:124–7.
48. Osio A, Fraitag S, Hadj-Rabia S, Bodemer C, de Prost Y, Hamel-Teillac D. Clinical spectrum of tufted angiomas in childhood: a report of 13 cases and a review of the literature. Arch Dermatol. 2010;146:758–63.
49. Leaute-Labreze C, Bioulac-Sage P, Labbe L, Meraud JP, Taieb A. Tufted angioma associated with platelet trapping syndrome: response to aspirin. Arch Dermatol. 1997;133:1077–9.
50. Fernandez-Pineda I, Lopez-Gutierrez JC, Ramirez G, Marquez C. Vincristine-ticlopidine-aspirin: an effective therapy in children with Kasabach-Merritt phenomenon associated with vascular tumors. Pediatr Hematol Oncol. 2010;27:641–5.
51. Nguyen JT, Koerper MA, Hess CP, Dowd CF, Hoffman WY, Dickman M, Frieden IJ. Aspirin therapy in venous malformation: a retrospective cohort study of benefits, side effects, and patient experiences. Pediatr Dermatol. 2014;31:556–60.
52. Comi A. Current therapeutic options in Sturge-Weber syndrome. Semin Pediatr Neurol. 2015;22:295–301.
53. Merskey C, Johnson AJ, Pert JH, Wohl H. Pathogenesis of fibrinolysis in Defibrination syndrome: effect of heparin administration. Blood. 1964;24:701–15.
54. Mazereeuw-Hautier J, Syed S, Leisner RI, Harper JI. Extensive venous/lymphatic malformations causing life-threatening haematological complications. Br J Dermatol. 2007;157: 558–63.
55. Ardillon L, Lambert C, Eeckhoudt S, Boon LM, Hermans C. Dabigatran etexilate versus low-molecular weight heparin to control consumptive coagulopathy secondary to diffuse venous vascular malformations. Blood Coagul Fibrinolysis. 2015;27(2):216–9.
56. Vandenbriele C, Vanassche T, Peetermans M, Verhamme P, Peerlinck K. Rivaroxaban for the treatment of consumptive coagulopathy associated with a vascular malformation. J Thromb Thrombolysis. 2014;38:121–3.
57. Randrianarisoa E, Kopp HG, Balletshofer BM, Jaschonek K, Kanz L, Haering HU, Rittig K. Management of disseminated intravascular coagulopathy with direct factor Xa inhibitor rivaroxaban in Klippel-Trenaunay syndrome. Blood Coagul Fibrinolysis. 2013;24: 766–70.
58. Mack JM, Richter GT, Crary SE. Effectiveness and safety of treatment with direct oral anticoagulant rivaroxaban in patients with slow-flow vascular malformations: a case series. Lymphat Res Biol. 2018;16:278–81.
59. Adams DM, Trenor CC 3rd, Hammill AM, Vinks AA, Patel MN, Chaudry G, Wentzel MS, Mobberley-Schuman PS, Campbell LM, Brookbank C, Gupta A, Chute C, Eile J, McKenna J, Merrow AC, Fei L, Hornung L, Seid M, Dasgupta AR, Dickie BH, Elluru RG, Lucky AW, Weiss B, Azizkhan RG. Efficacy and safety of Sirolimus in the treatment of complicated vascular anomalies. Pediatrics. 2016;137:e20153257. Epub 2016 Jan 18.
60. Wiegand S, Wichmann G, Dietz A. Treatment of lymphatic malformations with the mTOR inhibitor Sirolimus: a systematic review. Lymphat Res Biol. 2018;16:330–9.
61. Boscolo E, Limaye N, Huang L, Kang KT, Soblet J, Uebelhoer M, Mendola A, Natynki M, Seront E, Dupont S, Hammer J, Legrand C, Brugnara C, Eklund L, Vikkula M, Bischoff J, Boon LM. Rapamycin improves TIE2-mutated venous malformation in murine model and human subjects. J Clin Invest. 2015;125:3491–504.
62. Vlahovic AM, Vlahovic NS, Haxhija EQ. Sirolimus for the treatment of a massive capillary-lymphatico-venous malformation: a case report. Pediatrics. 2015;136:e513–6.

63. Kim D, Benjamin L, Wysong A, Hovsepian D, Teng J. Treatment of complex periorbital venolymphatic malformation in a neonate with a combination therapy of sirolimus and prednisolone. Dermatol Ther. 2015;28:218–21.
64. Salloum R, Fox CE, Alvarez-Allende CR, Hammill AM, Dasgupta R, Dickie BH, Mobberley-Schuman P, Wentzel MS, Chute C, Kaul A, Patel M, Merrow AC, Gupta A, Whitworth JR, Adams DM. Response of blue rubber bleb nevus syndrome to Sirolimus treatment. Pediatr Blood Cancer. 2016;63:1911–4.
65. McRae MY, Adams S, Pereira J, Parsi K, Wargon O. Venous malformations: clinical course and management of vascular birthmark clinic cases. Australas J Dermatol. 2013;54:22–30.
66. Hung JW, Leung MW, Liu CS, Fung DH, Poon WL, Yam FS, Leung YC, Chung KL, Tang PM, Chao NS, Liu KK. Venous malformation and localized intravascular coagulopathy in children. Eur J Pediatr Surg. 2017;27:181–4.
67. Leung YC, Leung MW, Yam SD, Hung JW, Liu CS, Chung LY, Tang MY, Fung HS, Poon WL, Chao NS, Liu KK. D-dimer level correlation with treatment response in children with venous malformations. J Pediatr Surg. 2018;53:289–92.

Practice Considerations for the Hematologist/Oncologist in Vascular Anomaly Clinics

14

Michael R. Jeng and Denise M. Adams

Introduction

With the increase in number of clinical centers focused on vascular anomalies, it is evident that a broad, interdisciplinary approach is optimal [1, 2]. This increased experience has demonstrated that hematology/oncology (H/O) is an integral specialty for a vascular anomaly team. These disorders may lead to clinical sequelae that are within the scope of practice for H/O. Familiarity with the nonvascular diagnoses (such as cancers) that are part of a differential diagnosis for vascular anomalies and malformations, experience with chemotherapy and developmental therapeutics, expertise with the management of coagulopathy and thromboses, and workup of anemia and thrombocytopenia are all expectations for H/O subspecialists. For some institutions, the incorporation of patients with vascular anomalies into the H/O program or a provider's clinical workflow can be challenging. Thoughtful consideration of the hematologist/oncologist's role in the context of the clinical infrastructure and available services at each center will promote optimal patient care and clinician well-being. This chapter reviews strategic practice considerations for the hematologist/oncologist in relation to their care of patients with vascular anomalies. The chapter is organized in order of increasing scope: from the individual, to clinical program, and then institution.

M. R. Jeng (✉)
Department of Pediatrics, Stanford University School of Medicine, Lucile Packard Children's Hospital, Palo Alto, CA, USA
e-mail: mjeng@stanford.edu

D. M. Adams
Dana-Farber Cancer Institute, Boston Children's Hospital, Boston, MA, USA

Division of Hematology/Oncology, Vascular Anomalies Center, Harvard Medical School, Boston Children's Hospital, Boston, MA, USA

C. C. Trenor III, D. M. Adams (eds.), *Vascular Anomalies*,
https://doi.org/10.1007/978-3-030-25624-1_14

Practice Considerations: Hematology/Oncology

Provider Perspective

Education and Clinical Experience

It is critical to educate oneself on the natural history and symptoms, common features and examination findings, diagnostic criteria, and important aspects of care, as well as treatment options and indications for intervention (may be domain of other specialties) in a range of vascular anomalies. An understanding of the current and historical classification systems is important and a good framework to begin to develop an understanding of vascular anomalies and malformations. The Hamburg classification system, based on the degree of blood flow (high or low flow), is used only by a limited number of investigators and providers [3]. The International Society for the Study of Vascular Anomalies (ISSVA) classification system is determined by an international expert consensus and is more widely adopted and regularly updated [4]. The ISSVA classification system provides a good framework for understanding and learning about the vascular anomalies by dividing the vascular anomalies into two primary groups: the vascular malformations and the vascular tumors. Because widespread adoption of a classification system with careful attention to adherence with diagnostic criteria and correct terminology has only recently occurred, any reading of the medical literature requires critical evaluation. Inaccurate information and conclusions exist in the peer-reviewed literature, and interpretation is sometimes needed in order to ensure meaningful clinical conclusions [5].

Tremendous discovery and increased understanding of vascular anomalies have occurred over the last 10 years. A detailed review of standard resources, such as Mulliken and Young's Vascular Anomalies [6], is prudent and is a logical step to pursue after classification systems. Providers should next develop a schedule of regular systematic updates of the literature, which should also include reviewing the recently published articles of the non-H/O specialties. For the neophyte "vascular anomalist," it may be helpful to visit an established vascular anomaly center for education and observation. General knowledge of pathology, radiology, and surgical services are helpful in making diagnostic and therapeutic decisions. Spending time with a pathologist reviewing the common features of each endothelial type (lymphatic, capillary, arterial, venous) can be helpful. In addition, observing interventional radiologists perform biopsies or sclerotherapy procedures with different sclerosing agents allows consideration of clinical options. An understanding of the types of laser therapy and outcomes from surgical debulking or resection will help with interdisciplinary discussion of cases. Therefore, it behooves the hematologist/oncologist to have a wide range of clinical experience and relevant knowledge [7, 8].

In recent years, physician and advanced practice providers established a group within the American Society of Hematology Oncology (ASPHO) called the Vascular Anomaly Special Interest Group (VA-SIG). Any member of ASPHO can participate in the VA-SIG depending on interest. Committees participate in activities that focus on different objectives, such as education, practice, or research. The ASPHO Annual Meeting often includes several educational sessions on vascular anomalies. Through the ASPHO VA-SIG, there are opportunities for developing mentor-mentee relationships and for patient consultations. Other meetings throughout the year with vascular anomaly educational programs include the annual Controversies in Vascular Anomalies Conference organized by Dr. Fran Blei et al. in NYC and ISSVA's Primer Course, which occurs on the first few days of the biennial research and administrative meeting. In addition, more extensive and specific post-hematology/oncology fellowship training opportunities, such as at the Cincinnati Children's Hospital Medical Center, are listed in the Post-PHO Fellowship Directory of ASPHO. In conclusion, because no formalized training exists for H/O in relation to diagnosis, treatment, and clinical care of patients diagnosed with vascular anomalies, the clinician should consider the development of a deliberate education plan, which may involve observation of other specialties.

Diagnostic and Therapeutic Interventions

The initial role of the hematologist/oncologist is to help establish and confirm the diagnosis. This is by taking a careful history, performing a complete physical examination, and review of radiologic imaging, laboratory results, and pathology, ideally in conjunction with the rest of the interdisciplinary team. Unlike the practice for much of oncology, which relies heavily on histologic determination of diagnosis, vascular anomalies often do not include pathologic evaluation, similar to some neuro-oncology cases. This is due to the frequent difficulty to perform the biopsy if in a difficult anatomic location and the potential for procedural-related complications. Due to the tissue heterogeneity in vascular tumors and malformations, the frequent ability to visualize the lesions, the presence of typical laboratory features, and a common clinical history, a specific diagnosis is often based on only a history, physical examination, blood work, and radiologic findings [7]. This change in diagnostic practice can be uncomfortable for the hematologist/oncologist and highlights the importance of interdisciplinary input. A regularly held, defined conference with the entire vascular anomaly clinical team is an optimal way to ensure interdisciplinary input and promote the most accurate diagnoses. This is also true in offering therapeutic options. H/O providers often attend and participate in tumor boards and should have familiarity with this type of multi-disciplinary clinical conference activity.

After the diagnosis is established, the hematologist/oncologist may participate in the development of a plan of care. Often, patient and family preferences, impact on quality of life, social factors, and the patients' desired outcomes, and both provider's and patient's own schedules, play a role in determining the plan. Often, this is due to the elective nature of the procedures and interventions. At first, this can be uncomfortable and unfamiliar for the hematologist/oncologist, whose practice usually involves offering the treatment that gives the best chance for long-term survival. The impact of each vascular anomaly on quality of life is subjective and multifactorial. Therefore, each medical provider's role is always first to determine the patient's desired outcome and then assess the best timing and intervention which will best meet their goals, outlining the risks and benefits. This can be very complex and may involve different specialties, each with their own clinics which may be physically in different locations. The hematologist/oncologist is often involved when medical intervention is part of the plan, and may determine the schedule of monitoring and follow-up visits, such as for cytopenias or coagulopathy, pain, or even anticoagulation. Due to the paucity of centers that provide a medical home for patients with vascular anomalies, patients frequently travel great distances. Early consideration of incorporating the primary care provider in the medical planning may be beneficial. Clear communication of care plans and educational material to the local provider is essential.

The clinical role may be that of a single consultation, part of several intermittent encounters, or a long-term provider of clinical care. It is important to be aware of each patient's resources and social situations, as these patients may be local, regional, national, or international and may need local physicians to help carry out the medical plan. After an inpatient admission, careful discharge planning is essential. Information for plans of care may include identification of emergency contacts, appropriate numbers, and service to call day and/or night, straightforward processes for admissions (admitting service qualifications), and identification of primary service attending. [The hematologist/oncologist's role and determination of primary service is discussed in the following section.] Along with patient education and contact information for each provider/specialty, clear identification of the roles for each subspecialty and for what indication to contact a specific provider/service must be included along with the comprehensive care plan. This information should not be given only to the patient but also to all of the patient's key providers. Many larger centers will have a program or clinical coordinator to help organize these processes. Clear and consistent communication is crucial, and an agreed-upon center template may be helpful.

Interdisciplinary Clinical Team

Infrastructure: Support and Leadership

Because of the complexity of the involvement of many specialties and the need to coordinate care, it is important to consider the clinical and administrative infrastructure for a vascular anomaly center. Important to a program's success is the identification of a support staff with identified roles. This staff includes schedulers, administrative assistants, program manager, nursing care coordinators, advanced practice nurses, social workers, child life specialists, psychologists, occupational and physical therapists, dieticians, and pharmacists. The incorporation of a clinical nurse specialist to provide patient and nursing education can also be beneficial. Available resources and size of the center will govern the number of dedicated staff to the program. Other clinical staff who may be involved include advanced practice providers (nurse practitioners and physician assistants) and hospitalists focused on inpatient care, residents, fellows, and other physicians from a range of specialties. Because vascular anomalies are not determined to be within the domain and scope of practice of a clinical specialty, it could be difficult to replace any of the providers or support staff. Thus, one may consider emphasis on educational opportunities for the entire clinical team and activities that promote professional reward and resilience. The importance of career longevity, wellness, and a maintained interest in the field should not be underestimated and should be cultivated. Another helpful consideration is if there is a commonly encountered language that requires a medical translator, it may be prudent to include them in some basic training so that they have a general understanding of the different concepts in vascular biology, an overview of the vascular malformations and anomalies, and some of the frequently encountered clinical scenarios. Regular re-evaluation of the structure and resource needs of the center, as well as the role of the hematologist/oncologist within the program, is encouraged.

It is important to determine the center's administrative structure and leadership. Perhaps in part due to the lack of an assignment to a subspecialty scope of practice, vascular anomaly centers can have their administrative center within an H/O program or under another specialty. Surgery, plastic surgery, dermatology, or interventional radiology are common subspecialties under which a vascular center may exist. Some centers are not formally established and consist of an informal group of subspecialists who care for vascular anomaly patients. They often function in a "virtual" manner. In this situation, it is advised to formalize the leadership and management structure. The program leadership should be responsible for oversight of the program, advocate for resources, be engaged in quality improvement, and help in organization and planning of clinical activities. For example, patient access and referrals may need planning. Referrals might occur in many different ways due to the multiple disciplines involved. New patient referrals might be made to the center directly or to a subspecialty clinic deemed appropriate by the primary care physician or referring provider. Due to the lack of a defined responsible specialty, patient self-referrals can occur frequently. A defined leadership team may help facilitate and oversee the referral process at for the program, which can be helpful. Another example is that clinical workflow differs at each center: some have one interdisciplinary clinic in which a team of different specialists sees the patients on the same day, while others may have a conference for discussion and then patients are seen within each subspecialty clinic. In some programs, clinics are organized by anatomic regions, allowing for the most specialized input. Thus, the clinical workflow may vary tremendously at each institution, and the hematologist/oncologist should consider this in determining their role. Clear delineation of the role with the expected provision of care will help to maintain professional boundaries and give the support staff the ability to provide the most effective support to both medical providers and patients.

Hematologist/Oncologist's Role

Depending on the center, H/O physicians can serve as a consultant, an intermittent provider for the team, or a primary physician who coordinates treatment plans and is the primary coordinator, serving to provide a medical home. The early determination of one's role is essential for success and satisfaction. A consistent role will help in promoting the expectations for support staff and effective team communication. Discussion should occur early with the vascular anomaly center's leadership team and with the leadership of the H/O program. Initial discussion of time commitment, needed resources, and clinical and academic expectations is important as patient volumes can increase quickly. Development of a formal business plan may be essential to success and provide adequate resources.

A reliance on the H/O service may occur organically and unintentionally as many similar issues exist in the care of patients with vascular anomalies and cancer. The complexity and diversity of the vascular anomalies leads to the need for a wide range of clinical services and resources. At diagnosis and for disease monitoring, the reliance on both radiographic and pathology services is similar to what is encountered in oncology. Coagulopathy, chemotherapeutic agents, subsequent immunosuppression, and the incorporation of genetic mutations as molecular drivers of disease to inform treatment decisions are frequent in the scope of practice for H/O. Care coordination and psychosocial support to patients with multidisciplinary needs, monitoring disease status, establishing adolescent/young adult (AYA) programs, evaluating for late effects from treatment, palliative care, and a continued focus on the quality of life are other activities familiar to the practice of H/O that will benefit the vascular anomaly clinical program. The management of patients requiring different levels of acuity is needed, which may be reflected in the subspecialty clinical privileges. Inpatient and outpatient care, possible transfusion or infusions therapies, frequent communication with emergency departments, and consultation with an intensive care team illustrate the wide-range (benign to life-threatening) clinical scenarios seen by H/O and vascular anomaly centers. These factors make H/O an logical specialty to be centrally involved in the care and coordination of care for patients followed by these centers. Because of the similarity in practice, it is easy to assume the role of primary care coordinator. Often this is unplanned and occurs by default. Thus, it is important to proactively define the roles within a program and set boundaries for expectations. This will ensure follow-through in patient care and communication and ultimately lead to the best patient outcomes. At academic centers, a discussion about the amount of allocated effort and expected revenue generation from the vascular anomaly program is encouraged. Finally, there should be some expectation for fluidity of this role with times for reassessment with leadership.

After one establishes expertise and experience in this field, it is important to educate your colleagues and institution to create awareness of the expertise of your vascular center. This may involve collaborating with your interdisciplinary team and presenting at multiple grand rounds throughout your institution (pediatric, surgery, orthopedic, ENT, dermatology, pathology, grand rounds). The goal is awareness and promotion of your specialty center to increase the referral base. Ultimately, this will enhance meaningful clinical research and allow the best academic scholarship in this arena.

Hematologist/Oncologist: Role Within the Team

Diagnostic Considerations: Clinical, Radiology, Pathology, and Genetic Testing

For every patient who presents with a vascular anomaly, the correct diagnosis is crucial. Unlike most patients cared for by an oncologist, vascular anomalies are not diagnosed by tissue pathology but rather a combination of history, clinical examination, radiologic evaluation, and only occasion pathology [4]. Thus, the hematologist/oncologist typically serves as a clinician who is knowledgeable about the clinical presentation and features and is familiar with the associated laboratory findings. Other clinicians who may serve in a similar capacity are dermatologists, interventional radiologists, and surgeons, including general surgeons, otolaryngologists, and plastic surgeons. A tissue biopsy is indicated to confirm or clarify the diagnosis and is an opportunity for genetic and research testing. Because a biopsy may only include a small area of the lesion, it is critical that the vascular anomaly team includes an experienced vascular pathologist or one that is willing to learn this field and consult with others. Ultrasonography and/or magnetic resonance imaging (MRI) may be frequently used to help establish a diagnosis. These two imaging modalities are often used in combination to determine the diagnosis. Thus, an experienced radiologist is very important to a vascular anomaly practice. Increasingly, common genetic mutations are associated with specific diagnoses, placing a higher emphasis on obtaining tissue biopsy. The practitioner should seek access to laboratories performing analysis for these genetic mutations. Finally, when contemplating the decision to obtain a tissue biopsy, a multidisciplinary debate may be facilitated to minimize any risks. There may be a high risk for adverse outcome, as in patients with coagulopathy or lymphatic malformation of the ribs. There are many considerations for the hematologist/oncologist and the vascular anomaly team when making a diagnosis in each patient, and individuality and clinical factors make standardization of care challenging.

Therapeutic Considerations

Patients with vascular anomalies require a wide range of subspecialists, procedures, medical interventions, and practice expertise for optimal care. Once a diagnosis is established, an interdisciplinary approach to interventional options should be outlined, with the inclusion of patient's and patient care providers' perspective. Medical, surgical, and supportive interventions should be individually determined for each anomaly. Medical interventions which may likely involve the hematologist/oncologist include observational monitoring with regular review of radiographic imaging, prescribing, and supporting patient engagement with dietary restrictions, anticoagulation, chemotherapy, and immune-modulating agents. The hematologist/oncologist may find that they are involved in the delivery of new biologic agents as genetics and personalized medicine become incorporated into the care of vascular anomalies. Other medical therapies that the hematologist/oncologist should be familiar with include holding immunosuppressive agents during infections, antibiotic therapy for active infections and possible prophylaxis, transfusion therapy, periprocedural supportive care, and pain management. Due to the life-threatening nature of some diagnoses, the hematologist/oncologist may be involved in helping families transition to palliative care, or even providing palliative care measures themselves in some circumstances.

Surgical interventions, such as resection, biopsy, sclerotherapy, pleurodesis, or endovascular embolization, should be available for optimal treatment of many vascular anomalies. Laser treatment may also be indicated. Depending on each center, surgeons, interventional radiologists, otolaryngologists, plastic surgeons, or dermatologists may be the most proficient in these procedures. Availability of anesthesia to aid in both procedures and in obtaining adequate radiologic studies especially helps in the care of the pediatric patients. In very rare cases, radiotherapy may need to be utilized, often on an emergent basis. Some nonmedical interventions which are used in the treatment and management of patients with vascular malformations include compression, massage, physical therapy, and psychosocial support. All interventions should be considered from a multidisciplinary approach, and the hematologist/oncologist would be prudent to identify the local resources available for their patients and the impact on their clinical practice [8, 9].

At minimum, an outpatient facility for the evaluation of patients and delivery of clinical care is necessary. An inpatient unit or day hospital may also be important to allow for safe delivery of interventions. For example, an infantile hemangioma in a neonate or premature infant may best be cared for with inpatient monitoring to begin propranolol therapy. Postoperative observation with monitoring for bleeding and pain post-sclerotherapy or post-biopsy may require admission to an inpatient unit. Centers caring for the most complex and aggressive vascular anomalies will require an on-call team for emergencies, an inpatient service, and access to an intensive care unit. Thus, for complex and aggressive vascular anomalies, care at a tertiary care center is likely to lead to the best outcomes. The hematologist/oncologist is typically familiar with inpatient care and nursing, and services such as dermatology or interventional radiology may not have an admitting service. Thus, the hematologist/oncologist may be tasked to develop a procedure for patients with emergent issues or those that require hospital admission. In one model, patients are admitted to a general medical service, with consultation from the required subspecialty services. In the centers where a hematologist/oncologist serves as the primary medical service, patients are admitted under their direct care. In this model, the expertise and familiarity of the entire H/O attending faculty should be considered. Finally, with enough volume and providers, independent vascular anomaly inpatient services may be an approprite care model. Thoughtful attention to these procedural details will help in the delivery of care and allow for the best patient experience and outcomes, and maximize chances for a rewarding and successful career.

Institutional Perspective: Business Planning

Program Financial Impact

From an institutional perspective, the financial health of any program is vital to resource planning and long-term success. Thus, members of the vascular anomaly clinic should familiarize themselves with the business aspects of clinical programs. A patient's overall impact, or clinical footprint which includes all of the different specialties, should be remembered in discussion of finances [10]. A method to accurately determine a program's volume and the overall clinical impact for the entire patient population is important, in order to justify a program and also to help use to gain resource allocation. The new ICD-10 code (discussed in next section) is designed to maximize billing and coding and is particularly helpful in vascular anomalies. ICD-10 includes attention to anatomic laterality and location, giving the ability to assign multiple independent diagnoses to a single patient, allowing for a higher degree of complexity and higher reimbursement. Due to the multispecialty involvement, high degree of non-face-to-face time in discussion of care, and involvement of patients in the decision-making process, it is important to be able to demonstrate a consistent picture of financial viability and health for any vascular anomaly program.

Billing, Scheduling, and Documentation

Several aspects about the most recent version (tenth version) of the International Classification of Diseases (ICD-10) may not be familiar to the hematologist/oncologist or the vascular anomaly team. Extra effort and careful attention to the documentation of the laterality of the vascular anomaly or tumor and its location should be made in the ICD-10 coding system. This will help localize the lesion and allow each billing encounters to focus on individual lesions and each specific clinical issue due to a lesion's anatomic location. For example, the specific vascular anomaly may be identified by the affected organ system, such as a hemangioma of the skin as opposed to the liver. In addition, recurrences of many types of vascular anomalies are common and may even occur in different organ systems or anatomic locations from those that were involved at diagnosis. As the provider becomes more familiar with the coding of vascular anomaly diagnoses, consistency in diagnostic coding will allow improved epidemiology and population studies to be performed.

Depending on the structure of the vascular anomaly clinic and the presence of a multidisciplinary evaluation, the billing and documentation may be approached differently at each center and specifically for the hematologist/oncologist. For example, at some centers, only a single service documents the clinic visit and patient examination for the entire multidisciplinary team. In some institutions, a nonsurgical or nonprocedural service documents and bills for the outpatient clinic visits, due to the higher reimbursement and wRVU allocated to procedures. Other systems may have the hematologist/oncologist admit the patients should inpatient care be warranted, as many services, such as dermatology and interventional radiology, may not have admitting service privileges. The hematologist/oncologist may need to demonstrate financial solvency in order to pursue this clinical interest, and with thoughtful planning there are several ways in clinical workflow that can help to maximize generation of wRVUs to illustrate clinical productivity. In conclusion, many areas exist for the hematologist/oncologist to consider as they embark on a career that encompasses vascular anomaly patients. Planning for the incorporation of these patients should be deliberate, because the H/O specialist is well suited to play a critical role in the care of any vascular anomaly patient and often is essential in the interdisciplinary care team.

References

1. Mattila KA, kervinen K, Kalajoki-Helmio T, Lappalainen K, Vuola P, Lohi J, Rintala R, Pitkaranta A, Salminen P. An interdisciplinary specialist team leads to improved diagnostics and treatment of pediatric patients with vascular anomalies. Acta Paediatr. 2015;104(11):1109–16.
2. Moneghini L, Sangiorgio V, Tosti D, et al. Head and neck vascular anomalies. A multidisciplinary approach and diagnostic criteria. Pathologica. 2017;109:47–59.
3. Belov S. Anatomopathological classification of congenital vascular defects. Semin Vasc Surg. 1993;6(4):219–24.
4. Wassef M, Blei F, Adams D, Alomari A, Baselga E, Berenstein A, Burrows P, Frieden IJ, Garzon MC, Lopez-Gutierrez JC, Lord DJ, Mitchel S, Powell J, Prendiville J, Vikkula M, ISSVA Board and Scientific Committee. Vascular anomalies classification: recommendations from the International Society for the Study of Vascular Anomalies. Pediatrics. 2015;136(1):e203–14.
5. Pahl KS, Kim K, Sams C, Alvarez H, Smith SV, Blatt J. Inconsistency in classification of vascular anomalies: what's in a name? Pediatr Blood Cancer. 2018;65(3):e26836.
6. Mullikan J, Burrows P, Fishman S. Mullikan and Young's vascular anomalies: hemangiomas and malformations. 2nd ed. Oxford, England, UK: Oxford University Press; 2013.
7. Lobo-Mueller E, Amaral JG, Babyn PS, John P. Extremity vascular anomalies in children: introduction, classification, and imaging. Semin Musculoskelet Radiol. 2009;13(3):210–35.
8. Meguid C, Ryan C, Edil B, Schulick R, Gajdos C, Boniface M, Schefter T, Purcell WT. Establishing a framework for building multidisciplinary programs. J Multidiscip Healthc. 2015;8:519–26.
9. Lerner S, Magrane D, Friedman E. Teaching teamwork in medical education. Mt Sinai J Med. 2009;76:318–29.
10. Ettinger AB, Blondell C. The clinician's guide to composing effective business plans. J Med Pract Manage. 2011;26(6):348–56.

Index

C. C. Trenor III, D. M. Adams (eds.), *Vascular Anomalies*,
https://doi.org/10.1007/978-3-030-25624-1

The manufacturer's authorised representative in the EU is Springer
Nature Customer Service Centre GmbH, Europaplatz 3, 69115 Heidelberg,
Germany. If you have any concerns regarding our products, please
contact ProductSafety@springernature.com

Printed and bound by CPI Group (UK) Ltd, Croydon, CR0 4YY
30/09/2026
02225705-0001